Oxford Textbook of

Global Health of Women, Newborns, Children, and Adolescents

Oxford Textbooks in Public Health

Oxford Textbook of
Global Health of Women, Newborns, Children, and Adolescents

Edited by

Delan Devakumar
Clinical Associate Professor in Child and Adolescent Health
Institute for Global Health, University College London, London, UK

Jennifer Hall
Principal Clinical Researcher
Institute for Women's Health, University College London, London, UK

Zeshan Qureshi
Academic Clinical Fellow in Global Child Health
King's College London, London, UK

Joy Lawn
Professor of Maternal, Reproductive and Child Health
London School of Hygiene and Tropical Medicine, London, UK

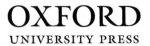
OXFORD
UNIVERSITY PRESS

UNIVERSITY PRESS

Great Clarendon Street, Oxford, OX2 6DP,
United Kingdom

Oxford University Press is a department of the University of Oxford.
It furthers the University's objective of excellence in research, scholarship,
and education by publishing worldwide. Oxford is a registered trade mark of
Oxford University Press in the UK and in certain other countries

Published in the United States of America by Oxford University Press
198 Madison Avenue, New York, NY 10016, United States of America

British Library Cataloguing in Publication Data
Data available

Library of Congress Control Number: 2018965054

ISBN 978–0–19–879468–4

Printed and bound by
CPI Group (UK) Ltd, Croydon, CR0 4YY

Foreword

Students have a pretty wide choice of clinical textbooks for the treatment of common maternal and child health conditions. But for those interested in global population health of mothers, newborns, children, and adolescents, with an emphasis on prevention and promotion, this textbook fills a surprising void. Drawing heavily upon course lecturers from Masters programmes at University College London and the London School of Hygiene and Tropical Medicine, it is organised using a lifecycle approach, with sections on the health of adolescents, women's reproductive and maternal health, newborns and stillbirths, and children. In keeping with the global burden and attention, this book focuses on reproductive and maternal mortality and morbidity, but recognises that women are more than just their reproductive role. Overall, it provides a concise, comprehensive, and long overdue review of the field.

The past two decades have seen a dramatic improvement in maternal and child survival. In most regions of the world death rates fell steadily. Malaria deaths declined, pneumonia case management improved, and diarrhoea and dehydration deaths fell with greater awareness of hygiene and early treatment. But demographic shifts, urbanisation, and humanitarian crises have created a new raft of challenges. Certainly, the survival agenda is not over. Death rates remain unacceptably high in marginalised populations, conflict is a daily threat to millions of families, and even if mothers and children have greater access to health facilities, the quality of care they receive is often suboptimal or lacking in dignity and respect. The newborn period has not seen as rapid a fall in deaths as later in childhood. And over medicalisation leads to new problems—antimicrobial resistance emerging from the widespread use and poor stewardship of antibiotics, and a pandemic of unnecessary caesarean sections, especially in the growing private sector.

As more children survive, attention shifts to their ability to grow, thrive, and flourish. In many countries exclusive breastfeeding rates have steadily fallen and infection rates in infancy mean stunting rates are stubbornly high. Stunting leaves a lifetime scar. Stunted children have poor cognitive development, poorer employment options and are more likely to have lower incomes as adults. At the same time, virtually all countries face a double burden of malnutrition. While we see less acute and chronic malnutrition, obesity rates in childhood have soared. Junk food, snacking, lack of opportunity to play and exercise, and increasing addiction to screens has created a new generation of overweight kids who face a future of diabetes and cardiovascular disease. For mothers, obesity and non-communicable diseases are replacing traditional causes of maternal mortality, even in the US, the only country to see a rise in maternal mortality rate since 1990.

Two areas of particular interest for policymakers are early child development and adolescent health. The Nobel Laureate, James Heckman, concluded that maximising the social and economic environment for early child development was among the most cost-effective policy decisions any government could make. Child maltreatment and abuse remains widespread, poorly studied, and rarely managed well. And we have barely researched how to engage with adolescents during the 10–18-year age period when they make choices about nutrition, diet, exercise, smoking, alcohol, and substance abuse, how to deal with stress and mental health, and the ontogeny of masculinity and adult sexual relationships.

Finally, we cannot be complacent. We face a burgeoning environmental and climate crisis which, in the lifetime of current students, could undo many of the gains we've made. The world economy remains volatile, with rising inequality within states. An emerging debt crisis could threaten the livelihoods in many low and middle-income countries. Corporate promotion of breastmilk substitutes, junk food, cigarettes, sugary drinks, and social media present new threats, as part of the global privatisation of childhood. Universal health coverage has a long way to go. New and emerging infectious threats are ever present.

This textbook is an invaluable introduction to the principles and practice of global women's, newborns', children's, and adolescents' health. It will help new students to be excited and challenged, to learn about the causes of ill health, and also the causes of the causes, and to become ever vigilant in health innovation, research, and advocacy. It is hoped that the book will help create a new generation of professionals and advocates who see the early years of life as pivotal to adult health, and to the achievement of the Sustainable Development Goals.

Anthony Costello
Former Director of Maternal, Child and
Adolescent Health at the World Health Organization.
Professor of Global Health and Sustainable Development,
University College London.

Acknowledgements

When this book was conceptualised, we were over optimistic about how long it would take. Looking back, it seems naïve to think it could have been otherwise. We would like to thank the many people who got us to this safe delivery. First, our sincere thanks to all our expert authors who made time despite their busy schedules to write such informative chapters. In particular we would like to credit Dr Hannah Blencowe and Dr Samantha Sadoo, who provided crucial inputs, especially in the newborn health section. We also appreciate the input of Mr Abdulkadir Elmi, Helena Qian and Dr Sruthi Mahadevan, who provided very useful comments on several sections of the book.

Finally, we would like to thank our long-suffering families, who have supported us throughout. As a group of editors, since starting work on this book, we have gained new family members, and also lost a much-loved one, with the death of Professor Stephen Lawn from a brain tumour in September 2016. Living out the themes of this book, we have also welcomed two new children into the world (with two more on the way), who are all both surviving and thriving, and looking forward to more attention.

Contents

Abbreviations

AAP	American Academy of Pediatrics		HEADSS	home, education, activities/employment, drugs, suicidality, sex
AIDS	acquired immune deficiency syndrome		HAI	hospital acquired infections
AMR	antimicrobial resistance		Hib	*Haemophilus influenzae* type b
ART	antiretroviral therapy		HIC	high-income countries
ASHA	accredited social health activist		HIE	hypoxic ischaemic encephalopathy
BCG	Bacillus Calmette-Guérin		HIV	human immunodeficiency virus
BEmOC	basic emergency obstetric care		HPV	human papilloma virus
BMGF	Bill and Melinda Gates Foundation		HRH	human resources for health
BMI	body mass index		HSP	health systems and policy
CDC	children in difficult circumstances		HSV	herpes simplex virus
CEmOC	comprehensive emergency obstetric care		IBFAN	International Baby Food Action Network
CMV	cytomegalovirus		ICBDMS	International Clearinghouse for Birth Defects Monitoring Systems
CNS	central nervous system		ICER	incremental cost-effectiveness ratio
COPD	chronic obstructive pulmonary disease		ICPD	International Conference on Population and Development
CPAP	continuous positive airway pressure		IAWG	Inter-Agency Working Group
CPR	contraceptive prevalence rate		iCCM	integrated community case management of childhood illness
CRP	C-reactive protein			
DALYs	disability-adjusted life-years		IFI	international finance institutions
DKA	diabetic ketoacidosis		IHD	ischaemic heart disease
DM	diabetes mellitus		ILO	International Labour Organization
DNA	deoxyribonucleic acid		IMAGE	Microfinance for AIDS and Gender Equity
DOHaD	Developmental Origins of Health and Disease		IMAI	integrated management of adolescent and adult illness
DOTS	directly observed treatment short-course			
DRC	Democratic Republic of Congo		IMCI	integrated management of childhood illness
ECD	early child development		IMNCI	integrated management of newborn and childhood illnesses
EFM	electronic foetal heart rate monitoring			
EPMM	ending preventable maternal mortality		IMF	International Monetary Fund
EUROCAT	European Concerted Action on Congenital Anomalies and Twins		IMR	infant mortality rate
			IPV	intimate partner violence
FGM	female genital mutilation		IUGR	intrauterine growth restriction
FGM/C	female genital mutilation/cutting		KMC	kangaroo mother care
GBS	group B streptococcus		LAC	Latin America and the Caribbean
GBV	gender-based violence		LARCs	long-acting reversible contraceptives
GDL	graduated driver licensing		LBW	low birthweight
GDP	gross domestic product		LCOR	International Liaison Committee on Resuscitation
GFATM	Global Fund to Fight AIDS, TB, and malaria		LIC	low-income countries
GHG	greenhouse gas		LMIC	low- and middle-income countries
GNI	gross national income		MDG	Millennium Development Goals
GPP	Global Public Private Partnership		MDR-GNB	multi-drug resistant gram-negative bacilli
GNI	gross national income			
GRADE	grading of recommendations, assessment, development, and evaluation			

MDSR	maternal death surveillance and response
MERS	Middle-East respiratory syndrome
MISP	minimum initial service package for reproductive health in crises
MMR	maternal mortality ratio
MMR	measles mumps and rubella
MNCH	maternal, newborn and child health
MNM	maternal near miss
MNP	micronutrients in powder
MTCT	maternal to child transmission
NCDs	non-communicable diseases
NGO	non-governmental organisation
NICU	neonatal intensive care unit
NTDs	neglected tropical diseases
ODA	official development assistance
OECD	Organisation for Economic Co-operation and Development
OOP	out-of-pocket payment
ORS	oral rehydration solution
PAHO	Pan-American Health Organization
PCR	polymerase chain reaction
PCV	pneumococcal conjugate vaccine
PI	ponderal index
PITC	provider-initiated testing and counselling
PJP	*Pneumocystis jirovecii* pneumonia
PLTC	potentially life-threatening condition or morbidity
PMNCH	Partnership for maternal, newborn, and child health
PMTCT	prevention of maternal to child transmission
POCSO	Protection of Children from Sexual Offences Act
PPH	postpartum haemorrhage
PPROM	preterm premature rupture of the membranes
pSBI	possible serious bacterial infection
PTSD	post-traumatic stress disorder
QALYs	quality-adjusted life-years
RCT	randomised controlled trial
RHD	rheumatic heart disease
RMNCH	reproductive, maternal, newborn, and child health
RMNCAH+A	reproductive, maternal, newborn, child health, and adolescents
RSV	respiratory syncytial virus

RUTF	ready-to-use therapeutic foods
SAM	severe acute malnutrition
SAMM	severe acute maternal morbidity
SARS	severe acute respiratory syndrome
SBA	skilled birth attendant
SBR	stillbirth rate
SGA	small for gestational age
SGBV	sexual and gender-based violence
SCD	sickle cell disease
SDG	Sustainable Development Goal
SDH	social determinants of health
SNEHA	Society for Nutrition, Education and Health Action
SRH	sexual and reproductive health
SRHR	sexual and reproductive health rights
SSA	sub-Saharan Africa
STIs	sexually transmitted infections (STIs)
T1DM	type 1 diabetes mellitus
T2DM	type 2 diabetes mellitus
TBA	traditional birth attendants
TFR	total fertility rate
TLTL	too little, too late
TMTS	too much, too soon
U5M	under-five mortality
UHC	universal health coverage
UN	United Nations
UNAIDS	Joint United Nations Programme on HIV/AIDS
UNCRC	United Nations Convention of the Rights of the Child
UNESCO	United Nations Educational, Scientific and Cultural Organization
UNFPA	United Nations Population Fund
UNHCR	United Nations High Commissioner for Refugees
UNICEF	United Nations Children's Fund
VLBW	very low birthweight
VZV	varicella zoster virus
WASH	water, sanitation, and hygiene
WCC	white cell count
WHA	World Health Assembly
WHO	World Health Organization
YLD	years lived with disability

Glossary and definitions

Absolute Risk (AR). Absolute risk or 'risk difference', is the risk of an outcome in one group minus the risk in another group.

Acquired immune deficiency syndrome. A spectrum of conditions that occur in the late stages of HIV infection, when the immune system is severely impaired.

Adaptation (in relation to climate change). Adaptions are actions that reduce the impacts of the effects of unavoidable climate change.

Adolescence. The World Health Organization defines adolescence as the period between ten and nineteen years (WHO, 2001). Many people now extend the upper age to twenty-four years, referring to adolescents and young adults (10–24 years). This period can be divided into early adolescence (10–14 years), late adolescence (15–19 years), and early adulthood (20–24 years).

Adulthood. The age that children and adolescents gain legal rights and accountabilities varies. Eighteen years is the legal age of the majority in many countries, although not universally. Different laws define adulthood at different ages depending on the activity in question (e.g. legal age of sexual intercourse, age of marriage, driving, voting, buying tobacco and alcohol).

Advocacy. The persuasive communication and targeted actions in support of a cause or issue that seek to change policies, positions, and programmes.

Alcohol and drug use disorders. This includes intoxication, harmful use, dependence or withdrawal, associated with psychosocial and health problems.

Antenatal care. Care provided to a woman once she becomes pregnant up until the point of delivery, designed to identify and minimise risk to the mother and the unborn baby. The WHO recommends that ANC should commence by the twelfth week of pregnancy and women should attend a minimum of eight times.

Antepartum stillbirth. Foetal death before the onset of labour.

Antimicrobial resistance. The ability of a microbe to resist effects of medication previously used to treat them.

Antiretroviral treatment. Combination of drugs commonly used in the management of HIV to suppress replication of the virus in the body.

Anxiety disorders (e.g. generalised anxiety, post-traumatic stress and obsessive-compulsive disorders). These are disorders characterised by feelings of apprehension, tension, worry, and physical symptoms (e.g. palpitations, difficulty breathing).

Asylum seeker. A person who has moved across an international border in search of protection under the 1951 Refugee Convention but whose claim for refugee status has not yet been determined.

Bias. A systematic error in measurement.

Bilateral donors. This refers to aid directly from one country government to the recipient country.

Birth asphyxia. A condition of impaired gas exchange that leads to hypoxia (low oxygen levels), hypercarbia (retention of carbon dioxide), and metabolic acidosis (low pH of the blood). 'Birth asphyxia' implies impaired oxygen delivery and decreased blood flow to the foetus, most frequently due to an acute event during childbirth (such as cord prolapse, placental abruption, uterine rupture).

Birth prevalence. The proportion of the number of persons with a condition at birth over the total number of livebirths.

Birthweight. The first weight of the foetus or newborn obtained after birth. For live births, birthweight should preferably be measured within the first hour of life, before significant postnatal weight loss has occurred.

Body mass index. A measure of obesity, calculated as weight (kg) divided by height (m) squared.

Catastrophic health expenditure. When out-of-pocket payments by a household exceed a defined threshold of household income.

Cerebrovascular accident. The sudden death of brain cells due to lack of oxygen from impaired blood flow. Also known as a stroke.

Child development. The process of emotional, physical, psychosocial, and cognitive change that occurs as a person ages from birth through to the end of adolescence.

Child maltreatment. This refers to all forms of physical and/or emotional ill-treatment, sexual abuse, neglect or negligent treatment or commercial or other exploitation, resulting in actual or potential harm to the child's health, survival, development or dignity in the context of a relationship of responsibility, trust or power. It is, first and foremost, a violation of a child's rights and includes witnessing domestic violence.

Child safeguarding. A broader concept encompassing child health and wellbeing, health promotion, advocacy, and injury prevention, in addition to protecting children.

Childhood behavioural disorders. These include attention deficit hyperactivity disorder (inattention, hyperactivity, and impulsiveness) and conduct disorder (antisocial and defiant behaviour).

Children in difficult circumstances. These are children who are exposed to intense multiple risks to their physical and mental health. A common characteristic of these children is that they lack proper adult care and protection and that they lead their lives outside mainstream society.

Chronic obstructive pulmonary disease. A lung disease characterised by chronic obstruction of the airways, impairing normal breathing that is non-reversible.

Civil society. The aggregate of non-governmental organisations and institutions that manifest interests and the will of citizens.

Clinical ethics. These are ethical principles guiding best practices in patient care. They are primarily focused on promoting the wellbeing, interests, and autonomy of patients and the ethical obligations that characterise the clinician-patient-family relationship.

Co-benefit. An ancillary benefit that results as an unintended side-effect from the primary intervention.

Confounder. A variable that is associated both with the intervention and the outcome, and is not on the causal pathway. Its presence may explain the observed effect rather than the intervention or exposure itself.

Cognitive behavioural therapy. A psychological talking therapy that examines how feelings, thoughts, and behaviours are connected and aims to break negative thought-behaviour cycles.

Coincidental death. Incidental or accidental deaths of pregnant women from causes unrelated to or unaffected by the pregnancy, such as motor vehicle accidents, homicides, or unrelated malignancies. These deaths are *not* included in most maternal death statistics.

Communicable disease. An infectious illness that can be transmitted from one infected source to another, for example malaria, HIV/AIDS, and influenza.

Complementary feeding. The provision of nutrient-containing foods or liquids other than breast milk during the period of breastfeeding.

Congenital anomalies (birth defects, congenital disorders, or congenital malformations). Structural or functional anomalies that occur during intrauterine life (before birth), and can be identified antenatally, at birth, or sometimes later in infancy.

Continuum of care. The connection between essential reproductive, adolescent, maternal, newborn, and child health packages through 'time'. It also describes the links between level of care (through 'place'); between community settings and facility settings.

Contraceptive prevalence rate. The percentage of women married or in-union aged 15–49 who are using, or whose sexual partner is using, at least one modern method of contraception.

Co-payments. These are fixed payments made by individuals with health insurance, at the point of receiving a covered service.

Costs. The value of resources used to deliver an intervention or associated with its consequences (e.g. increased healthcare use).

Deoxyribonucleic acid. Repeat sequence molecule that form chromosomes and carries the genetic information.

Depressive disorder. Defined as at least two weeks of low/irritable mood, low energy, and loss of interest, potentially with sleep or appetite disturbances, physical complaints, and psychomotor retardation (slowing of physical activity).

Developmental Origins of Health and Disease. The concept that early life environmental exposures can influence health outcomes and health trajectories later in life.

Developmental potential. The achievements across different developmental domains that a child is expected to make given an optimal environment. This can be estimated based on developmental progress in peers conceived, born, and raised in an environment that provides optimal physical (e.g. nutrition), emotional and cognitive support (e.g. stimulation through play).

Developmental trajectory. The sequence of developmental changes as they occur within an individual child; often based on timing of acquiring specific skills ('milestones').

Diabetes mellitus. A disease related to impaired functioning or production of insulin, leading to high glucose levels.

Type 1 diabetes mellitus is related to absolute deficiency of insulin, with usual onset in children. Type 2 diabetes mellitus is related to insulin resistance, usually acquired in adulthood, and associated with lifestyle factors such as obesity.

Direct maternal death. A death that occurs during pregnancy or up to forty-two days afterwards resulting from obstetric complications, interventions, omissions, or incorrect treatment.

Disability. The presence of a physical or mental impairment which has a substantial and long-term adverse effect on the ability to carry out normal day-to-day activities.

Disability-adjusted life years. A measure of disease burden, where one DALY equates to one healthy year lost due to the disease through ill health, disability, or premature death.

Discount rate. This is a weighting attached to cost and benefits occurring in the future that accounts for the fact that people value present costs and benefits more highly.

Early onset (neonatal) disease. Neonatal infection with onset on days 0–6.

Early stillbirth. Foetal death with a birthweight of 500 g or more, gestational age of twenty-two weeks or more, or length of 25 cm or more.

Eclampsia. The combination of pre-eclampsia with seizures.

Economic cost. The value of all resources used to produce an intervention, expressed in terms of their 'opportunity cost'.

Economic evaluation. The comparative analysis of alternative courses of action in terms of their costs and consequences.

Effects. The consequences of a health intervention; either outputs (activities) or impacts (health effects).

Endemic. When an infection is constantly present within a geographically-defined human population without the need for external inputs

Enzootic. When an infection is constantly present within a geographically-defined animal population without the need for external inputs

Epidemiological transition. The replacement of infectious diseases by chronic non-communicable diseases over time due to expanded public health and sanitation.

Epigenetics. A change in the phenotype (physical appearance and characteristics) of an organism due to a change in the expression of DNA and subsequent protein formation, rather than a change in the DNA code itself.

Epilepsy. The persistent predisposition to seizures caused by abnormal electrical activity in the brain, as well as the neurobiological, cognitive, psychological, and social consequences of this condition.

Evidence-based. The conscientious, explicit, and judicious use of current best evidence in making decisions about the care of communities and populations in the domain of health protection, disease prevention, health maintenance, and improvement.

Exclusive breastfeeding. When the infant receives only breast milk, without any other liquids or solids, except for oral rehydration solution, or drops/syrups of vitamins, minerals or medicines.

Extremely preterm. Babies born alive before twenty-eight completed weeks of pregnancy

Family planning. The way individuals and couples can achieve their desired number of children and the spacing of their births, using contraceptive methods and/or assisted reproduction.

Female genital mutilation/cutting. Partial or total removal of external female genitalia, or other injury to the genital organs for non-medical reasons.

Financial cost. The actual expenditure on the resources used to produce an intervention.

Financial protection. The ability of a health system to safeguard people against financial hardship associated with paying for health services.

Gender equality. This refers to equal treatment of all genders in laws and policies, and equal access to resources and services within families, communities, and society at large.

Gender equity. This refers to fairness and justice in the distribution of benefits and responsibilities between people of all genders.

Gender. The socially constructed characteristics of women and men—such as norms, roles, and relationships of and between groups of women and men.

Gender based violence. Violence resulting from the normative roles, inequalities, and power relationships associated with gender

Global public private partnerships and organisations. These bodies were established to mobilise both public and private resources to achieve global health goals

Gravida. The number of times that a woman has been pregnant.

Gross domestic product. The monetary value of all goods and services produced within a country.

Gross national income. Domestic plus foreign output from residents of a country.

Health and human rights. An approach to health ethics which argues that the promotion and advancement of health and wellbeing in the broader social sense must also attend to the promotion of human rights and dignity—rights and protections owed universally to all persons by virtue of being human and part of the global community, irrespective of nationality or geographic location.

Healthcare professional. A person who has completed accredited training in a healthcare profession such as medicine, nursing, or midwifery, licenced by a government agency and/or certification by a professional organisation.

Healthcare system. The organisation of people, institutions, and resources to improve the health of a population.

Healthcare worker. A person engaged in the promotion, protection, or improvement of the health of a population.

High-income countries. Countries with a gross national income per capita of more than US$12,235.

Hospital-acquired infection. Infection in a patient hospitalised for at least the preceding forty-eight hours

Human papilloma virus. A group of over one hundred viruses that affect the skin and moist areas, including the mouth, cervix, and anus. It is the most common sexually transmitted infection. Nearly all sexually active people acquire it at some point in their lives. Some types of HPV cause genital warts and cancers, particularly cervical cancer.

Human immunodeficiency virus. The retrovirus that causes AIDS, and is a major cause of mortality and morbidity worldwide.

Human resources for health. The global health workforce.

Humanitarian crisis. A humanitarian crisis occurs in a country, region, or society where there is a total or considerable breakdown of authority resulting from internal or external conflict and which requires an international response that goes beyond the mandate or capacity of any single agency and/or the ongoing UN country programme.

Hypoxic ischaemic encephalopathy. A neonatal encephalopathy which follows a hypoxic insult during labour/delivery, frequently associated with multi-system dysfunction. However, as the aetiology of encephalopathy is often unknown, most now prefer to use the general term neonatal encephalopathy, and then specify if there is an association with intrapartum injury.

Immediately postpartum. The time period up to twenty-four hours post-delivery.

Immunosuppression. The suppression of the immune response resulting in reduced ability to fight infection.

Impoverishing health expenditure. When out-of-pocket payments push a household below or further below the poverty line.

Improved drinking water. Water that has come from a source that has been actively or naturally protected from contamination, particularly from faecal matter.

Incremental cost-effectiveness ratio. The difference in costs divided by the difference in effects of two competing interventions.

Indirect maternal death. Deaths that occur during pregnancy or within forty-two days of pregnancy, as a result of a pre-existing condition exacerbated by pregnancy, for example cardiovascular disease, or a disease acquired during pregnancy but not related to it, such as malaria.

Infant mortality rate. The probability of dying between birth and one year of age, expressed per 1000 live births.

Injuries. The physical damage that results when a human body is suddenly subjected to energy (mechanical, thermal, or radiated) in amounts that exceed the threshold of physiological tolerance—or else the result of a lack of one or more vital elements, such as oxygen.

Integrated management of childhood illness. An integrated approach to child health from the WHO that focuses on the wellbeing of the whole child.

International Monetary Fund. A coalition of 189 countries aiming to foster global monetary cooperation, international trade, financial stability, high employment rates, poverty reduction, and sustainable economic growth.

Intentional injuries. These are injuries resulting from intended actions by oneself or others. It commonly includes self-harm, interpersonal violence, collective violence, and legal intervention.

Internally displaced person. A person who has been forced to flee their home but remains within the border of their country of residence.

Intimate partner violence. Physical, sexual, or psychological harm by a current or former partner/spouse, not requiring sexual intimacy

Intrapartum care. Care provided to women during labour and childbirth.

Intrapartum period. This refers to childbirth, from the onset of labour to the end of the third stage of labour (after the baby and placenta have been delivered).

Intrapartum stillbirth. Foetal deaths after the onset of labour but before birth.

Intrapartum-related neonatal deaths (previously called 'birth asphyxia' deaths). This refers to deaths in the first twenty-eight days of life in full-term babies with neonatal encephalopathy or who cannot be resuscitated (or for whom resuscitation is not available). Where possible, other causes (such as congenital malformations) should be excluded.

Ischaemic heart disease. Disease of the heart related to impaired blood supply from blockage/narrowing of the arteries.

Intrauterine growth restriction. The failure of a foetus to achieve their genetic growth potential. Most will also be small for gestational age.

Late maternal deaths. The deaths of women from direct or indirect causes more than forty-two days, but less than one year, after the end of pregnancy.

Late onset (neonatal) disease. Neonatal infection with onset on days 7–27.

Late postpartum period. The time period from forty-two days post-delivery until one year.

Late stillbirth. The ICD-10 and the WHO definition is foetal death with a birthweight of 1000 g or more, gestational age of twenty-eight weeks or more (i.e. third trimester), or length of 35 cm or more.

Lifetime risk of maternal death. The probability that a woman will die from a maternal cause, assuming the age-specific risk of maternal mortality for a given population in a given year.

Long-acting reversible contraceptives. LARCs are contraceptives that are effective for an extended period without requiring user action, for example intrauterine devices.

Low- and middle-income countries (LMICs). An economic categorisation of countries devised by the World Bank. It encompasses both low-income countries with per capita incomes lower than US$1005 and middle-income countries with per capita incomes lower than $12,236. Seventy per cent of the world's poor (earning less than $1.90 a day) live in middle-income countries.

Low birthweight. A birthweight <2500 g, independent of gestational age.

Macronutrients. These include proteins, carbohydrates, and fats.

Malnutrition: The lack of proper nutrition, caused by eating a diet in which nutrients and energy are either lacking or in excess. Malnutrition may also be caused by conditions that impair absorption of nutrients or illness.

Maternal death. The death of a woman while pregnant or within forty-two days of termination of pregnancy, irrespective of the duration and the site of the pregnancy, from any cause related to or aggravated by the pregnancy or its management, but not from accidental or incidental causes. These deaths are subdivided into direct and indirect maternal deaths.

Maternal health. The health of women during pregnancy, childbirth, and the postnatal period.

Maternal morbidity. Any condition attributed to, or aggravated by, pregnancy or childbirth, which has a negative impact on the woman's wellbeing and/or functioning.

Maternal mortality rate. The number of maternal deaths in a population of women of reproductive age during a specified period; expressed per 1000 per year.

Maternal mortality ratio. The number of maternal deaths per 100,000 live births during the same period.

Maternal or perinatal mental health. This describes the emotional health and wellbeing of women from conception until the end of the first postnatal year.

Maternal or perinatal psychiatric disorder. Any mental illnesses as defined by the WHO International Classification of Disease (ICD-10), occurring during the perinatal period.

Meningitis. An inflammation of the meninges, caused by infection.

Meta-analysis. A summary calculation combining the information from more than one study to produce an overall effect estimate.

Micronutrients. These include vitamins and minerals that are essential for physiology.

Mid-level provider. These are qualified healthcare workers who have less formal training than health professionals and a more restricted scope of practice.

Millennium Development Goals. The eight goals agreed by the international community, under the auspices of the United Nations in 2000. They focused on low- and middle-income countries and there were three goals directly related to health—including reducing child and maternal mortality significantly by 2015.

Mitigation related to climate change. Actions that limit the extent of climate change, by reducing greenhouse gas emissions.

Moderate to late preterm. Babies born alive at 32–37 weeks of pregnancy.

Multilateral organisations. These are international organisations (e.g. WHO/UNICEF/World Bank) which provide advice and/or money to address global, regional and national concerns.

Natural reservoir. The long-term host organism of a pathogen, who often do not get the disease caused by the pathogen.

Neglect. This includes both isolated incidents, as well as a pattern of failure over time on the part of a parent or other family member to provide for the development and well-being of the child—where the parent is in a position to do so—in one or more of the following areas: health, education; emotional development; nutrition; shelter and safe living conditions.

Neglected tropical diseases. A group of seventeen chronic infections that disproportionately affect poorer populations.

Neonatal death. the death of a liveborn baby at 0–27 days of age (early: 0–6 days, late: 7–27 days).

Neonatal encephalopathy. A clinically-defined syndrome of disturbed neurological function in the earliest days of life in the term infant, manifested by difficulty with initiating and maintaining respiration, depression of tone and reflexes, subnormal level of consciousness, and, often, seizures. It may follow an intrapartum hypoxic insult, or be due to another cause.

Neonatal mortality rate. The number of neonatal deaths per 1000 live births.

Neonatal period. The first twenty-eight days of life.

Non-communicable disease. A non-infectious and non-transmissible medical condition or disease.

Non-governmental organisations. and civil society organisations. These are generally non-profit entities addressing particular issues or groups of people (like children or humanitarian emergencies) through projects or awareness raising.

Nulliparous. A woman who has never given birth.

Obesity. Defined as a BMI>30 kg/m^2

Obstetric fistula. A hole between the vagina and rectum and/or bladder that is caused by prolonged obstructed labour, leaving a woman incontinent of urine or faeces or both.

Obstetric transition. A concept describing the transition from high maternal mortality to low maternal mortality and from direct obstetric causes to indirect causes of maternal mortality, alongside increasing age at first pregnancy.

Obstructed labour. When it is not possible for a baby to be born vaginally. It may be because the baby is not in an appropriate position to progress through the birth canal or the baby is too big to pass through the pelvis.

Odds. Those with the outcome divided by those without the outcome.

Odds Ratio (OR). The odds of an outcome in one group divided by the odds of the same outcome in another group.

Opportunistic pathogens. Microbes that only cause clinical infection in individuals with a weakened immune system.

Opportunity cost. The value of the next best alternative use of the resources used by an intervention.

Out-of-pocket payments. Any direct outlay by households to healthcare providers, including healthcare workers, healthcare facilities, and pharmacies.

Organisation for Economic and Co-operation and Development. An intergovernmental organisation of thirty-seven mainly high-income countries with the aim to stimulate economic progress and world trade.

Overweight. Defined as a BMI>25 kg/m^2. It is also defined as weight for height ≥2 z-scores (standard deviations) adjusted for age and sex for children under five years old and BMI-for-age >1 z-score above the median (WHO Child Growth Standards).

Parity. The number of times the woman has given birth to a foetus with a gestational age of 24 weeks or more, regardless of whether the child was born alive or was stillborn.

Particulate matter. Fine particles emitted from the combustion of fossil fuels, among other things, that cause disease.

Partogram/partograph. A chart which is filled in for women in labour. It pictorially represents her progress through her labour and alerts staff if there is a problem with her progress so that they can act.

Perinatal period. The time from twenty-two completed weeks of gestation to seven completed days after birth (except with regard to mental health—see Maternal or Perinatal mental health).

Perspective (economic). A statement of whose costs or effects should be valued.

Physiological changes of pregnancy. There are normal adaptations of a pregnant woman's body that optimise conditions for the developing baby, but which mean that she responds differently to communicable or non-communicable diseases.

Pneumonia. An infection in the lungs.

Policy adoption. The process by which a policy is discussed, developed, and endorsed by authorised stakeholders.

Policy implementation. When adopted policies are put into effect.

Policy. This refers to decisions, plans, and actions that are undertaken to achieve specific healthcare goals within a society.

Ponderal index. The ratio of weight to length of a baby.

Possible serious bacterial infection. Clinically defined based on the presence of any one of the following clinical signs in infants aged <2 months: history of difficulty feeding, history of convulsions, respiratory rate >60 breaths per minute, severe chest in drawing, temperature >37.5ºC or <35.5ºC, movement only when stimulated.

Postnatal. The forty-two days (six weeks) following childbirth.

Postpartum care. Care provided to women following delivery and up until one-year post delivery.

Postpartum haemorrhage. Blood loss of 500 ml or more after birth.

Potentially life-threatening condition or morbidity. This refers to clinical conditions or diseases that can threaten a woman's life during pregnancy, labour, or after termination of pregnancy. Also known as 'severe maternal complications'.

Pre-eclampsia. A condition specific to pregnancy comprising high blood pressure, alongside other abnormalities such as protein in the urine or abnormal blood tests of the liver or kidney. If untreated it can lead to strokes or even progress to fits (eclampsia).

Preterm birth. Birth before thirty-seven completed weeks of gestation.

Preterm prolonged rupture of membranes. When the cervical membranes have been ruptured for >18 hours before birth at a gestation <37 weeks.

Primary prevention. This refers to preventing illness/injury before it occurs.

Prolonged rupture of membranes. When the cervical membranes ruptured for >18 hours before birth

Public health ethics. These are ethical principles guiding the evaluation of health interventions, programmes, or policies, primarily appealing to the overall good or benefit to the health of a population as a whole or key public health outcomes. Considerations of justice at the population level also attend to the fair distribution of health benefits and minimising health burdens, particularly for the worst off.

Quality-adjusted life-years. A measure of health status, which adjusts length of life to reflect quality of life.

Recessive inheritance. In recessive inheritance, a mutation has to be inherited from both parents in order for a person to be affected. Such parents are often unaffected carriers because they only have a single copy of the mutant gene.

Refugee. According to the UN Convention (1951), a refugee is a person who owing to a well-founded fear of being persecuted for reasons of race, religion, nationality, membership of a particular social group or political opinion, is outside the country of their nationality and is unable, or owing to such fear, is unwilling to avail themselves of the protection of that country; or who, not having a nationality and being outside the country of their former habitual residence, as a result of such events, is unable to or, owing to such fear, is unwilling to return to it.

Reliable. Reliable measures give the same result when repeated in the same circumstances.

Reproductive health. A state of complete physical, mental and social wellbeing in relation to the reproductive system, and to its functions and processes. It entails the ability to reproduce and have the freedom to choose if, when, and how often to do so. It also includes access to a range of information, methods, facilities, and services to enable informed, free, and responsible decision making about reproductive behaviour.

Resilience. The product of a combination of coping mechanisms.

Rheumatic heart disease. Permanent damage to the heart as a result of rheumatic fever.

Risk. Those with the outcome divided by the total population.

Risk Ratio (RR). The risk of an outcome in one group divided by the risk of the same outcome in another group, also known as 'relative risk'.

Road traffic injuries. A fatal or non-fatal injury incurred as a result of a collision on a public road involving at least one moving vehicle.

Secondary prevention. The immediate response to an illness/injury to minimise the impact.

Self-harm. Intentional self-inflicted injury or poisoning. There is an increased risk of suicide when associated with ongoing stressors (e.g. interpersonal issues, physical abuse) and other mental disorders.

Sensitivity analysis. An assessment of sensitivity of the main findings to the assumptions made, to the structure of a model, and to uncertainty in the data.

Sepsis. Infection in the bloodstream, it can occur as a result of infection in the perinatal period.

Severe acute malnutrition. When weight for height z-score is <−3 or when malnutrition is associated with oedema.

Severe acute maternal morbidity. A woman who nearly died but survived a complication that occurred during pregnancy, childbirth or within forty-two days of termination of pregnancy. Also known as 'maternal near miss'.

Sex. The biological characteristics that define humans as female or male.

Sexual health. A state of complete physical, mental and social wellbeing in relation to sexuality. It requires a positive and respectful approach to sexuality and sexual relationships, as well as the possibility of having pleasurable and safe sexual experiences, free of coercion, discrimination, and violence.

Sickle cell disease. A disease of the blood caused by abnormal shaped haemoglobin.

Skilled birth attendant. An accredited health professional such as a midwife, doctor, or nurse who has been educated and trained to proficiency in the skills needed to manage normal (uncomplicated) pregnancies, childbirth, and the immediate postnatal period, and in the identification, management, and referral of complications in women and newborns.

Small for gestational age. Infants with a birthweight below the tenth percentile for their gestational age and sex.

Social determinants of health. Social determinants of health are 'the conditions in which people are born, grow, live, work, and age. These circumstances are shaped by the distribution of money, power, and resources at global, national, and local levels.'

Soil transmitted helminth infections. Nemotodal worm infections transmitted via ingestion of soil contaminated with human faeces, or skin penetration.

Stakeholders. Individuals or groups with a vested interest or power in decision making relating to an overall goal.

Stillbirth rate. The number of late stillbirths per 1000 births (live and stillbirths).

Strategy. A plan of action designed to achieve a vision or putting a plan into operation in a skilful way.

Stunting. Defined as a height-for-age z-score ≤−2, taken in the standing position in children >2 years of age and lying down in children <2 years.

Sustainable Development Goals or the 'global goals'. These constitute seventeen goals agreed by the international community, again under the auspices of the United Nations, in 2015. There is one health goal (goal 3), but many others have implications for health. Some targets are directly related to women's, children's, and adolescents' health, including ending preventable child mortality. The target date for their achievement is 2030.

Systematic Review. A review of a clearly formulated question using explicit methods to identify and critically appraise relevant research to answer it.

Task-shifting. The systematic delegation of tasks to less specialised health workers.

Tertiary prevention. The long-term care to lessen the morbidity/mortality associated with an illness/injury.

Time horizon. The time period over which costs and effects are measured and valued.

Total fertility rate. The average number of children a woman will have during her reproductive life.

Traditional birth attendant. A person who assists the mother during childbirth and who initially acquired her skills by delivering babies herself or by working with other TBAs.

Trial. A test of an intervention. Randomised controlled trials (RCTs) involve random allocation to intervention and control groups to balance out both measured and unmeasured potential confounders.

United Nations Convention of the Rights of the Child. An international declaration that forms the bedrock of children's rights internationally.

Under-five mortality rate. The probability of dying between birth and exactly five years of age, expressed per 1000 live births.

Unintentional injuries. Injuries that occur without intent of harm; intentional injuries occur with the intent to harm.

United Nations. An international organisation formed in 1945 to confront common challenges amongst member states.

United Nations Children's Fund. A UN body aimed at providing humanitarian and developmental assistance to children and mothers internationally.

United Nations Educational, Scientific and Cultural Organization. An agency set up to promote peace and security through international collaboration in the above domains

United Nations Population Fund. A UN body initially set up to address rapid global population growth. It aims to improve reproductive health, supporting wanted pregnancies, improving pregnancy related care, and ensuring every young person's potential is fulfilled.

Universal health coverage. This includes financial risk protection, access to quality essential healthcare services and access to safe, effective, quality and affordable essential medicines and vaccines for all.

Unmet need for family planning. Women (usually married) who are fertile and sexually active but are not using contraception, despite not wanting more children.

Unsafe abortion. The termination of a pregnancy by people lacking the necessary skills, or in an environment lacking minimal medical standards, or both.

User fees. Direct payment by patients at the point of service delivery.

Valid. Valid measures give results that have the intended meaning in the research context.

Very low birthweight. A birthweight <1500 g.

Very preterm: Babies born alive at 28–32 weeks completed weeks of pregnancy

Violence against women. Violence involving men and women, in which the female is usually the victim; and which is derived from unequal power relationships between men and women.

Violence is directed specifically against a woman because she is a woman, or it affects women disproportionately. It includes, but is not limited to, physical, sexual, and psychological harm (including intimidation, suffering, coercion, and/or deprivation of liberty within the family, or within the general community).

Wasting. Defined as a weight-for-height z-score ≤ -2.

Willingness to pay. A measure of the monetary value placed on a programme's benefits.

World Health Assembly (WHA). The key decision-making body of the WHO, attended by a delegate from all member states.

World Health Organization. The WHO directs international health within the UN, aiming for the highest attainable level of health in all countries.

Years lived with/lost to a disability. The number of healthy years lost due to disability and is a measure of the burden of a disease.

Young people. A more general term that commonly refers to the 10–24-year-old age group.

Youth. The United Nation defines youth as people aged 15–24 years.

Contributors

Aula Abbara, Department of Infection, Imperial College London, UK

Suraya Abdul-Razak, Centre for Adolescent Health, Murdoch Children's Research Institute, Melbourne, Australia; Universiti Teknologi MARA, Malaysia

Saima Aftab, Department of Pediatric Newborn Medicine, Brigham and Women's Hospital, Boston, US

Mags Beksinska, University of the Witwatersrand, Johannesburg, South Africa

José Belizán, Institute for Clinical Effectiveness and Health Policy, Buenos Aires, Argentina

Hannah Blencowe, London School of Hygiene and Tropical Medicine, London, UK

Josephine Borghi, London School of Hygiene and Tropical Medicine, London, UK

Helen Brotherton, London School of Hygiene and Tropical Medicine, London, UK

Marly Cardoso, University of São Paulo, São Paulo, Brazil

Beatrice Chikaphonya-Phiri, Dowa District Hospital, Dowa, Malawi

Takondwa Chimowa, University of Malawi, Zomba, Malawi

Kelly Clarke, University College London, London, UK

Tim Colbourn, University College London, London, UK

Gabriela Cormick, Institute for Clinical Effectiveness and Health Policy, Buenos Aires, Argentina

Geoff Debelle, Birmingham Children's Hospital, Birmingham, UK

Delan Devakumar, University College London, London, UK

Caroline Fall, University of Southampton, Southampton, UK

Rashida Ferrand, London School of Hygiene and Tropical Medicine, London, UK

Lian Folger, Department of Pediatric Newborn Medicine, Brigham and Women's Hospital, Boston, US

Selena Gleadow Ware, NHS Lothian and University of Edinburgh, Edinburgh, UK

Anu Goenka, University of Manchester, Manchester, UK

Jennifer Hall, University College London, London, UK

Kara Hanson, London School of Hygiene and Tropical Medicine, London, UK

Dougal Hargreaves, University College London, London, UK

Therese Hesketh, University College London, London, UK

Michelle Heys, University College London, London, UK

Adnan A Hyder, George Washington University, Washington DC, US

Martha Kamanga, University of Malawi, Kamuzu, Malawi

Raymond Kanthiti, Mitundu Community Hospital, Lilongwe, Malawi

Maureen Kelley, University of Oxford, Oxford, UK

Kalyanaraman Kumaran, University of Southampton, Southampton, UK

Hannah Kuper, London School of Hygiene and Tropical Medicine, London, UK

Joy Lawn, London School of Hygiene and Tropical Medicine, London, UK

Anne CC Lee, Department of Pediatric Newborn Medicine, Brigham and Women's Hospital, Boston; and Department of International Health, Johns Hopkins Bloomberg School of Public Health, Baltimore, US

Mark Lee, Northwick Park Hospital, London, UK

Qingfeng Li, Johns Hopkins University, Baltimore, US

David Lissauer, University of Birmingham, Birmingham, UK

Tom Lissauer, Imperial College, London, UK

Heather Lytle, Baylor College of Medicine, Houston, US

Dan Magnus, Bristol Royal Hospital for Children, Bristol, UK

Address Malata, previously of International Confederation of Midwives; University of Malawi, Zomba, Malawi; and Malawi University of Science and Technology, Thyolo, Malawi

Blerta Maliqi, World Health Organization, Geneva, Switzerland

Kate Mandeville, London School of Hygiene and Tropical Medicine, London, UK

Fred Martineau, London School of Hygiene and Tropical Medicine, London, UK

Elizabeth Mason, University College London, London, UK

Mary McCauley, Liverpool School of Tropical Medicine, Liverpool, UK

Abi Merriel, University of Bristol, Bristol, UK

Nicole Minckas, Institute for Clinical Effectiveness and Health Policy, Buenos Aires, Argentina

Elizabeth Molyneux, University of Malawi, Zomba, Malawi

Sowmiya Moorthie, PHG Foundation, Cambridge, UK

Chelsea Morroni, Liverpool School of Tropical Medicine, UK; Botswana UPenn Partnership, Botswana; University of Cape Town, Cape Town, South Africa; University of the Witwatersrand, Johannesburg, South Africa

Sarah Moxon, London School of Hygiene and Tropical Medicine, London, UK

Saiqa Mullick, University of the Witwatersrand, Johannesburg, South Africa

Jessica Mvula, University of Malawi, Zomba, Malawi

Bernadette O'Hare, University of Malawi, Zomba, Malawi

Miriam Orcutt, King's College London, London, UK

David Osrin, University College London, London, UK

Shefali Oza, London School of Hygiene and Tropical Medicine, London, UK

George C Patton, Centre for Adolescent Health, Murdoch Children's Research Institute, Australia; University of Melbourne, Australia

Lavanya Pillay, University of the Witwatersrand, Johannesburg, South Africa

Jacqueline Pitchforth, University College London, London, UK

Catherine Pitt, London School of Hygiene and Tropical Medicine, London, UK

Melanie Pleaner, University of the Witwatersrand, Johannesburg, South Africa

Zeshan Qureshi, London School of Paediatrics, London, UK

Mopo Radebe, University of the Witwatersrand, Johannesburg, South Africa

Atif Rahman, University of Liverpool, Liverpool, UK

Patricia Rondó, University of São Paulo, São Paulo, Brazil

Richard Rosch, University College London, London, UK

David A Ross, London School of Hygiene and Tropical Medicine, London, UK; and World Health Organization, Geneva, Switzerland

Mike Rowson, University College London, London, UK

Samantha Sadoo, London School of Hygiene and Tropical Medicine, London, UK

Susan M Sawyer, Centre for Adolescent Health, Royal Children's Hospital, Australia; Murdoch Children's Research Institute, Australia; and University of Melbourne, Australia

Lauren Schaeffer, Department of Pediatric Newborn Medicine, Brigham and Women's Hospital, Boston, US

Anna Seale, London School of Hygiene and Tropical Medicine, London, UK

Clare Shortall, Doctors of the World, London, UK

Jenni Smit, University of the Witwatersrand, Johannesburg, South Africa

Robert Stewart, NHS Lothian, Edinburgh, UK; and University of Manchester, Manchester, UK

Cally Tann, London School of Hygiene and Tropical Medicine, London, UK

Sebastian Taylor, Royal College of Paediatrics and Child Health, London, UK

Nynke van den Broek, Liverpool School of Tropical Medicine, Liverpool, UK

Tony Waterston, Retired

Nicholas Watts, University College London, London, UK

Jonathan Wells, University College London, London, UK

Bhanu Williams, Northwick Park Hospital, London, UK

Ingrid Wolfe, King's College London, London, UK

Zhou Xudong, Zhejiang University School of Public Health, China

Sílvia Shikanai Yasuda, Barnet Enfield and Haringey Mental Health Trust, Enfield Town, UK

SECTION 1

Introduction

CHAPTER 1

Women's, children's, and adolescents' health in a changing world

Mike Rowson

This chapter sets the scene for the book, providing an overview of the dominant trends in global health over the last twenty years, with particular reference to women's, children's, and adolescents' health. It shows how various transitions are challenging the global health agenda. It highlights the continuing relevance of health systems and the social determinants of health to the women's, children's, and adolescents' health agenda going forward and references 'big picture' issues that should concern all global health advocates.

Key points

♦ On a global scale, investments in women's, children's, and adolescents' health have led to large improvements in outcomes in the last two decades. However, at the national and sub-national level there is a more diverse picture. In particular the rural poor in low- and middle-income countries (LMICs) still face high levels of preventable mortality. Within cities, women, children, and adolescents face a broad range of health and social issues with the poorest groups having worse health outcomes.

♦ A new set of issues driven by a range of transitions taking place in both developed and developing countries will force a new women's, children's, and adolescents' health agenda. This will need to focus on equity, health systems, non-communicable diseases, and mental health and be less centered on the interests of rich donor nations.

Background

Global health is defined by Koplan as an 'area of study, research and practice that places a priority on improving health and achieving health equity for all people worldwide'. It has evolved from its initial focus on tropical medicine in the era of colonial rule in the nineteenth century—measures largely focused on protecting the colonisers rather than people living in those countries—to promoting health and development through aid investment (though again largely focused on infectious diseases) since the Second World War. More recently the emphasis has shifted to addressing the social determinants of health and equity and global threats such as climate change, uncontrolled tobacco promotion, and emerging and re-emerging infections. Humanitarian crises and responses to epidemics are important too. Some argue that we are now in a new era where LMICs are taking more control of their own health policy agendas.

The scope of women's, children's, and adolescents' health has gone through a similar evolution. Concern with protecting women, children, and adolescents has led to significant investments by aid donors over the last century, including global campaigns such as the United Nations Children Fund's (UNICEF's) Child Survival Revolution of the 1980s. These continued in the era of the Millennium Development Goals (MDGs) but there is also acknowledgement of the importance of underlying issues such as poverty and inequality in shaping women's, children's, and adolescents' health outcomes and of the need to tackle these. The scope of women's, children's, and adolescents' health has gradually been refined to encompass its different population sub-groups more explicitly, such as neonates and adolescents, and there is greater consideration of issues beyond preventable mortality, such as mental health.

Progress

Since 1990, the world has seen significant declines in child and maternal mortality (52% and 44% reductions respectively in 2015). Yet both figures are below the desired targets (66% and 75% reductions) set out in the MDGs and agreed by the international community in 2000. Annual aid funding from public and private donors for maternal, newborn, and child health was estimated to have increased from approximately $3 billion in 1990 to $11 billion in 2016. Half (52%) of all countries increased their annual rate of reduction in child mortality over the 1990–2000 period. By 2015, the improvements, when looked at on a global scale, represented an estimated 48 million additional lives saved than if the global child mortality rate had remained at the level it was in the year 2000. However, the contribution made by aid, as opposed to other factors such as rising living standards and increased health expenditures by developing country governments, is still to be determined. Additionally, it is clear that certain groups have been left behind. For example, although stillbirths and neonatal deaths are declining, it is at a much slower rate than under-five mortality overall, partly due to relatively little policy focus on this demographic. Adolescent health was also under prioritised and their needs are currently gaining traction amongst health and policy professionals.

Now, a new set of global targets have been agreed upon—the Sustainable Development Goals (SDGs) to be achieved by 2030. Of the seventeen SDGs, which range across subjects such as poverty, the environment and women's empowerment, eleven contain targets

Table 1.1 Sustainable Development Goals which contain specific women's, children's, and adolescents' health targets

SDG goal	Associated women's, children's, and adolescents' health target
Goal 2: End hunger, achieve food security, and promote sustainable agriculture	'By 2030, end all forms of malnutrition, including achieving, by 2025, the internationally agreed targets on stunting and wasting in children under five years of age, and address the nutritional need of adolescent girls, pregnant and lactating women and older persons.'
Goal 3: Ensure health lives and promote wellbeing for all ages	'By 2030, reduce the global maternal mortality ratio to less than 70 per 100,000 live births.'
	'By 2030, end preventable deaths of newborns and children under five years of age with all countries aiming to reduce neonatal mortality to at least as low as 12 per 1000 live births and under-five mortality to at least as low as 25 per 1000 births.'
	'By 2030, ensure universal access to sexual and reproductive healthcare services, including for family planning, information, and education, and the integration of reproductive health into national strategies and programmes.'
	'Achieve universal health coverage, including financial risk protection, access to quality essential health-care services and access to safe, effective, quality and affordable essential medicines and vaccines for all.'
Goal 5: Achieve gender equality and empower all women and girls	'Eliminate all forms of violence against all women and girls in the public and private spheres, including trafficking and sexual and other types of exploitation.'
	'Eliminate all harmful practices, such as child early and forced marriage and female genital mutilation.'
	'Ensure universal access to sexual and reproductive health and reproductive rights as agreement in accordance with the Programme of Action of the International Conference on Population and Development and the Beijing Platform of Action and the outcome documents of their review conferences.'
Goal 6: Ensure availability and sustainable management of water and sanitation for all	'By 2030, achieve access to adequate and equitable sanitation and hygiene for all and end open defecation, paying special attention to the needs of women and girls and those in vulnerable situations.'

related to health, including universal health coverage. Specific child and maternal health targets in the SDGs (Table 1.1) remain as ambitious as they were for the MDGs but now include absolute, rather than relative, targets. The World Health Organization (WHO) notes that 'achieving the SDG target of a global maternal mortality ratio (MMR) below seventy will require reducing global MMR by an average of 7.5% each year between 2016 and 2030'. This is about triple the annual rate of reduction achieved between 1990 and 2015.

The situation of the poorest and other vulnerable groups needing most help is not captured by these trends. Globally, inequalities are increasing. In 1990, a pooled average of the maternal mortality ratio in the ten countries with the highest MMR was one hundred times greater than in the ten countries with the lowest. That gap

had increased to 200 times greater in 2015. According to the WHO, Finland had an MMR of 3/100,000 in 2015, while Sierra Leone had an MMR of more than 1300. Within countries, there are huge inequities too, with women, children, and adolescents living in rural areas and/or from lower socioeconomic groups facing the greatest health burdens. The health systems in place are simply inadequate to support required equity improvement in many of the poorest countries of the world.

Any further outcome improvement is dependent on coming to grips with a range of transitions faced by all countries and, in the women's, children's, and adolescents' health space, the new challenges of maternal morbidities, childhood obesity and non-communicable diseases, as well as emerging infectious diseases, such as Zika virus. The specific women's, children's, and adolescents' health targets in the SDGs are illustrative of this increasing range of issues, but are not comprehensive. There are also SDG goals with no specific women's, children's, and adolescents' health targets (such as goal 1 on poverty reduction or goal 4 on education)—but whose achievement are vital for improvement of women's, children's, and adolescents' health.

Challenges

Currently, the world is experiencing four major transitions—all interlinked—which are likely to reconfigure priorities in the next two decades, including for women's, children's, and adolescents' health.

An epidemiological transition is underpinned by a dramatic demographic shift. As death rates of under-fives fall, there is an upsurge of adolescents and young people in the developing world population implying greater attention is needed upon this underserved group. Widespread migration has also meant they are increasingly urbanised. In cities, they face the problems of modernity—exposure to sexual health risks, road traffic accidents, and the risk factors underpinning non-communicable diseases (NCDs). Urban contexts, particularly cities with large slum populations, are places where women, children, and adolescents from the poorest groups are vulnerable to disease, discrimination, and abuse.

These changes are themselves underpinned by an economic transition. Economic growth drives urbanisation and simultaneously moves more countries from a low-income economy bracket to a middle-income economy one. As economic growth does not always translate into poverty reduction, there are huge numbers of poor people living in fast-growing economies like India and China. A billion people (about 70% of the world's poor) now live in middle-income countries. This also means that the far greater part of the global burden of disease now rests in these countries too, not the poorest ones. Yet aid donors may not prioritise interventions in these countries, and there is a persuasive argument that as developing economies grow, they themselves have greater ability to address their own problems.

Economic shifts also create a political transition, with increased weight in global affairs gradually accruing to the richer developing countries (e.g. Brazil, Russia, India, and China). Domestic political reaction to economic stagnation in rich countries has changed the political discourse to a nationalist one, manifest in Britain's decision to leave the European Union and Donald Trump's election victory in the United States in 2016. This imperils not only the aid agenda, but also efforts to address cross-border threats such as infectious diseases and climate change, and may yet hold consequences for institutions of global health governance like the WHO, as they become viewed with ever greater scepticism by their more wealthy nation funders.

Finally, an increasingly visible environmental transition—human-induced climate change—also has current and predicted health impacts. These impacts will manifest directly through the ramifications of extreme weather on health and indirectly through dynamic distribution of disease compounded by environmental changes. The population's response to climate change consequences (e.g. migration) may also be significant. Whilst positive effects may arise, women, children, and adolescents are a particularly vulnerable population and likely to be impacted by the negative outcomes.

Notwithstanding these shifts, Jamison et al. (2013) point to the persistence of 'hotspots of preventable mortality', that now, because of the economic transition, do not fall solely within the poorest countries, but which are concentrated in rural areas across LMICs. They estimate that child mortality rates are 92 deaths per 1000 live births in rural areas and 56 per 1000 in large urban ones. Similarly, a major review of the burden of maternal poor health by Graham et al. (2016) notes a pattern of 'diversity and divergence ... reflecting inequities in wealth, rights and access to care'.

Another persistent challenge of particular relevance to women's, children's, and adolescents' health is failing health systems in LMICs. One shared characteristic amongst numerous health systems is their extraordinary degree of commercialisation. According to Lagarmasino et al., (2009) in Pakistan, India, Bangladesh, China, and Nigeria (countries where the bulk of the world's poor live), out-of-pocket expenditures on health care make up more than half of total health expenditures. This can lead people to delay or forgo treatment, get into debt or be pushed further into poverty. When people do access care, it may not be of high quality in either public or private sector. In sub-Saharan Africa, the World Bank's International Finance Corporation notes that 50% of the poorest population quintile are accessing care from private providers, whereby healthcare services from shops, pharmacies and traditional healers is often completely unregulated. A recent review of private sector provision by Mackintosh et al. (2016) cited evidence from Malawi, Ghana, and Tanzania which revealed a general increase in private sector engagement for the treatment of children with diarrhoea (especially shops and pharmacies) over the past twenty years.

The reasons for these persistent challenges are diverse. They are related to poor national governance, including corruption, underfunding of public services, and discrimination and lack of rights for women, children, and adolescents. It may also be true that the international community has picked the 'low-hanging fruit' of preventable mortality in easier-to-reach groups through increased investment in the MDG era; now a new approach is needed to tackle upcoming challenges.

Conclusions

What do these global health transitions mean for action on women's, children's, and adolescents' health in the future?

First, the quick shifts in epidemiology and demography we are experiencing make the SDGs inadequate for capturing the complexity of the emerging women's, children's, and adolescents' health agenda. The seventeen separate goals also arguably encumbers joint action and goals set at the global level may resonate less at the national level. The UN's Global Strategy on Women's, Children's, and Adolescents' Health (2016–2030) is a step forward, but advocates acting both at global and national levels and will have to carefully analyse the issues of highest priority and form the coalitions needed to achieve their own targets. A retreat from aid by the rich nations, coupled with increasing ownership of the policy agenda by poor countries will make action by civil society in developing countries even more important.

Second, as fewer and fewer women's, children's, and adolescents' health issues are addressed without improved and sustainable healthcare systems (rather than top-down interventions funded by donors), the WHO's vision of Universal Health Coverage (UHC) will become more relevant for women, children, and adolescents. UHC seeks to improve the coverage of quality health services across populations as well as the range of interventions; and to do this in a way which does not lead people into financial difficulty. Historical experience indicates that governments invest more in health systems as they get richer, and so there is reason for hope here. However, attention will still be needed to address the hardest-to-reach groups. The way people are treated by health providers—particularly women and adolescents from poorer populations who often face discrimination and abuse—speaks not just to needed improvements in the clinical quality of care, but in the human dimension as well.

Third, tackling poverty, inequality, environmental challenges, and discrimination—the social determinants of health—implies a research agenda which is not so much focused on addressing 'preventable mortality' or 'saved lives' but on the causes of inequity, the failure of so many countries to address the social determinants of health, poor decision making on the part of individuals and families, and on poor health system performance. This will require a multi-disciplinary approach to understanding why—despite the existence of many successful interventions for women's, children's, and adolescents' health—the burden of illness remains so great, especially among poor and other vulnerable groups.

Case study: The Global Strategy for Women's, Children's, and Adolescents' Health (2016–2030)

Parallel to the launch of the SDGs in 2015, the then UN Secretary General Ban Ki-moon announced a new US$25 billion, fifteen-year Global Strategy for Women's, Children's and Adolescents' Health. Involving multistakeholder groups including developing country governments, major charities, philanthropists and the private sector, the strategy underpins the ambitions of the SDGs to end preventable child mortality and goes further to focus on the need for women, children, and adolescents everywhere to not just survive but 'thrive and transform the world'. It acknowledges the need to take a multi-sectoral approach to achieving these goals, in recognition of the wide range of underpinning health threats.

Questions

1. Do you feel that the global goal of ending preventable child mortality by 2030 is achievable? Why or why not?

2. Which of the transitions described above do you think will have the most impact on the lives of women, children, and adolescents in the coming decade, and why?

3. Will achieving UHC be the single most important contribution to achieving global commitments to women, children and adolescents? Why or why not?

Key publications

Jamison D, Summers L, Alleyne G, et al. (2013). Global health 2035: a world converging within a generation. *Lancet* 382: 1898–1955.
An agenda-setting look into the future of global health.

Sumner A (2016). *Global Poverty, Deprivation, Distribution and Development Since the Cold War*. Oxford University Press: Oxford, UK.
Understanding the changes in global poverty in recent years, and the underlying causes of these changes.

United Nations (2017). Sustainable Development Goals: 17 goals to transform our world. Available at: http://www.un.org/sustainabledevelopment/sustainable-development-goals/
Find out the full range of goals that will set the development and global health agendas until 2030.

Bibliography

Glassman A, Duran D, and Sumner A (2011). Global health and the new bottom billion. Center for Global Development Working Paper 270. Center for Global Development: Washington, DC. Available at: https://www.cgdev.org/publication/global-health-and-new-bottom-billion-what-do-shifts-global-poverty-and-global-disease

Graham W, Woodd S, Byass P, et al. (2016). Diversity and divergence: the dynamic burden of poor maternal health. *Lancet* 388: 2164–75.

Institute for Health Metrics and Evaluation (2017). *Financing Global Health 2016: Development Assistance, Public and Private Health Spending for the Pursuit of Universal Health Coverage*. IHME: Seattle, WA.

International Finance Corporation (2011). Healthy partnerships: how governments can engage the private sector to improve health in Africa. IFC: Washington, DC. Available at: https://openknowledge.worldbank.org/handle/10986/2304

Koplan J, Bond T, Michael H, et al. (2009). Towards a common definition of global health. *Lancet* 373: 1993–5.

Lagomarsino G, Nachuk S, and Singh Kundra S (2009). Public stewardship of private providers in mixed health care systems. Development and Rockefeller Foundation: Washington, DC. Available at: https://www.r4d.org/wp-content/uploads/Public-Stewardship-of-Private-Providers-in-Mixed-Health-Systems.pdf

Lancet Maternal Health Series (2016). Available at: http://www.thelancet.com/series/maternal-health-2016

Mackintosh M, Channon A, Karan A, et al. (2016). What is the private sector? Understanding private provision in the health systems of low-income and middle-income countries. *Lancet* 388: 596–605.

Save the Children (2015). The urban disadvantage: state of the world's mothers 2015. Save the Children Federation: Fairfield, CT. Available at: https://resourcecentre.savethechildren.net/library/state-worlds-mothers-2015-urban-disadvantage

Watts N (2015). Health and climate change: policy responses to protect public health. *Lancet* 386: 1861–1914.

World Health Organization (2015). Trends in maternal mortality: 1990 to 2015. Geneva, WHO. Available at: http://apps.who.int/iris/bitstream/handle/10665/194254/9789241565141_eng.pdf;jsessionid=7C2B435A1A8E17A9A8677F9558C8C85D?sequence=1

You D, Hug L, Ejdemyr S, et al. (2015). Global, regional and national levels and trends in under-five mortality between 1990 and 2015, with scenario-based projections to 2030: a systematic analysis by the UN Inter-agency Group for Child Mortality Estimation. *Lancet* 386: 2275–86.

CHAPTER 2

Strategies through the lifecourse to improve maternal, newborn, child, and adolescent health

Joy Lawn and Samantha Sadoo

This chapter explores shifts from 'maternal and child health' (MCH) to many issues that may compete, notably reproductive, maternal, newborn, child, and adolescent health, and onwards towards the lifecourse and continuum of care. We discuss what this shift means for programmatic services and integrated essential packages of care, and the implementation challenges in reality.

Key points

◆ Women's, children's, and adolescents' health has been at the heart of global primary health care and national health services since these were established in the post-World War Two era. With expanding global health funding, in particular for infectious diseases, and fragmentation, this cohesion has been lost and specific aspects neglected, notably newborns, stillbirths, and adolescents.

◆ Adopting a lifecourse approach brings attention to these target populations that have previously been overlooked in the Millennium Development Goal (MDG) era.

◆ Two-thirds of maternal, newborn, and child deaths and stillbirths could be prevented with essential, integrated packages of care. Integrating packages of care by time and place enhances cost-effectiveness, increases uptake of services and health promotion, and is more convenient for patients.

◆ The biggest gaps in coverage, equity, and quality of care are around the time of birth when the risk of death and disability are the highest. Progress depends on more predictable health systems building and overcoming supply barriers (especially financing) and demand barriers (especially affecting women and girls).

◆ More focus is needed on routine data to track progress, especially programmatic coverage. Implementation research and discovery science investments are also key.

Background

Since the formation of the World Health Organization (WHO) in the 1940s, global and national programmes have used women's, children's, and adolescents' health as the foundation. In the 1970s the focus was particularly on family planning, with a population control paradigm. During the 1980s, with the first child survival revolution led by the United Nations Children's Fund (UNICEF), there was increasing focus on the child, particularly immunisation, and primary healthcare level interventions. An influential paper in 1985 'Where is the M in MCH?' called for more attention to maternal health. Over the next two decades, there was competition between maternal and child health programmes, missing the increasing burden of newborn deaths and stillbirths that was dropped between them.

A decade after the MDGs were set in 2000, there was recognition that almost half of under-five deaths were in the neonatal period, that these deaths would not be reduced by traditional child health programmes focused on infectious conditions and under nutrition, and that addressing the main causes of neonatal deaths would involve more cohesive programmes for women and their babies. This concept was termed the 'continuum of care', and led to a shift from MCH to Maternal, Newborn, and Child Health (MNCH), and then Reproductive, Maternal, Newborn, and Child Health (RMNCH) to underline the crucial importance of reproductive health, especially with the emergence of family planning investments in 2012. Since the end of the MDGs in 2015 there has been an increasing spotlight on the neglected area of adolescent health (RMNCH+A), which is a crucial time of transition, with risks and opportunities for healthy behaviours and adverse outcomes.

The lifecourse approach (Figure 2.1) highlights the importance of the various stages but also those factors that run through the lifecourse and even from generation to generation, notably nutrition. The lifecourse could be considered to start at various points, but for this book we start with the adolescent girl.

A functioning health system requires effective community services, primary, and facility based care. Community services reach the most vulnerable populations, and can promote behaviour change and provide preventive care, as well as improve the demand for facility care. Yet the highest impact care, such as emergency obstetric care and care for small and sick newborns, can only be provided at scale in facilities. This may seem obvious, but over the last decades the policy pendulum has swung between major investment in hospitals, to focusing on primary care and community workers, and now back to a recognition that both are needed and must be well linked.

Interventions organised by a lifecourse approach

The continuum of care includes the two dimensions through the lifecourse (Figure 2.1A), and between levels of care (community, primary, and facility) (Figure 2.1B). At each point in the lifecourse different services are required, and can be provided at different levels of care. This results in a matrix of integrated packages involving different types of care, including curative and palliative care (Figure 2.2).

More than 200 evidence-based interventions for RMNCH+A are outlined in this book, which would be difficult to scale up in isolation. In 2007 a *Lancet* paper outlined a series of integrated,

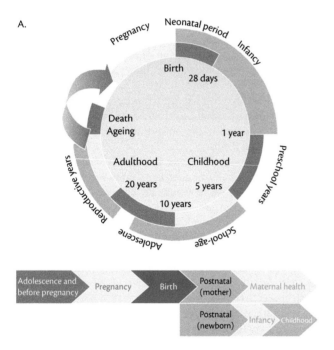

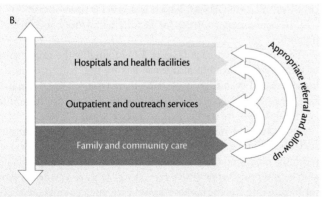

Figure 2.1A–B Connecting care during the lifecycle (A) and at places of caregiving (B).

healthcare packages. Most of these packages are present in almost every country, with some being fairly standard care, such as antenatal and promotive child health, but may vary in the number of visits or complexity of interventions offered. Others are still new or are less widely available, such as facility-based newborn care.

At each point in the lifecourse a package of care is required at different levels of the healthcare system: clinical care (typically facility-based care providing individual case management of illnesses), outpatient and outreach services, and family and community care. It is crucial that communication and transport systems are well established between the levels of care; women with obstetric emergencies can die within hours, and newborns can die in minutes.

We provide an overview of packages ordered by point in the lifecourse, in the same way that this book is ordered: starting from the adolescent girl, through sexual and reproductive health, pregnancy, postnatal/newborn care, and child health. The detailed evidence-based interventions and delivery strategies will be discussed further in the relevant chapters and can be adapted to a given health systems context.

Adolescent health

Outpatient and outreach services: The family and community are important settings particularly for encouraging positive development and healthy behaviours. With the main determinants of adolescent health being outside the remit of the health sector, interventions must also involve sectors relating to education, social protection, employment, media and technology, the environment and infrastructure, and law. The provision of high-quality and accessible education has the potential for the greatest impact on adolescent health and wellbeing.

Clinical care package: This includes the management of the major causes of adolescent morbidity and mortality, including unintentional injury, violence, communicable diseases such as respiratory infections and diarrhoea, non-communicable diseases including obesity, mental health, and sexual and reproductive health.

Reproductive health

Outpatient and outreach services: These can deliver many interventions as well as importantly provide health education and promotion. The unmet need for family planning remains high; an estimated 13% of all maternal deaths are caused by unsafe abortion. Also highly cost-effective is the management of sexually transmitted infections including prevention and early detection for both men and women. Reproductive health can also be improved by enhancing the general health and wellbeing of women, through education, nutrition, and services addressing gender-based violence, alongside clinical care.

Clinical care package: This includes the management of clinical problems affecting women of reproductive age, such as sexually transmitted infections or human immunodeficiency virus (HIV), other gynaecological conditions, safe abortion, or post-abortion care.

Care during pregnancy, labour, and childbirth

Outpatient services: These can be utilised to provide antenatal care. The WHO now recommend that every woman receive at least eight antenatal visits during her pregnancy, at specific times with specific content. Essential components include screening and prompt

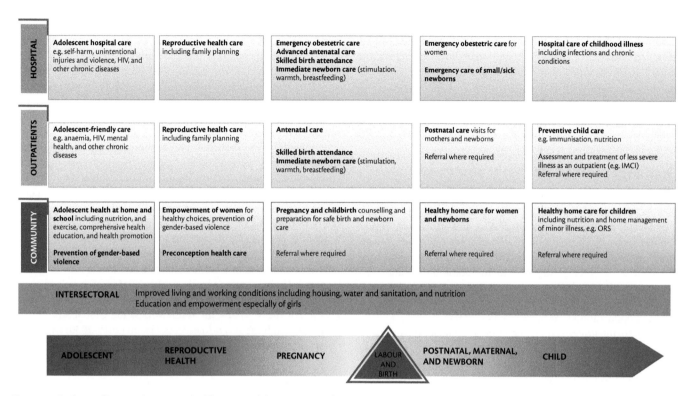

Figure 2.2 Packages of interventions across the lifecourse and the continuum of care.
Source: data from Kerber, KJ. et al. Continuum of care for maternal, newborn, and child health: from slogan to service delivery. *The Lancet* (370):135–1369. Copyright © 2007 Elsevier Inc. All rights reserved.; and Every Newborn Study Group. Every Newborn; An Executive Summary for The Lancet's Series. *The Lancet*. May 2014. Copyright © 2014 Elsevier Inc. All rights reserved.

treatment for infection, high blood pressure and anaemia; preventive interventions such as tetanus immunisation and insecticide-treated bednets; and counselling on various topics, including nutrition, hygiene, HIV status, birth, and care of the newborn.

Clinical care package: This comprises skilled attendance at birth, the availability of emergency obstetric care, and basic newborn care. Skilled attendance at birth has been scaled up at varying rates globally; progress has been slower in South Asia and sub-Saharan Africa. Twenty-four-hour access to quality facilities which can offer safe instrumental delivery and Caesarean sections is vital for women experiencing complications around delivery; barriers to access may be geographical, financial, and cultural.

Postnatal maternal and newborn care

Outpatient services: Postpartum haemorrhage and infection cause the majority of maternal deaths, and around two million babies die in their first week of life; high quality and comprehensive coverage of postnatal care will significantly reduce maternal and newborn mortality. A routine visit in the first few days after birth is recommended, aiming to promote healthy behaviours, support feeding, identify complications, and refer if necessary. Some will require additional support, such as for preterm babies. Postnatal care should also link the woman to family-planning services, and the baby to child health care.

Clinical care package for women: Emergencies such as postpartum haemorrhage or infection require rapid and skilled obstetric services, with additional support (e.g. transfusion facilities).

Clinical care package for small and sick newborns: Twenty-four-hour care must be available for acutely sick and small newborns. Newborns may die quickly, for example due to intrapartum-related complications shortly after birth, or complications of prematurity or infection. Care in hospitals for these vulnerable newborns is a recent programmatic focus for low- and middle-income countries, and requires more skilled nursing and medical care as well as more complex equipment.

Child health care

Outpatient outreach services: Routine immunisation has achieved high coverage, significantly improving child survival. Other preventive interventions include nutrition, of which there have been varying levels of success, and exclusive breastfeeding, of which rates are still low worldwide. Traditionally, integrated management of childhood illness (IMCI) has focused on case management in an outpatient setting, though more recently it has been used at community and referral level as well, and has added care of the sick newborn.

Clinical care: Children can become seriously ill from infections such as malaria, pneumonia, or meningitis. Globally injuries and non-communicable disease account for a higher proportion of post-neonatal deaths. Hospital care for children, including surgery, may only be available in larger urban centres and with cost barriers.

Intersectoral family and community care package

Women, adolescents, and children spend most of their lives at home and in the community, for example at school. Healthy behaviours such as hygiene, nutrition, early and exclusive breastfeeding, are all paramount at home. In addition, access to care such as the demand for skilled care at birth or early recognition of illness are dependent on knowledge and empowerment. Social determinants of health have a major impact on women, children, and adolescents, conversely, community approaches and especially empowerment and education of girls and women can be transformative for health outcomes and society more broadly.

Challenges

Universal coverage of care for women and children through these essential packages has been estimated to prevent around two-thirds of maternal, newborn, and child deaths, and stillbirths (Figure 2.2). Yet ongoing short-termism and unpredictability in health financing, both from country governments and donors, impedes systematic scale up of these packages. In addition, ongoing competing priorities between groups and agencies focused on the various target populations, or very specific interventions may result in missed opportunities for more rapid progress.

A shift to integrated implementation is crucial, with data to measure the gaps in coverage, equity, and quality of care. More investment and focus on improving and using the data for programme improvement is key. Both discovery and implementation research are required to drive innovation, but research investments need to be better aligned to burden of disease.

Conclusions

Women's health and that of their children are intricately linked and dependent on one another, and the lifecourse of the girl, and her education are especially critical. This book is structured around that lifecourse, starting with the adolescent (Table 2.1).

Case study: Partnership for Maternal Newborn and Child Health and rising focus on adolescent health

In 2005, global attention was brought to the significant burden of neonatal mortality with the publication of the *Lancet Neonatal Series*, and also the ongoing burden of maternal and child deaths, with only

Table 2.1 Summary of target populations through the lifecourse, linked to sections in this book

Target population through the Lifecourse	Number of deaths	Section in this book
Adolescents	1.2 million	4
Women of reproductive age	—	5
Pregnant women	0.30 million	5
Postnatal women	0.30 million	5
Stillbirths	2.6 million	6
Newborns	2 million	6
Children (1 month - 5th birthday)	3.2 million	7
Families and social context	—	Throughout

ten years left before the end of the MDGs. Three existing organisations agreed that a united voice would be more effective and these merged: the Partnership for Safe Motherhood and Newborn Health (hosted by the WHO), the Healthy Newborn Partnership (based at Save the Children USA), and the Child Survival Partnership (hosted by UNICEF, New York). This merger gave birth to the Partnership for Maternal Newborn and Child Health (PMNCH), to support accelerated progress towards MDGs 4 and 5, through enhanced accountability. The Partnership's conceptual framework the continuum of care covering sexual, reproductive, maternal, newborn, child, and adolescent health. Its four strategic objectives are: advocacy, alignment, analysis and accountability. Currently it comprises over 700 organisations, spanning 77 countries, which include intergovernmental organisations, non-governmental organisations; academic, research, and training institutions, healthcare professional associations private sector partners, UN agencies, and global financing mechanisms. The Partnership led to the UN Secretary General's Global Strategy from 2010 to 2015, which helped more than double global funding for women's, children's, and adolescents' health. For the SDG era, the framework is the Global Strategy for Women's Children's and Adolescents' Health (2016-2030) with three pillars: survive, thrive, and transform.

Questions

1. Summarise the concept of the continuum of care.

2. Describe the evolution from 'maternal and child health' to the lifecourse approach, including target groups that have been previously neglected.

Key publications

Kerber K, de Graft-Johnson J, Bhutta Z, et al. (2007). Continuum of care for maternal, newborn, and child health: from slogan to service delivery. 2007, *Lancet* 370(9595): 1358–69.
Comprehensive overview of the continuum of care.

PMNCH website
http://www.who.int/pmnch/en/
The main website of the Partnership for Maternal Newborn, and Child Health, describing its key activities and opportunities to get involved.

The Global Strategy for Women's, Children's, and Adolescents' Health (2016–2030)
www.who.int/pmnch/media/events/2015/gs_2016_30.pdf
This document sets out the UN's strategy to improve women's children's, and adolescents' health by 2030.

Bibliography

Countdown to 2015 final report: http://countdown2030.org/reports-and-articles/2015-final-report
Lancet Ending Preventable Stillbirth Series (2016), 387.
Lancet Every Newborn Series (2014), 384.
Lancet Maternal Health Series (2016), 388.
Lancet Neonatal Survival Series (2005), 365.
Lawn J, Tinker A, Munjanja S, and Cousens S (2007). Where is maternal and child health now? *Lancet* 368: 1474–77.
The World Health Report (2005). Make every mother and child count.
Stenberg K, Axelson H, Sheehan P, et al. (2014). Advancing social and economic development by investing in women's and children's health: a new Global Investment Framework. *Lancet* 383(9925): 1333–54.

CHAPTER 3

Agencies and actors in women's, children's, and adolescents' health

Mike Rowson

This chapter reviews the relevant institutions of global health governance, how they are governed and financed, and examines how these have evolved over the past seventy years.

Key points

◆ Global health governance represents a delicate balance between competing party interests, including the organisations set up to manage it (like the World Health Organization (WHO), United Nations Children's Fund (UNICEF)), the rich nations that largely fund them, and the poor nations where much of their advice and resources are directed.

◆ Global health governance has grown over the last seventy years. New actors like philanthropists, civil society organisations, and the private sector exist and their influence is both praised and criticised. In response, global health has moved from an agenda driven by United Nations (UN) agencies, to one driven by funders and coalitions of interested parties, and this is particularly visible in the area of women's, children's, and adolescents' health. But this raises new issues of fragmentation and accountability.

◆ The number of new issues coming onto the agenda—and in global health more broadly—suggest that governance arrangements will evolve further. But there may still be a role for a coordinator of this new interconnected world. Will the World Health Organization prove up to the challenge?

Background

The past century has seen a solid set of organisational structures evolve to manage the challenges of global health. These were set up initially under the auspices of the UN, but now all kinds of actors, public and private, local, national, and international are contributing to the governance of global health. These changes have implications for how and who sets the agenda for women's, children's, and adolescents' health, and for management and daily financing of on-the-ground interventions.

Global health governance 1.0: the WHO in the lead

The UN was established in response to the breakdown of international order that had occurred from the 1920s onwards,

culminating in World War Two. The nation states that agreed to set up the new body did not see this as a 'world government'. Instead the UN represented a delicate balance between the interests of individual nation states and their recognition that many global problems could not be solved by any one of them acting alone, no matter how powerful. War was one such problem—global poverty and disease were others. The UN's specialised health agency, the WHO, its children's charity, UNICEF, and the United Nations Population Fund (UNFPA) dominated the aid landscape for child wellbeing during the second half of the twentieth century.

The WHO has a staff of 7000 people and an annual budget of around US$2–2.5 billion. Its supreme decision-making body is the World Health Assembly (WHA) who ratify the organisation's policies and its budget and other organisational matters. All 194 member states of the WHO are represented by ministers of health or senior government officials responsible for public health. All member countries have to make a financial contribution to the WHO, but most of the budget comes from additional, voluntary contributions from rich nations.

The WHO has widespread respect among low- and middle-income countries (LMICs), as an important forum where their concerns can be heard. An important moment for the organisation came in 1978, when it produced the 'Health for All by the year 2000' Alma-Ata Declaration on Primary Health Care. The declaration set out a comprehensive vision of a functioning health system, including the need to address the determinants of health outside the health sector, such as education and improvements in water and sanitation. Much of the practical focus of the declaration was on addressing the burden of high mortality—especially among children—which weighed upon developing countries.

UNICEF also took a leading role in this period. The organisation, which today has an annual budget of around US$5 billion (financed on a voluntary basis from governments, the private sector, civil society, and individual donations) addresses a wide range of children's issues (not just health). It collaborated with WHO to produce the Alma-Ata Declaration, but subsequently backed a slimmed-down version of primary health care which focused on specific interventions which were thought to have the biggest impact on child health, including growth monitoring, oral rehydration therapy, breastfeeding, and immunisation, coupled with attention to family planning, food supplementation, and female education. This became known as the 'child survival revolution' and it received massive backing from donors, though it had run out of steam by the mid-1990s. UNICEF also backed the UN Convention on the Rights of the Child (1989), a human rights instrument which quickly gained international acceptance.

UNFPA was set up in 1969 to address global concerns with rapid population growth. More broadly, it aims to support reproductive health care for women and youth in more than 150 countries and tackle issues such as child marriage, female genital mutilation, and gender-based violence. In doing so, it is guided by the 1994 Programme of Action of the International Conference on Population and Development (a hugely influential UN Summit), in which UNFPA played a leading role. It is a relatively small agency with an annual budget of about US$1 billion, mainly financed on a voluntary basis by high-income country government donors.

The WHO's relative power declined in the 1990s, as a result of funding challenges and poor leadership. The leadership of global health policy passed to the World Bank, who made major policy interventions and backed them with massive spending power. The WHO was also slow to act on the acquired immunodeficiency syndrome (AIDS) crisis which began to decimate African populations in the 1990s. This paved the way for a transformation of global health governance.

Global health governance 2.0: growth in actors and funding

The Human Immunodeficiency Virus (HIV)/AIDS crisis and the continuing scourge of other infectious diseases gripped the international community in the run-up to the new millennium, and led to the founding of the Global Fund to Fight AIDS, tuberculosis and malaria in 2002. The Global Fund represented a new type of organisation (dubbed a Global Public Private Partnership (GPPP)) meant to mobilise both government and private sector support for health objectives. Donors also set up the Global Alliance on Vaccines and Immunisations (now known as Gavi, the Vaccine Alliance) as another GPPP to galvanise international action in this area once more. These organisations had governing bodies that were much smaller than the WHA, and included representation beyond governments.

This resulted in renewed energy for global health. Financial resources from international donors increased six-fold from the 1990s to the present day, and stood at over US$37 billion in 2016. Despite attempts to encourage the private sector, much of this funding came from existing bilateral donors—such as the UK and US governments. Where the private sector was involved, most resources came from private philanthropy, notably the Bill and Melinda Gates Foundation, as well as international non-governmental organisations such as Save the Children. The private commercial sector has not provided great resources. Funding for maternal and child health saw a particularly large rise, increasing from about US$3 billion in 2003 to US$11 billion. Two thirds of this funding is for child health, particularly more 'vertical' programmes such as immunisation, HIV/AIDS, and malaria. Annual rates of reduction in child mortality improved substantially after 2000, as did those for maternal mortality, albeit to a lesser extent. Neonatal mortality rates reduced much more slowly, with few mentions in donor funding prior to 2005.

Increased resources were, however, accompanied by increased fragmentation in the global governance of maternal and child health which resulted in clashing mandates, gaps, and inefficiency. There was an attempt to bring together actors and agencies separately concerned with different aspects of the maternal-child health continuum, in order to mobilise support for Millennium Development Goals

(MDGs) 4 and 5, which were focused on child and maternal health. This resulted in the Partnership for Maternal, Newborn and Child Health (Chapter 2), which eventually burgeoned into a network of over 700 actors, including governments, non-governmental organisations, health professional associations, academic departments, private foundations, and companies, attempting to set a common agenda for women's, children's, and adolescents' health, shifting the paradigm to Maternal, Newborn and Child Health (MNCH).

Yet fragmentation remains within such broad coalitions, and the partnership has arguably marginalised consideration of controversial issues, such as stillbirths, abortion, and sexual and reproductive rights. Targeted approaches to improving quality of life of specific populations still dominate over broader health systems and social determinants of health approaches which might benefit wider populations. There is concern over the influence of private actors on decision-making processes, and the accountability of these groups.

Global health governance 3.0: a new approach

Some commentators are now suggesting that further innovation is needed in global health governance. The realities of globalisation and technological change make nation states less important than before, and global health needs organisations that work with many partners who can bring information, influence, and resources to the table. The old decision-making processes, it is said, are not up to the challenge of responding to a fast-changing world.

Challenges

As Chapter 1 demonstrated, there is also a new agenda for women's, children's, and adolescents' health emerging which moves beyond 'lives saved' to thinking about how children might thrive into adolescence and adulthood, and about new issues such as mental health, non-communicable diseases (NCDs), and the effects of climate change and war.

Nonetheless, the likeliest outcome may be more of the same. New issues are likely to come onto the global agenda in a haphazard way. Developing countries may become the trailblazers for a more joined up approach, as they expand their health systems, and address a fuller range of women's, children's, and adolescents' health concerns as time passes. Advocacy by civil society organisations may also be needed to refocus the health agenda—however, the strength of these actors, and their willingness to challenge existing paradigms remains to be seen.

Conclusions

This chapter has shown that powerful nation states, and their resources, have been key at every stage of the governance of maternal and child health globally. It is certain that their interests will continue to exert a major influence. We may have a more pluralistic system today, but there is an argument that we need a strong coordinating body to give this system a steer. An 'upgraded' WHO, setting the new policy agenda, engaging with the realities of global health governance 3.0, and reaching out to wider networks of actors may be the organisation to do this. But it will need to keep the support of its nation state members in doing so, in particular the rich and influential ones (Table 3.1).

Table 3.1 Who's got the power? Key actors in global health and their governance and financing

Agency (year established)	Remit	Sources of funding	Role in women's, children's, and adolescents' health	Total funding for all activities (2015 or 2016)
Multilateral agencies				
World Health Organization—WHO (1948)	The WHO is a rule creator and agenda setting organisation.	A levy proportional to GDP from all member states and voluntary contributions from, mainly, rich nation governments.	Identifies research priorities and sets guidelines for improving women's, children's, and adolescents' health for national governments and other stakeholders. Responsible for health data and estimates.	Programme budget approximately US$2 billion on annual basis (more commonly expressed as approx US$4 billion on biennial basis)
United Nations Children's Fund— UNICEF (1946)	Promotes children's rights worldwide and takes action to improve their livelihoods, and leading implementor in almost all countries. Upholds the UN Convention on the Rights of the Child.	Voluntary donations from member governments and fundraising from private sources.	Promotes and funds programmes in countries to improve child health, including large scale notably for immunisation, HIV, malaria. Provides data and policy perspectives on child health worldwide.	US$5 billion in contribution income
United Nations Population Fund— UNFPA (1969)	Supports reproductive health worldwide.	Governments and the private sector.	Supports reproductive health care worldwide for women and young people; promotes the health of pregnant women; supports prevention of FGM, child marriage.	US$979 million in contribution income
World Bank (1944)	Provides grants, loans and policy advice to promote long-term development and poverty reduction.	Governments, interest on World Bank loans, money raised on stock market.	Funds projects to support child health, as well as broader health systems strengthening at country level.	US$45 billion Combined IDA and IBRD lending
Donor governments (three biggest women's, children's, and adolescents' health contributors among rich nation governments)				
Agency (year established)	Remit	Sources of funding	Role in women's, children's, and adolescents' health	Total funding for all activities (2015 or 2016)
USA—United States Agency for International Development—USAID (1961) and other agencies.	Lead US government aid agency tackling global poverty and promoting economic development and democracy.	American taxpayers.	Funds projects in 25 priority countries to tackle family planning, maternal and child health, malaria, and nutrition.	US$33.5 billion
United Kingdom— Department for International Development—DfID (1964, renamed in 1997)	Lead UK government department tackling poverty in developing countries and other global challenges.	British taxpayers.	Funds research and programmes in priority countries to reduce maternal, newborn, and child deaths. Also focuses on family planning and FGM.	US$18 billion
Canada—Global Affairs Canada (formerly Canadian International Development Agency (1968))	Promotes international development efforts on behalf of the Canadian government.	Canadian taxpayers.	Funds interventions to promote maternal and child health, with priority given to child nutrition and development.	US$4 billion

(continued)

Table 3.1 Continued

Global public—private partnerships				
Agency (year establ,ished)	**Remit**	**Sources of funding**	**Role in women's, children's and adolescents' health**	**Total funding for all activities (2015 or 2016)**
Gavi, the Vaccine Alliance (2000)	Aims to improve access to new and underused vaccines for children in the world's poorest countries by pooling public and private sector resources and expertise.	Kick started by major donation from Bill and Melinda Gates Foundation, mainly funded by rich country governments (with contribution from poor countries) and private sector donations.	Funds vaccine investment (including in systems), improves markets for vaccines and other immunisations, promotes access to vaccines.	US$1.6 billion in contribution income
Global Fund to Fight AIDS, tuberculosis, and malaria (2002)	Funding (not implementing) agency, aimed at addressing the three diseases.	Mainly funded by rich nation governments, though some developing country governments also invest. PRODUCT (RED) also raises funds from popular consumer brands. Bill and Melinda Gates Foundation has provided significant resources.	Provides financing for projects to tackle HIV for adolescents and young women and other aspects of women's, children's, and adolescents' health affected by the three diseases.	US$5.2 billion in contribution income
Philanthropy and non-governmental organisations (examples)				
Bill and Melinda Gates Foundation (2000)	Philanthropic agency funding development and health priorities in poorer countries and vulnerable groups and education in the United States.	Investment assets from Bill and Melinda Gates, with contributions from financier Warren Buffett.	Invests in the development and delivery of interventions that can improve the health and survival of women, newborns, and young children.	US$4.3 billion in grantee support
Save the Children (1919)	International non-governmental organisation with international office and 28 high income country members.	Donations from government and the private sector, fundraising from the general public.	Provide interventions and support community health systems in developing countries. Undertakes policy advice and advocacy on child health.	US$2.1 billion turnover

Source: data from the WHO, UNICEF, UNFPA, World Bank, USAID, DfID, Global Affairs Canada, Gavi, Global Fund to Fight AIDS, Tuberculosis and Malaria, Bill & Melinda Gates Foundation and Save the Children. Please note there may be significant funding fluctuations from year to year.

Questions

1. Has the increasing number of actors involved in women's, children's, and adolescents' health, especially since 2000, been a good thing?

2. With increased global funding for women's, children's, and adolescents' health, and a much bigger proportion coming from private philanthropy, what is the role for national governments in funding their own health care systems?

Key publications

Frenk J and Moon S (2013). Governance challenges in global health. *New Eng J Med* 368(10): 936–42.
    Good overview of global health governance in general.

Lawn J, Rohde J, Rifkin S, et al. (2008). Alma-Ata 30 years on: revolutionary, relevant, and time to revitalise. *Lancet* (372)9642: 917–27.
    This paper shows the power of the original Alma-Ata declaration and its relevance to the current era.

Bibliography

Grollman C, Arregoces L, Martinez-Alvarez M, Pitt C, Mills A, and Borghi J (2017). Eleven years of tracking aid to reproductive, maternal, newborn and child health: estimates and analysis for 2003–13 from the Countdown to 2015. *Lancet Global Health* 5: e104–14.

Institute for Health Metrics and Evaluation (2017). *Financing Global Health 2016: Development Assistance, Public and Private Health Spending for the Pursuit of Universal Health Coverage.* IHME: Seattle, WA.

McDougall L (2016). Discourse, ideas and power in global health policy networks: political attention for maternal and child health in the Millennium Development Goal era. *Globalization and Health* 12: 21.

Pitt C, Grollman C, Martínez-Álvarez M, Arregoces L, Lawn J, and Borghi J (2017). Countdown to 2015: an analysis of donor funding for prenatal and neonatal health, 2003–2013. *BMJ Global Health* 2: e000205

Smith R and Lee K (2017). Global health governance: we need innovation not renovation. *BMJ Global Health* 2: e000275.

Storeng K and Behague D (2016). 'Lives in the balance': the politics of integration in the Partnership for Maternal, Newborn and Child Health. *Health Policy and Planning* 31: 992–1000.

SECTION 2

Research methods

CHAPTER 4

Research methods and evidence-based medicine

Tim Colbourn

This chapter provides an overview of research methods used to build the evidence base for global maternal and child health. It covers primary data collection, secondary data analysis, systematic reviews, and meta-analysis and provides tips on how to interpret the scientific literature. This chapter should be read in conjunction with Chapter 5 on economic evaluation and Chapter 44 on converting research into policy to put the use of research evidence into context.

Key points

- Clearly define a research question before deciding what study type is best suited to answer it.

- Designing a research study involves detailed attention to practical details, including how groups are going to be defined.

- Scientific studies are sometimes published with incorrect conclusions. Critically appraise each study, and define appropriate conclusions that are based on the data and methodology.

Background

Rigorous research is necessary to understand problems in global women's, children's, and adolescents' health and to design and evaluate interventions to overcome them. Different research methods are suitable for different ends, that is, case reports and case-control studies are more suitable for discovery and explanatory research, whereas randomised controlled trials (RCTs) are more suitable for evaluation of interventions. Rather than using intuition or best guesses from basic science, policy and practice should be based on rigorous evidence, using methods and avoiding common study limitations described in this chapter. This is evidence-based medicine and involves basing decisions on systematic reviews and critical appraisal of published research studies.

Recommendations

Use EQUATOR network reporting guidelines http://www.equator-network.org/. To ensure research is reported well, guidelines for different study types have been created, for example PRISMA for systematic reviews and meta-analyses, and STROBE for observational studies.

Primary research

The first step in research is to clearly define your question—what are you investigating? in what population? where? when? compared to what? For example: 'what is the effect of having four antenatal care visits compared to no antenatal care on maternal mortality in pregnant women giving birth to their first child in rural Zambia in 2018?' To answer this question, you would need to collect data on a representative sample of pregnant women in rural Zambia after clearly defining rural Zambia, antenatal care visits, pregnant women, and maternal mortality. You could use a variety of study designs to answer this question. Some common designs and their pros and cons are listed in Table 4.1.

Research data can be qualitative (words) or quantitative (numbers). Data are collected to answer a research question, either seeking to understand a problem, or design or test an intervention to overcome a problem. Qualitative research involves conducting interviews or focus group discussions with people who are affected by the problem or who are involved in intervention delivery. Quantitative research involves use of standardised, reliable and valid measurements to determine the relative or absolute size and distribution of a problem and the relative or absolute effect of an intervention on the problem as characterised by an outcome of interest.

In global women's, children's, and adolescents' health, epidemiological studies seek to understand the distribution and determinants of problems such as maternal mortality, premature birth, or childhood under-nutrition. Studies from other allied health disciplines such as anthropology, demography, health psychology, and economics may shed further light on such problems. Taking one such problem, maternal mortality, formative research studies may then seek to develop interventions to reduce maternal mortality by targeting the causes and antecedent conditions discovered by the epidemiological and other descriptive studies. The intervention can then be tested in a trial to determine if it can reduce maternal mortality. An example of a trial to reduce maternal mortality is Lewycka et al. (2013), who trialled women's groups practising participatory learning and action to reduce maternal and newborn mortality in Malawi.

Primary research studies can be summarised and pooled in secondary research. Figure 4.1 provides an overview of different types of research and their functions through to policy and practice.

Table 4.1 Types of research design

Type of research	Description	When it is used	Advantages	Disadvantages
Case report/ case series	Report(s) on disease presentation or treatment effect in individual(s).	For rare diseases, rare presentations of diseases, new treatments, or new reactions to known treatments.	◆ Low cost ◆ Quick ◆ Easier follow-up	◆ Less representative of population ◆ Inferences about prevalence or causality difficult to establish
Cross-sectional study	Representative population sample studied at one time point.	To measure disease prevalence and risk factors.	◆ Relatively cheap ◆ Results generalisable to source population	◆ Most severe/fatal disease presentations often excluded ◆ Causality difficult to establish
Case control study	Comparison of people with the disease/outcome (e.g. neonatal sepsis) to those without the disease/outcome (controls) in terms of exposure to risk factors.	To establishing associations between a disease and risk factor(s).	◆ Can study uncommon diseases ◆ Relatively quick and cheap	◆ Identification of suitable controls—matched with cases on important variables—may be difficult ◆ Less strong causal evidence than cohort studies as difficult to establish that exposure preceded outcome
Cohort study	A population with a range of risk factors is followed up at multiple time points and the outcome(s) of interest are measured.	Good for identifying premorbid disease markers, measuring disease prevalence and incidence, and determining risk factors.	◆ Information about exposures (risk factors) is collected before outcomes happen, so temporal relation of exposure and outcome is clearer	◆ Expensive and time-consuming ◆ Difficult to prevent loss-to-follow-up
Randomised controlled trial	One group in the trial receives an intervention (e.g. new medical treatment) and the other group—the control group—receives current treatment or a placebo. Individuals have an equal random chance of being allocated to each group, and participants, investigators, and analysts may be blinded to the allocation.	Excellent for looking at effects of a new treatment on a known disease, or looking at primary preventative measures.	◆ Randomisation means that groups should be similar in both measured and unmeasured confounders, allowing a causal estimate of the effect of the new intervention on the outcome ◆ Allows blinding of participants, so results cannot be affected by knowledge of the intervention	◆ Expensive ◆ Logistically difficult to recruit sufficient numbers, ensure adequate blinding, and complete follow-up
Systematic review/ meta-analysis	Combines information from multiple independent studies to answer a research question. Systematic reviews do this in a descriptive manner; meta-analysis estimates an overall effect.	To answer a research question using all available evidence. Meta-analysis can determine overall effect size when some studies reject the null hypothesis and others do not.	◆ Relatively cheap ◆ Can provide strong evidence ◆ Can qualify and quantify inconsistencies across similar studies ◆ Results generalisable to large population(s), and also, via subgroup analysis, to population subsets	◆ Publication bias: negative/ insignificant results are less often published (though there are methods to assess this) ◆ Meta-analysis results can be manipulated by cherry picking favourable studies

Measures of effect and statistical significance

Quantitative results are often reported as risk ratios (RR) or odds ratios (OR). These can both be derived from a two-by-two table of the numbers of people who have, and do not have the outcome of interest each subdivided by those who were exposed to the environmental hazard (in observational epidemiology) or the intervention of interest. The case study provides an example and shows the calculations. The absolute risk (AR) may be very small even though the RR or OR is large, that is, a RR of two (one group having

twice the risk of another) would apply to an increase in risk from 0.0001% to 0.0002%.

OR and RR effects are usually reported with a 95% confidence interval (95% CI), which provides a range that we can be 95% confident that the true effect lies within. The larger the sample size the narrower the confidence interval and the more sure we can be of the effect size. Statistical significance is directly related to the 95% CI—at the commonly used 5% level of significance (p<0.05) the 95% CI of a RR or OR will not span 1 (no difference between groups), that

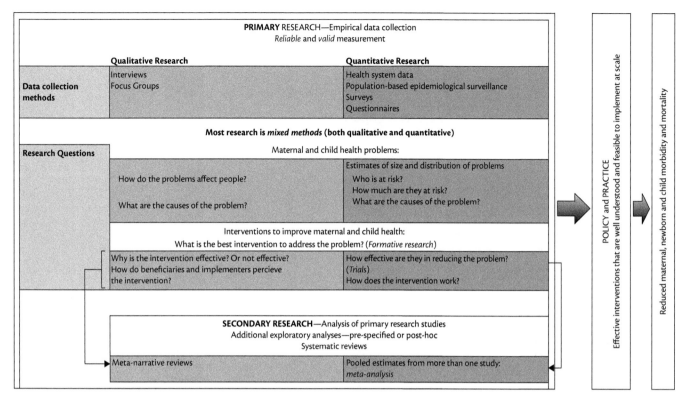

Figure 4.1 Overview of research methods.

is, we are 95% confident in our rejection of the null hypothesis of no difference between groups—either the effect is an increase in risk or odds (RR or OR above 1), or a decrease (RR or OR below 1).

Secondary research

Secondary research involves further analysis of data collected in primary research studies. Exploratory analyses use data to answer questions that the primary study may not have been originally designed to answer. Such post-hoc analyses are prone to bias, therefore should be confirmed by further prospective primary studies specifically designed to answer the question.

Trials can be pooled in a meta-analysis to calculate an overall measure of effect. Meta-analyses are often informed by systematic reviews. Figure 4.2 shows results of a systematic review and meta-analysis of the effect of women's groups practising participatory learning and action. The pooled effect estimate from the four high-coverage studies indicates a 33% (95% CI: 25–40%) reduction in neonatal mortality.

Interpreting the literature—common study limitations

When reading research literature it is important to critically assess the study methods and reporting of results in order to be sure the results and conclusions are robust. Some common study limitations are:

Insufficient sample size—small sample sizes lead to uncertain effects (large confidence intervals) and studies that may not be able to answer the question.

Confounding and incorrect attribution—the results of observational studies, or trials with inadequate random allocation, may be confounded by other causal factors. When such variables are measured it is possible to adjust the intervention effect for their presence by including them in the analysis. Studies measuring changes in outcomes over time without a comparison group may be subject to attribution bias, too, if plausible secular trends (background changes) unrelated to the intervention are responsible for outcome changes.

Unreliable or invalid measurement—pilot testing can ensure the questionnaire results in consistent responses in the same population. Validation is required to ensure the questions or measurements measure the construct, concept, or outcome they are intended to.

Challenges

There needs to be a greater focus on applied population-based research, trialling of interventions in real-life settings, and understanding how they work via implementation science (investigation of how interventions are implemented) and theory-based evaluation studies. Too great a proportion of biomedical research funding is spent on basic laboratory science and not enough is spent on population-based interventions, which could have a much larger impact in the short to medium term.

Research funding is also too often wasted on poor-quality research or research that is not reported, or reported badly, hindering its translation to policy and practice, and lessening impact on health. Adhering to reporting standards and providing incentives

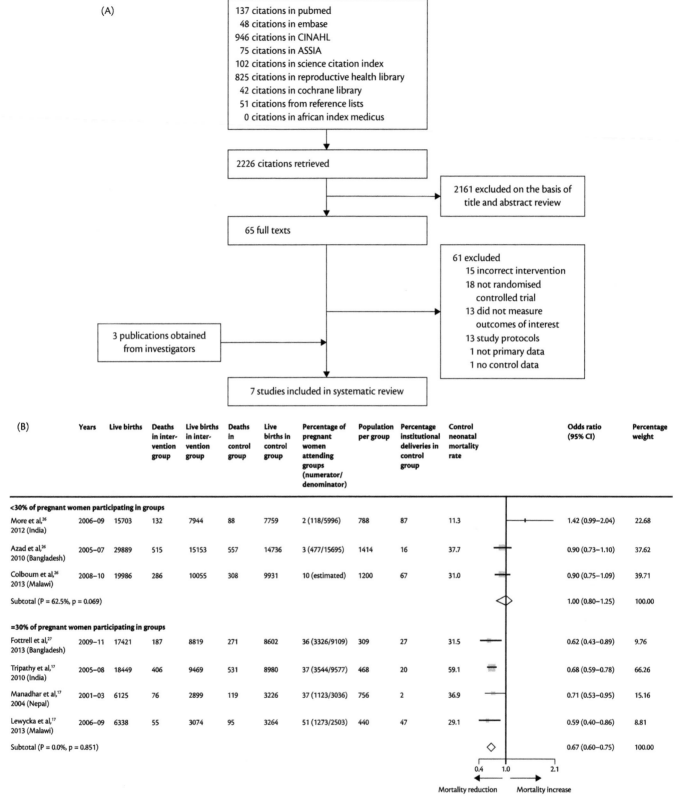

Figure 4.2 (A) Systematic review results. (B) Meta-analysis results for the effect of women's groups on neonatal mortality.

(A) Reproduced from Prost et al. Women's groups practising participatory learning and action to improve maternal and newborn health in resource-limited settings: systematic review and meta-analysis. *The Lancet*, 381 (9879), 1736–1746. Copyright © 2013 Elsevier Ltd. Open Access.

(B) Reproduced from Prost et al. Women's groups practising participatory learning and action to improve maternal and newborn health in resource-limited settings: systematic review and meta-analysis. *The Lancet*, 381 (9879), 1736–1746. Copyright © 2013 Elsevier Ltd. Open Access.

to peer reviewers and journal editors should increase the quality of scientific reporting.

Future priorities

♦ Negative/insignificant results are less often published, leading to distortion in reviews of evidence, and leading to publication bias. Dealing with publication bias is important, and initiatives such as AllTrials (www.alltrials.net) are working to ensure the results of all trials are freely available.

♦ Data collection and interventions using mobile phones present opportunities for more efficient research and interventions with potentially greater reach. Such technology enables people to be involved in research as citizen scientists, and behaviours can change via such active participation. The exponential increase in data generation presents opportunities for linking large datasets ('big data') towards answering research questions requiring large sample sizes.

♦ Larger collaborations of researchers and implementers spanning multiple disciplines are increasingly needed to address population-based research challenges. Future research priorities involve measuring the poorest and most vulnerable populations to ensure no one is left behind, and tackling the 'know-do' gap to improve front-line implementation and mechanisms ensuring sustainability of interventions.

Conclusions

Research, carefully undertaken and correctly applied, can transform policy and practice to achieve better outcomes for mothers and children in all settings.

Case study: two-by-two table calculations

		Outcome		Total
		Premature delivery	Term delivery	
Exposure	Antenatal care	60	540	600
	No antenatal care	90	310	400
	Total	150	850	1000

Odds of premature delivery with antenatal care = 60/540 = 11.1%

Odds of premature delivery without antenatal care = 90/310 = 29.0%

Odds ratio = 11.1/29.0% = 0.38

The odds of premature delivery in those with antenatal care are 0.38 times the odds in those without antenatal care.

Odds ratios are used in case control studies where the total population size is unknown, and are also, due to the mathematical properties of statistically modelling binary outcomes, the results of logistic regression analyses.

Risk of premature delivery with antenatal care = 60/600 = 10.0%

Risk of premature delivery without antenatal care = 90/400 = 22.5%

Risk ratio = 10.0/22.5% = 0.44

The risk of premature delivery in those with antenatal care is 0.44 times the risk in those without antenatal care.

Risk ratios are used when the total population is known, and are more intuitively interpretable than odds ratios.

Absolute risk = 10.0% – 22.5% = –12.5%

The absolute risk of premature delivery in those with antenatal care is 12.5% less than the risk in those without antenatal care.

Absolute risks should also be presented in addition to relative measures of effect (OR or RR) to give an indication of the size of the population affected and the public health significance of the findings.

Questions

1. What kinds of questions can primary research answer?

2. Why are systematic reviews important and how can they help policy makers?

3. What does a risk ratio of 0.75 (95% CI: 0.45–1.05) mean in terms of:

   a) The percentage reduction in risk?

   b) The statistical significance

   c) The likely sample size (small or large)

4. Describe a common problem in maternal or newborn health, specify a research question aimed at tackling the problem and design a research study to answer the question.

Key publications

Bonita R, Beaglehole R, and Kjellström T (2006). *Basic Epidemiology,* second edition. World Health Organization. http://whqlibdoc.who.int/publications/2006/9241547073_eng.pdf
   A highly recommended introduction to epidemiology.

Kirkwood B and Sterne J (2003). *Essential Medical Statistics.* Wiley-Blackwell: London, UK.
   Excellent introductory textbook on medical statistics—covers all the methods you will need in undergraduate and postgraduate study.

Pope C and Mays N (2008). *Qualitative Methods in Healthcare Research,* third edition. BMJ Books: London, UK.
   Good introductory textbook detailing how to conduct and interpret qualitative research.

Porta M (2014). *A Dictionary of Epidemiology,* sixth edition. Oxford University Press: Oxford, UK.
   Contains detailed definitions and illustrated examples of concepts and topics from basic through to more advanced epidemiology.

Bibliography

Chalmers I, Bracken M, Djulbegovic B, et al. (2014). How to increase value and reduce waste when research priorities are set. *Lancet* 383: 156–65.

Chan A-W, Song F, Vickers A, et al. (2014). Increasing value and reducing waste: addressing inaccessible research. *Lancet* 383: 257–66.

Damschroder L, Aron D, Keith R, Kirsh S, Alexander J, and Lowery J (2009). Fostering implementation of health services research findings into practice: a consolidated framework for advancing implementation science. *Implement Sci* 4: 50.

Evidence-Based Medicine Working Group 1992. Evidence-based medicine. A new approach to teaching the practice of medicine. *JAMA* 268: 2420–5.

Glasziou P, Altman D, Bossuyt P, et al. (2014). Reducing waste from incomplete or unusable reports of biomedical research. *Lancet* 383: 267–76.

Greenhalgh T, Howick J, and Maskrey N (2014). Evidence-based medicine: a movement in crisis? *BMJ* 348: g3725.

Ioannidis J, Greenland S, Hlatky M, et al. (2014). Increasing value and reducing waste in research design, conduct, and analysis. *Lancet* 383: 166–75.

Lewycka S, Mwansambo C, Rosato M, et al. (2013). Effect of women's groups and volunteer peer counsellors on rates of mortality, morbidity and health behaviours in mothers and children in rural Malawi (MaiMwana): a factorial, cluster-randomised controlled trial. *Lancet* 381: 1721–35.

Prost A, Colbourn T, Seward N, et al. (2013). Women's groups practising participatory learning and action to improve maternal and newborn health in resource-limited settings: systematic review and meta-analysis. *Lancet* 381: 1736–46.

Rogers P, Petrosino A, Huebner T, and Hacsi T (2000). Program theory evaluation: practice, promise, and problems. *New Directions for Evaluation* 87: 5–13.

Sondaal S, Browne J, Amoakoh-Coleman M, et al. (2016). Assessing the effect of mHealth interventions in improving maternal and neonatal care in low- and middle-income countries: a systematic review. *PLoS ONE* 11: e0154664.

Vandenbroucke J (2008). Observational research, randomised trials, and two views of medical science. *PLoS Med* 5: e67.

CHAPTER 5

Economic evaluation in global health

Catherine Pitt, Josephine Borghi, and Kara Hanson

This chapter introduces key concepts and terminology used in the economic evaluation of strategies to improve health in a global context. It should be read in conjunction with Chapter 4 on research methods and evidence-based medicine, Chapter 8 on health workers and health systems, and Chapter 44 on translating research into policy.

Key points

♦ Economic evaluation provides a framework for systematically comparing the costs and effects of healthcare interventions to help choose which interventions to invest in.

♦ The cost of an intervention is the value of the resources used to produce it and associated with its consequences; valuing these resources requires recognition that resources are scarce, and that they have alternative uses.

Background

Given the scarcity of resources to fund the health sector, choices must be made as to where to invest. Each time a choice is made, alternative possible choices are foregone. Economic evaluation aims to inform policy decisions about whether to invest (or disinvest) in specific activities by comparing the relative costs and effects of two or more interventions.

Recommendations

Economic evaluations should be conducted and reported in standardised ways to enable the comparison of results across studies, to assess generalisability of findings, and to determine the study quality. Generic reporting guidelines and critical appraisal checklists recommend the types of information that should be presented in a research article. A reference case for conducting economic evaluations in low- and middle-income countries has been developed by the International Decision Support Initiative.

What is health economic evaluation?

Economic evaluation is a systematic comparison of the costs and consequences of two or more alternative courses of action. Economic evaluation involves carefully setting out the decision problem; framing the economic evaluation; measuring and valuing the costs and effects associated with an intervention relative to

alternatives; and bringing these data together with other evidence, often with modelling.

How is a health economic evaluation conducted?

The following steps should be undertaken:

1. Frame the evaluation: define the scope of the study, considering who the decision makers are, the decision problem(s) they face, and resource availability.

2. Define the intervention and comparator: consider who does what to whom, when, in what setting, and with what resources. For a new intervention, at least one of the comparisons should reflect current practice, to determine whether a change is warranted.

3. Choose the study perspective: for example a healthcare provider perspective, a third-party payer perspective, or a societal perspective (Table 5.1). The perspective can also apply to effects; for example, an insurance company may only consider the effects of an intervention on its policyholders.

4. Determine the time horizon: it should be long enough to capture all expected differences in costs and effects between the interventions under study. Time horizons depend on the nature of the intervention, and can be, for example, the duration of a programme (e.g. bed nets), or remaining life expectancy (e.g. treatment for a chronic condition).

5. Set the discount rate: to account for the fact that people place a higher value on costs and effects now rather than in the future, a discount rate is applied to future costs and effects. This is usually 3% per year.

Once these steps have been completed, the next step is to measure and value the costs and effects.

Measuring and valuing costs

The value of all resources that contribute to the delivery of the interventions and its associated effects (such as changes in utilisation) should be estimated, with a focus on the costs that are expected to differ between the interventions compared. Economic cost refers to the full value of resources consumed, determined by their opportunity cost. Researchers sometimes also measure 'financial costs', which refer to the monies paid for a given resource. Costs can

Table 5.1 Study perspectives

Perspective	Description
Healthcare provider perspective	Only the costs incurred by the programme provider are included.
Third-party payer perspective	Only the costs incurred by the health insurance agency are included.
Societal perspective	Includes all costs, regardless of who bears them, and is recommended for analysis in low- and middle-income countries.

be classified by type of input (e.g. staff time, medicines, transport, buildings, and equipment associated with the intervention), by the intervention activity (e.g. training, service delivery, monitoring), or by the source of payment (e.g. households, national government, donor agency).

Measuring and valuing health effects

The choice of effect measure determines the type of economic evaluation (Table 5.2) as well as the usefulness of the analysis. Condition-specific effects, such as a reduction in blood pressure, are often measured in clinical trials. Unless interventions are evaluated with the same measures of effects, their relative benefits cannot be compared. For example, it is not possible to compare vaccination and obstetric care unless an outcome that is common to both can be measured, such as deaths averted. Equally, studies presenting the cost per death averted or cost per life-year saved cannot be compared directly with interventions that reduce morbidity or improve quality of life.

To help compare interventions with different outcome profiles, composite measures such as disability-adjusted life-years (DALYs) and quality-adjusted life-years (QALYs) combine measures of length and quality of life into a single measure. One DALY reflects a year of life in full health lost, while one QALY reflects a year in full

Table 5.2 Types of economic evaluations

Evaluation type	Definition	Possible summary measures
Cost-effectiveness analysis	Health effects measured in 'natural units'.	◆ Cost per life-year saved ◆ Cost per death averted ◆ Cost per case of malaria averted ◆ Cost per unwanted pregnancy averted
Cost-utility analysis	Health effects measured using a generic measure combining length and quality of life.	◆ Cost per DALY averted ◆ Cost per QALY gained
Cost-benefit analysis	Health effects valued in monetary terms.	◆ Incremental net benefit (i.e. value of health effects less costs)

Source: adapted from Drummond, M.F. et al. *Methods for the economic evaluation of health care programmes.* Oxford, UK: Oxford University Press. Copyright ©2015 Oxford University Press.

health gained. Both measures use weights to adjust for time spent in less than perfect health. For each health state, a universal DALY weight can be applied to all populations, while QALY weights vary across populations because they reflect local population preferences regarding that health condition. DALYs are more frequently used in low- and lower-middle-income countries; QALYs are more frequently used in high- and upper-middle-income countries. They cannot be compared directly with one another.

Analysis

Once costs and effects have been measured, valued, and discounted for each of the interventions under study, they are typically combined into a summary measure, the incremental cost-effectiveness ratio (ICER), in which the difference in costs of a given intervention (e.g. social marketing to promote modern contraceptive use) relative to an alternative (e.g. no social marketing) is divided by the difference in their effects:

$$ICER = \frac{Costs_{social\ marketing} - Costs_{no\ social\ marketing}}{Effects_{social\ marketing} - Effects_{no\ social\ marketing}}$$

The ICER reflects the additional cost per additional unit of effect achieved by an intervention compared with an alternative. If the ICER is below a given threshold, then the intervention of interest (in this case social marketing), would be considered cost-effective with respect to the alternative (no social marketing), for that threshold. The World Health Organization used to state that interventions costing less than a country's per capita gross domestic product (PCGDP) per DALY averted are 'highly cost-effective' and those costing less than three times PCGDP per DALY averted are 'cost-effective', but these thresholds are now agreed to be too high. In the United Kingdom, the National Institute for Health and Care Excellence uses a threshold of £20,000–30,000 per QALY gained.

Modelling

Models help to communicate the decision problem and to synthesise data from multiple sources. They can also be used to project costs and outcomes over longer time frames than clinical studies. Decision trees, the simplest model type, are particularly useful for simple interventions with linear pathways to outcomes, and illustrate the decision problem visually (Figure 5.1). Markov models are used when costs and consequences vary over time and/or when patients move back and forward between health states, such as for chronic conditions. Transmission models are less widely used, but are important for infectious diseases like measles because they account for how diseases spread between people.

Sensitivity analysis

Sensitivity analysis is used to assess how sensitive the main findings are to the assumptions made, to the structure of a model, and to uncertainty in the data. A first step is to vary one parameter at a time, such as the intervention's effectiveness or the unit cost of staff, considering its lowest and then highest plausible value based on the literature and/or local information, and then re-estimate the ICER. Probabilistic sensitivity analysis is used to account for

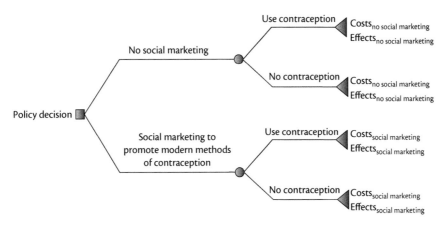

Figure 5.1 A simplified decision tree.

uncertainty in multiple parameters simultaneously. Assessing and communicating uncertainty to decision makers is an important aspect of a robust analysis. If the main decision recommendation remains the same for all sensitivity analyses, then it can be said to be 'robust'.

Using economic evaluation evidence in decision making

If an intervention is both more costly and more effective than its alternative, decision makers must decide whether the extra effects are worth the extra cost. This can be determined by whether the ICER lies below ICERs for alternative interventions or agreed thresholds.

Cost-effectiveness is not and should not be the only criterion on which policy makers base their decisions. Considerations of the budget impact, affordability, and equity effects of competing interventions, as well as their social acceptability and feasibility given health system constraints (such as the availability of human resources), are also important. For example, an intervention in pregnancy may cost less per DALY averted than agreed thresholds, but may not be funded if not acceptable to women or if the resource requirements exceed the available health budget.

Challenges

The conduct and reporting of economic evaluations are often not standardised. This makes it difficult to compare results across studies. Assessing the transferability and generalisability of economic evaluation findings from one setting to another is particularly important where funding for local research is scarce. It is very difficult, however, because it is often unclear how to account for the impact that differences between settings in demography, epidemiology, socioeconomic conditions, and health systems, including patient and provider behaviour, may have on costs, effects, and cost-effectiveness.

Comprehensively assessing the effects of interventions on women's, children's, and adolescents' health within economic evaluations can present challenges. Stillbirth and miscarriage, for example, are not captured in DALYs and are only reflected in QALYs in their impact on the mother's health. Early analyses of interventions to prevent malaria in pregnancy only examined effects on newborn outcomes

and did not include the consequences for mothers of reduced maternal anaemia and malaria morbidity. Lack of data makes it difficult to model how poor foetal, neonatal, and child health may impact lifelong health effects and their associated costs.

In all settings, commonly used thresholds for judging whether an intervention is cost-effective may be too high and lead to recommendations that are unaffordable.

Future priorities

To increase the conduct and use of economic evaluation to inform decision-making in low- and middle-income countries (LMICs), it is important to:

♦ Improve the availability of routine programme monitoring data on costs and effects.

♦ Increase the quality and comparability of economic evaluations conducted.

♦ Improve decision makers' ability to understand and appraise evidence.

♦ Strengthen national and regional health policymaking institutions.

Conclusions

Economic evaluations compare the relative costs and effects of two or more interventions to help guide policy decisions and investment choices. Their increased conduct and use in LMICs will help optimise the use of limited resources to improve health.

Case study: cost-effectiveness data can stimulate the scale-up of interventions

Cost-effectiveness data can be important in advocating for increased investment and scale-up of a given programme. For example, at just $US3 per DALY averted, hygiene promotion (such as handwashing with soap) was found to be the most cost-effective method of reducing diarrhoeal disease and associated mortality in children in low-income settings. This finding was instrumental in making the case for the scale-up of this intervention in low-income countries.

Questions

1. What are the main effect measures used in cost-effectiveness analyses and what are their strengths and weaknesses?

2. Alongside the incremental cost-effectiveness ratio, what other types of evidence might policymakers want to consider when deciding whether to implement a new strategy?

3. Identify the inputs and activities for an intervention which distributes insecticide treated bednets for malaria prevention to pregnant women during antenatal care. What data sources might you use to measure resource quantities consumed and how might you value them?

Key publications

Creese A and Parker D (1994). *Cost Analysis of Primary Health Care: a Training Manual for Programme Managers.* World Health Organization: Geneva.
  A practical set of guidelines for collecting and analysing cost information.

Drummond M, Sculpher M, Claxton K, et al. (2015). *Methods for the Economic Evaluation of Health Care Programmes*, fourth edition. Oxford University Press: Oxford, UK.
  The standard textbook for economic evaluation. http://info.worldbank.org/etools/docs/library/48284/20603.pdf.

Husereau D, Drummond M, Petrou S, et al. (2013). Consolidated Health Economic Evaluation Reporting Standards statement. *Cost Effective Resource Allocation* 11: 6.
  The most widely used guidelines for reporting economic evaluations, to support standardization and comparability.

International Decision Support Initiative. IDSi reference case for economic evaluation. http://www.idsihealth.org/resource-items/idsi-reference-case-for-economic-evaluation/
  This outlines a set of principles for undertaking economic evaluations of health interventions in low- and middle-income countries.

Mangham-Jefferies L, Pitt C, Cousens S, et al. (2014). Cost-effectiveness of strategies to improve the utilization and provision of maternal and newborn health care in low-income and lower-middle-income countries: a systematic review. *BMC Pregnancy Childbirth* 14: 243.
  A review of the evidence on cost-effectiveness of maternal and child health interventions.

Bibliography

Black R, Laxminarayan R, Temmerman M, and Walker N (2016). *Disease Control Priorities*, 3rd edition: volume 2. Reproductive, Maternal, Newborn, and Child Health. Washington, DC: World Bank. https://openknowledge.worldbank.org/handle/10986/23833

Briggs A, Claxton K, and Sculpher M. (2006). *Decision Modelling for Health Economic Evaluation.* Oxford University Press: Oxford UK.

Devlin N and Parkin D (2004). Does NICE have a cost-effectiveness threshold and what other factors influence its decisions? A binary choice analysis. *Health Econ* 13(5): 437–52.

Gomes M, Grieve R, Nixon R, and Edmunds W. (2012). Statistical methods for cost-effectiveness analyses that use data from cluster randomized trials: a systematic review and checklist for critical appraisal. *Med Decis Making* 32: 209–20.

Greco G, Lorgelly P, and Yamabhai I (2016). Outcomes in economic evaluations of public health interventions in low- and middle-income countries: health, capabilities and subjective wellbeing. *Health Econ* 25 Suppl 1: 83–94.

Griffiths U, Legood R, and Pitt C (2016). Comparison of economic evaluation methods across low-income, middle-income and high-income countries: what are the differences and why? *Health Econ* 25 Suppl 1: 29–41.

ISPOR (2016). *ISPOR Good Practices for Outcomes Research Index* (Online). International Society for Pharmacoeconomics and Outcomes Research. Available: http://www.ispor.org/workpaper/practices_index.asp.

Petrou S and Gray A (2011). Economic evaluation alongside randomised controlled trials: design, conduct, analysis, and reporting. *BMJ* 342.

Petrou S. and Gray A. (2011). Economic evaluation using decision analytical modelling: design, conduct, analysis, and reporting. *BMJ* 342.

Pitt C, Vassall A, Teerawattananon Y, et al. (2016). Foreword: health economic evaluations in low- and middle-income countries: methodological issues and challenges for priority setting. *Health Econ* 25 Suppl 1: 1–5.

Salomon J, Haagsma J, Davis A, et al. (2015). Disability weights for the Global Burden of Disease 2013 study. *The Lancet Global Health* 3: e712–23.

Walker D and Kumaranayake L (2002). Allowing for differential timing in cost analyses: discounting and annualization. *Health Policy Plan* 17, 112–118.

SECTION 3

Important concepts across the lifecourse

CHAPTER 6

Social determinants of health

Sebastian Taylor and Bernadette O'Hare

Key points

◆ Social determinants—the social, economic, political, cultural, and environmental conditions in which we are born, grow, learn, work, and age—systematically influence individual and collective health. This means that discussion around improving any aspect of health requires a debate on how to address its social determinants.

◆ Children are particularly susceptible to the influence—positive or negative—of social determinants, due to their dependency on others, and the sustained effect of determinants from before birth across the lifecourse.

Background

Life expectancy at birth varies dramatically by country and region of birth; from 84 years in Japan to 46 in Sierra Leone, shaped broadly by a country's level of socioeconomic development. In London there is a 16-year difference in life expectancy at birth for males born between 2010–2014, between the wealthiest and poorest neighbourhoods.

Since the early 1980s, an upsurge in interest and research using social determinants of health (SDH) models has built a global evidence base supporting the scientific consensus that health outcomes and life chances are significantly determined by the material conditions in which families and communities live. Within rich and poor countries alike, a child's life chances are shaped by a hierarchy of interacting factors—from biology and genetics, through behaviour, education, and access to health care, to household income and parental social and economic status. Social and economic status of individuals and families are mediated by opportunities for education, employment, and income, themselves influenced by norms of gender, ethnicity, class, or caste. Finally, the way social norms and policies enable healthy growth are shaped by national (and increasingly global) systems of governance—power over policy-setting and revenue, which determines how and to whom the benefits of resources and growth flow. These are the SDH (Figure 6.1).

Childhood health and wellbeing is a powerful determinant of adult health. Childhood illnesses can have lifelong impact on societal participation and economic productivity. Persistent exposure to malaria in children, for example, can reduce adult earning potential by as much as 50%. Childhood nutrition is a critical determinant of cognitive and physical development, educational performance, lifetime earnings potential, and intergenerational

risk of persistent household poverty. Conversely, reductions in child mortality (and related reductions in household fertility) were estimated to account for 30–50% of the rapid economic growth experienced in the East Asian 'miracle' countries between 1965 and 1990. Stenberg et al. (2013) estimated a benefit-cost ratio for interventions in reproductive, maternal, neonatal, and child health in low- and middle-income countries (LMICs) of 8.7 by 2035.

Wealth and health

There is little dispute that national wealth and household assets are important to improving families' health, in all countries. Equally, the role of enhanced health care—universally and equitably accessible—is a vital component of countering social inequality and reducing mortality and morbidity. However, the SDH model makes a powerful argument, with equal clarity, that neither rising wealth, nor an increasingly sophisticated health sector is, on its own, an adequate solution.

Poverty is often viewed as the preeminent determinant of health. Lack of disposable income clearly inhibits ability to finance vital health goods from adequate family food to quality health care and education. But economic poverty is itself the manifestation of underlying social status, insofar as gender, ethnicity, caste, and class all shape individuals' opportunities to access education, find employment, and earn income.

Improvement in aggregate economic wealth alone does not translate automatically into better child health (Figure 6.2 and Figure 6.3). Although it is clear from the graph that countries with a higher per capita income have lower levels of child mortality, the relationship is non-linear and, by implication, mediated by other factors. The clustering in the lower left-hand corner suggests a number of countries with low levels of both per capita gross national income (GNI) and under-five mortality. Clearly, in these countries other factors, such as social policies, independent of economic resources, appear to be having a significant positive effect.

National and global influences on the social determinants of health

Underlying and shaping the economic and social status of households and communities are deep-seated societal, political, and cultural norms, laws and policies that favour some over others. Reforming these requires deep-rooted political change. Inequality and household disadvantage, with all the familiar consequences for children's chances of survival, growth, and opportunity to flourish,

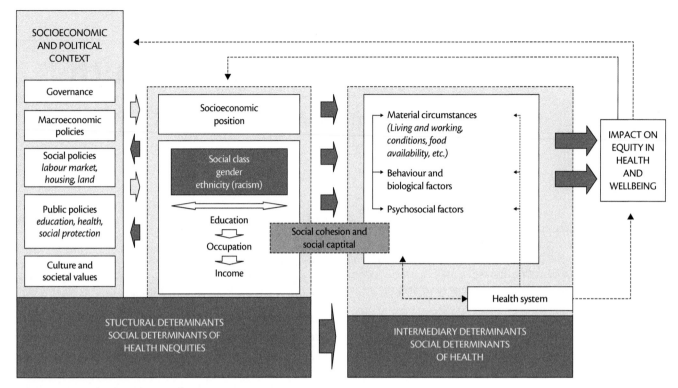

Figure 6.1 A conceptual framework for social determinants of health.
Reproduced with permission from Solar, O. et al. Conceptual framework for action on the social determinants of health. Social Determinants of Health Discussion Paper 2 (Policy and Practice). Geneva: World Health Organization. Copyright © 2010 World Health Organization.

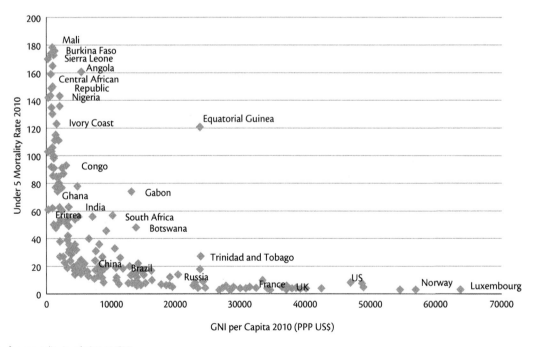

Figure 6.2 Under-five mortality in relation to GNI.
Reproduced with permission from Bell, R., Donkin, A., and Marmot, M. (2013). Tackling structural and social issues to reduce inequities in children's outcomes in low- to middle-income countries, Office of Research Discussion Paper No.2013-02, UNICEF Office of Research, Florence.

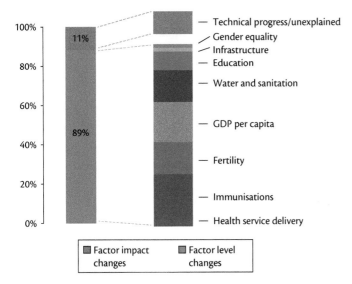

Figure 6.3 Proportional impact of factors on under-five mortality change, 1990–2010.

Reproduced from Bishai, D.M. et al. Factors Contributing to Maternal and Child Mortality Reductions in 146 Low- and Middle-Income Countries between 1990 and 2010, *PLoS One*, 11(1): e0144908, 2016. Copyright © 2016 Bishai et al. This is an open access article distributed under the terms of the Creative Commons Attribution License, which permits unrestricted use, distribution, and reproduction in any medium, provided the original author and source are credited.

is heavily determined by a country's distinct forms of social hierarchy and intersecting discriminations based on gender, ethnicity, religion, caste, or class. It is the willingness of governments, in countries at all levels of economic development, to confront and challenge the operation of these embedded hierarchies that lies further upstream towards the source of social inequality and poor and inequitable health.

LMICs—particularly the poorest, including those classed as 'fragile or conflict-affected'—a basic lack of resources to invest in SDH. They are often hard-pressed to raise revenue through domestic channels such as taxation. Personal income tax, which tends to be progressive, makes up almost a quarter of government revenue in Organisation for Economic Cooperation and Development (OECD) countries, but less than 10% in low-income countries (LICs) (Moore, 2013). This increases reliance on indirect tax income, for example versions of value-added tax, which tends to be regressive, and on international trade transactions, and hence on the tax behaviour of multinational enterprises. Corporate income tax contributes 12% to government revenues in LICs compared to 7% in high-income countries (HICs). Corporate tax avoidance, therefore, has a very significant impact in poorer countries, and consequently the health of their populations. Further, missed opportunities for domestic resource mobilisation include difficulties in effectively taxing often large informal sectors, as well as problems of corruption and perverse tax incentives, all significantly reducing the potential of these countries to invest in SDH.

At the multilateral level, international finance institutions (IFI)—principally the World Bank and International Monetary Fund (IMF)—exercise significant influence over resource flow to LICs. In effect, they operate a gatekeeping function with regard to LICs' ability to access concessionary and other international finance.

Donors and international investors tend to follow IFI country fiscal policy approval. Thus powerful stakeholders in the IMF have considerable impact on the global development agenda.

In the 1980s and 1990s structural adjustment loans, designed and managed by the IMF and World Bank as a fiscal response to the global debt crisis, came with the conditionality of liberalisation, including reducing import tariffs on trade, and liberalising foreign direct investment policy. Trade liberalisation weakened tax revenues for all categories of countries since the 1970s, but precipitately for poorer countries in South Asia and sub-Saharan Africa. The reduction in import taxes resulted in loss of government revenue and most LIC have only managed to replace 30%.

Official development assistance (ODA) allocations to global health—including maternal, newborn, and child health—have increased substantially over the last 20 years. For all its problems and shortfalls, there is a significant body of evidence affirming a positive correlation between aid income, improvements in global health, and investment in SDH. That said, international aid flows can be highly volatile, distorted by donors' domestic politics and foreign policy agendas. Aid volatility and external agenda-setting reduce the ability of aid-recipient governments to pursue the long-range planning necessary for addressing structural health determinants, and to directing investments to national and local priorities.

The proportion of aid provided direct to recipient government remains small, with considerable amounts bypassing government and going to independent non-governmental organisation (NGO) or other aid contractors. This can actively weaken, or fail to strengthen, government capacity in LMICs, which is vital to building national leadership and coordinating capability—political leadership and policy coordination being especially important in building a coherent, integrated approach to integrated SDH action. Further, donors may undermine their own aid efforts by sustaining an international financial system which enables corporations to shift profit out of poor countries using financial opacity and enabling corrupt elites to hide state assets in HIC banks.

Ultimately, the ability of LMICs to invest in improving the social determinants of child health is heavily influenced, far upstream, by the institutional structures of power which set the rules for global finance and trade. Presently, rule-setting is dominated by a small number of HICs. Reconfiguring the system of global governance for finance and trade to rebalance in favour of health outcomes and protection and promotion of health determinants will be key to sustainable improvement in the structural drivers of child health and, hence, to the achievement of the SDGs.

Challenges

It is estimated that the upstream or structural determinants of health account for two-thirds of health outcomes. However, there is a distinct tendency, across academic, research, media, and policy sectors to give primacy to proximal, that is, biological, genetic factors, and behavioural choices, rather than distal causes of poor health.

Future priorities

◆ The SDH agenda invokes clear political priorities: future SDH action will depend on supporting coherent, integrated national strategies, including for countries currently struggling with weak governance and resource-scarcity.

♦ Under current processes of globalisation, more research is needed to elucidate, with equivalent rigour to biomedical studies, the influence of the global and multilateral systems, and international actors, on the SDH.

Conclusions

The SDH agenda points to the growing global evidence base of a systematic association between material circumstances and child health outcomes, and the underlying forces that distribute those conditions hierarchically and inequitably. Child health has improved in the last quarter-century, but disparities between and within countries remain large and unacceptable. Social, economic, political, cultural, and environmental conditions exercise a very substantial influence on children's life chances and ability to grow and develop. The healthy development of children into productive adolescents and adults is itself one of the most powerful determinants of a country's ability to grow its way out of national poverty. Poverty—understood as multidimensional rather than simply economic—constitutes a powerful driver of mortality and morbidity. But poverty is not a naturally-occurring phenomenon. Local conditions of poverty and ill-health must be viewed through the lens of wider norms, policies, and programmes at both national and global levels.

Case study: early child development and long-term impact of poor childhood nutrition

Early child development (ECD) incorporates three interlinking domains of intervention: physical, social/emotional, and language/cognitive. Intervention in ECD is a means of improving population health through the lifecourse, associated with better child, adolescent and adult health, and enhanced impact on individuals' social and economic participation.

Conditions in the first years of life strongly determine a child's subsequent chances of growth and development. In 2011, just over a quarter of all children under five years old were stunted—the result of chronically inadequate nutrition. Stunting is associated with suboptimal brain development, with lifelong consequences for their potential to benefit from education, develop skills, and earn income which drives household poverty into the next generation. Inequitable distribution of the effects of nutritional poverty may also be determined within families, households or regions, by underlying social, political, and cultural norms of gender, ethnicity caste, or class.

Improving nutritional status of children—for example through supplementary feeding programmes or through subsidy to poor households' income—can substantially mitigate the effects of malnutrition. But interventions which couple improvement of nutritional access with wider social/emotional and cognitive growth, such as activities enhancing child stimulation, have considerably greater positive impact on development of children's cognitive and language capabilities. ECD policies to improve households' material conditions relating to income and food access, may do better when implemented in conjunction with more structural national family-friendly policies and programmes supportive of social/emotional and cognitive stimulation in the home.

Questions

1. How does the SDH conceptual framework help us to understand child health and what are its principal weaknesses?

2. Why might national governments struggle to implement an SDH approach to child health?

3. Is it feasible to trace causal pathways from processes of globalisation to localised child health outcomes?

Key publications

Bishai D, Cohen R, Alfonso Y, Adam T, Kuruvilla S, and Schweitzer J (2016). Factors contributing to maternal and child mortality reductions in 146 low- and middle-income countries between 1990 and 2010. *PLoS* 11(1): e0144908.

The authors reviewed the main interventions which are associated with the reduction in child mortality in LMIC and found that more than half of the gains were due to interventions outside the health sector. (Note GDP per capita is included in this model, but the impact of GDP or income is mediated via these determinants of health, i.e. water, sanitation, education, and health care.)

WHO/Commission on Social Determinants of Health. *Closing the gap in a generation: health equity through action on the social determinants of health.*

The Commission calls on the WHO and all governments to lead global action on the social determinants of health with the aim of achieving health equity.

Bell R, Donkin A, and Marmot M (2013).Tackling structural and social issues to reduce inequities in children's outcomes in low- and middle-income countries. Office of Research Discussion Paper; Perspectives on Equity, UNICEF.

This paper provides a conceptual and operational framework along the SDH approach and generates important insights that we can now apply to broader outcomes for children.

Bibliography

Baum F, Sanders D, Fisher M, et al. (2016). Assessing the health impact of transnational corporations: its importance and a framework. *Global. Health* 12(1): 27.

Clements B, Gupta S, and Nozaki M (2013). What happens to social spending in IMF-supported programmes? *Appl. Econ.* 48(November): 4022–33.

Currie J and Vogl T (2012). Early-life health and adult circumstance in developing countries. NBER Working Paper No. 18371, September.

Fjeldstad O (2013). *Taxation and development. A review of donor support to strengthen tax systems in developing countries.* UNU-WIDER: Helsinki, Finland. p. 30

Moore M (2013). Obstacles to increasing tax revenues in low-income countries, ICTD Working Paper 15, December.

Solar O and Irwin A (2010). A conceptual framework for action on the social determinants of health. Social Determinants of Health Discussion Paper 2 (Policy and Practice).

Stenberg K, Axelson H, Sheeham P, et al. (2013). Advancing social and economic development by investing in women's and children's health: a new global investment framework. *Lancet* 383 (9925): 1333–54.

Taylor S and Rowson M (2009). Global financing for health: aid and debt relief in Labonte R, Schrecker T, Packer C, Runnels V (eds). *Globalization and Health: Pathways, Evidence and Policy*. Routledge: Abingdon, UK.

Taylor S, Perez-Ferrer C, Griffiths A, and Brunner E (2015). Scaling up nutrition in fragile and conflict-affected states: the pivotal role of governance. *Social Science & Medicine* 126: 119–27.

UNICEF (2015). *State of the World's Children*. UNICEF: New York, US.

Woodward D (2013). A high price to pay: IMF governance, management of developing country financial crises, and health impacts, Oslo-Lancet Commission on global governance for health. https://www.med.uio.no/helsam/english/research/global-governance-health/background-papers/imf-governance-health.pdf

World Bank (2016). *Poverty and Shared Prosperity 2016: Taking on Inequality*. Washington, DC: World Bank.

CHAPTER 7

Developmental origins of health and disease

Caroline Fall and Kalyanaraman Kumaran

This chapter sets out the evidence that adverse environmental exposures during foetal and early postnatal life create a lifelong vulnerability to common non-communicable diseases.

Key points

- Sub-optimal nutrition during foetal and infant development is associated with an increased risk of non-communicable diseases (NCDs) in adult life.

- Animal experiments show that this is due to permanent effects on the structure and function of tissues and hormone systems, and may be mediated by epigenetic changes.

- NCD risk is increased further by excess adiposity gain, and/or unhealthy lifestyles, in later life.

- Intervention studies are ongoing to identify ways to improve early development and prevent later disease.

Background

The concept that foetal under-nutrition is an important contributor to the risk of NCDs in adult life was developed by David Barker and colleagues in the 1990s. He showed that people of lower birth or infant weight had an increased risk of adult hypertension, heart disease, type 2 diabetes, and metabolic syndrome, and that comparable disorders could be induced in experimental animals by under-nourishing mothers during pregnancy. Foetal undernutrition impairs the development of the pancreas, liver, kidneys, skeletal muscle, and adipose tissue, and alters the sensitivity of hormone systems. This leads not only to cardio-metabolic disease, but also to renal and lung disease, osteoporosis, and mental ill health. Although foetal undernutrition may be transient, these changes become permanent or 'programmed' because they occur during critical periods of early plasticity, and therefore cannot be reversed later.

Other environmental influences can programme later disease. These include foetal 'over-nutrition' as in maternal diabetes or obesity, exposure to maternal smoking or environmental pollutants, pregnancy complications, and the woman's metabolism, physical activity, and lifestyle. The effects of these on foetal tissues, not birthweight itself, are thought to be responsible for later disease (Figure 7.1); however, birth weight is a crude summary of the effect of these factors on the foetus. Epigenetic changes, induced by the

foetal nutritional environment, may be important mediating mechanisms. These include stable alterations to DNA (such as methylation), which affect the *expression* of genes without altering their structure (base pair sequences).

Postnatal weight gain and growth

Cohort studies have shown that greater weight gain in the first 1–2 postnatal years is either unrelated to adult NCD risk or protective. It may be beneficial because of better lean mass accrual, or because some plasticity remains at this age, enabling the continuing development of tissues. Greater infant weight gain in low- and middle-income countries (LMICs) reduces infant mortality and improves childhood cognitive ability, leading to the suggestion that the first 1000 days (from conception to the end of infancy) is a critical time to achieve optimal nutrition as a means of improving human capital without increasing the risk of later NCDs.

In contrast to infant weight gain, greater weight or body mass index (BMI) gain in later childhood or adolescence is consistently associated with an increased risk of heart disease, hypertension, and type 2 diabetes. The highest risk is found in individuals who were light at birth but became heavy, or developed other unhealthy lifestyles, as older children or adults (Figure 7.2). Possible explanations are that more rapid postnatal weight gain may indicate greater severity of foetal growth restriction, or that accelerated weight gain is disadvantageous in itself, placing excessive demands on organs that are incapable of compensatory hyperplasia, such as the pancreas or kidneys. It may increase adiposity; fat maintains its capacity for growth throughout life, while muscle loses the capacity for cell division soon after birth. Another possibility is that the hormones driving compensatory weight gain (e.g. insulin-like growth factors) have adverse long-term cardio-metabolic effects.

Other early life exposures

Compared with formula feeding, breastfeeding has been associated with less obesity and diabetes, and lower blood pressure and lipids, in later life. Maternal smoking is associated with increased obesity in children. Stressful experiences in early life, and environmental pollutants, may also have a role in the programming of adult disease.

Evidence from intervention studies in humans

Unlike the robust demonstration of cardio-metabolic programming using interventions in experimental animals, the evidence for

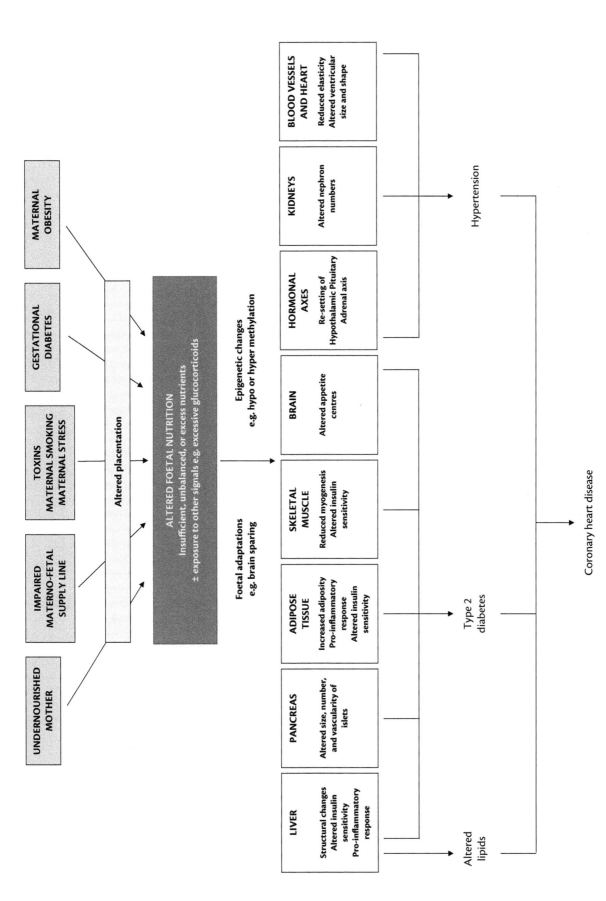

Figure 7.1 Foetal programming of adult disease.

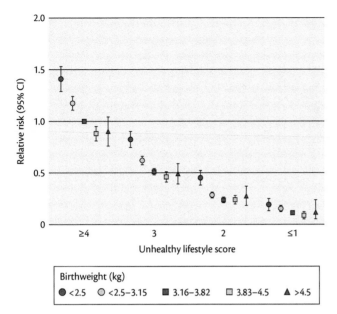

Figure 7.2 Risk of type 2 diabetes according to birthweight and unhealthy adult lifestyle score. Data from the Health Professionals Follow-up Study and Nurses' Health Study (three million person years of follow-up).

Note: the lifestyle score was based on diet (alternate healthy eating index 2010), current smoking (no/yes), physical activity (time spent in moderate/vigorous activity), alcohol consumption and BMI.

Reproduced with permission from Li et al. Birth weight and later life adherence to unhealthy lifestyles in predicting type 2 diabetes: prospective cohort study *BMJ*.2015; 351. doi: https://doi. org/10.1136/bmj.h3672. Copyright © 2015 BMJ. Open Access.

programming in humans comes mainly from observational research. Some studies have examined cardio-metabolic risk markers in children whose mothers took part in nutritional supplementation trials during pregnancy, trials of intensive management of gestational diabetes, or trials to reduce maternal obesity or excessive gestational weight gain. None have demonstrated sustained improvements in cardio-metabolic risk markers in the children. However, all these interventions probably started too late to influence first trimester processes such as placentation, organogenesis, and peri-conceptional epigenetic changes, which are crucial to foetal programming. Research on the Developmental Origins of Health and Disease (DOHaD) in humans is currently focusing on preconception intervention studies, powered for long-term follow-up of the offspring, which will test DOHaD concepts rigorously and examine mechanisms (e.g. epigenetics).

Public health implications

NCDs are a leading cause of death and disability globally, and are rising rapidly in prevalence in LMICs. Current preventive strategies focus on adults with pre-existing risk factors. The DOHaD concept offers the potential for an alternative prevention strategy of optimising early development, which may also benefit human capital and subsequent generations. Potential interventions include improving the lifestyle, health, and nutrition of women and their partners before pregnancy, maintaining this throughout pregnancy, supporting breastfeeding, and optimising childhood nutrition. Maternal mortality has fallen in many high-income countries to the extent that preconception health and lifestyle factors, such as obesity and pre-existing physical and mental health issues, are now

the most important risk factors for maternal death. Addressing these issues therefore has significant potential benefits for maternal mortality and morbidity, as well as the long-term benefits for the child and society.

Challenges

Evidence that nutritional and other exposures during early development make an important contribution to adult NCD risk currently relies mainly on observational research. Proof from intervention studies is required. The need for preconceptional interventions in mothers and fathers, and long-term follow-up of the offspring, makes this research challenging.

Future priorities

- Research planning should take a long-term view and enable the follow-up of high quality trials to obtain hard disease outcomes in later life. Follow-up decades after initial exposure to childhood insults will clarify further disease risk in the long term.
- Surrogate markers of early-life programming at young ages are needed; the field of epigenetics offers this potential. This will enable a better understanding of both when early-life programming has occurred, and where to focus interventional strategies.
- Interventions to reduce childhood adiposity should consider upward movement across centiles as well as frank obesity, as this is also associated with increased risk

Conclusions

The concept that improving the nutrition and health of parents before and during pregnancy may prevent common NCDs has important public health implications. More robust interventional evidence is required in order to quantify the importance of these early life exposures, delineate the mechanisms involved, and stimulate public health action.

Case study: crossing upward centiles in weight is associated with risk

A consistent finding in all populations is that upward crossing of weight or BMI centiles in childhood or adolescence, on a background of low birthweight, is associated with an increased risk of adult cardiovascular disease and diabetes. In LMICs, increasing childhood BMI does not necessarily equate to obesity. In Delhi, India, Bhargava et al. (2004) found that children who later developed diabetes had a low mean childhood BMI (around the 15th percentile of the WHO growth reference) but were on an upward trajectory. This is likely to be a common growth pattern in LMICs.

Questions

1. Why is rapid weight gain in childhood associated with an increased risk of adult cardiovascular disease and type 2 diabetes?
2. What type of research in humans would provide the best evidence for or against the 'developmental origins' hypothesis?

3. What maternal and paternal factors are associated with an increased risk of obesity and diabetes in the offspring?

Key publications

Armitage J, Khan, Taylor, Nathanielsz, and Poston L (2004). Developmental programming of the metabolic syndrome by maternal nutritional imbalance: how strong is the evidence from experimental models in mammals? *J Physiol* 561: 355–77.
A review of evidence for developmental programming in experimental animals.

Barker D, Gluckman P, Godfrey K, et al. (1993). Foetal nutrition and cardiovascular disease in adult life. *Lancet* 341: 938–41.
A review of fetal programming written by those who conceived the DOHaD hypothesis.

Dabelea D and Pettitt D (2001). Intrauterine diabetic environment confers risks for type 2 diabetes mellitus and obesity in the offspring in addition to genetic susceptibility. *J Pediatric Endocrinol Metab* 14: 1085–91.
Evidence that gestational diabetes programmes diabetes in the offspring.

Godfrey K, Costello P, and Lillycrop K (2015). The developmental environment, epigenetic biomarkers and long-term health. *J Dev Orig Health Dis* 6: 399–406.
A review of epigenetis in developmental programming of disease.

Li Y, Ley S, Tobias D, et al. (2015). Birth weight and later life adherence to unhealthy lifestyles in predicting type 2 diabetes. *BMJ* 351: h3672.
Evidence that foetal under-nutrition adds to the NCD risks associated with unhealthy adult lifestyles.

Bibliography

Adair L, Fall C, Osmond C, et al. (2013). Disentangling how relative weight gain and linear growth during early life relate to adult health and human capital in low- and middle-income countries. *Lancet* 382: 525–34.

Armitage J, Khan I, Taylor P, Nathanielsz P, and Poston L (2004). Developmental programming of the metabolic syndrome by maternal nutritional imbalance: how strong is the evidence from experimental models in mammals? *J Physiol* 561: 355–77.

Barker D, Gluckman P, Godfrey K, Harding J, Owens J, and Robinson J (1993). Foetal nutrition and cardiovascular disease in adult life. *Lancet* 341: 938–41.

Bhargava S, Sachdev H, Fall C, et al. (2004). Relation of serial changes in childhood body mass index to impaired glucose tolerance in young adulthood. *New Eng J Med* 350: 865–75.

Dabelea D and Pettitt D (2001). Intrauterine diabetic environment confers risks for type 2 diabetes mellitus and obesity in the offspring in addition to genetic susceptibility. *J Pediatric Endocrinol Metab* 14: 1085–91.

Devakumar D, Fall C, Sachdev H, et al. (2016). Maternal antenatal multiple micronutrient supplementation for long-term health benefits in children: a systematic review and meta-analysis. *BMC Med* 14(1): 90.

Eriksson J, Forsen T, Tuomilehto J, Barker D (2001). Early growth and coronary heart disease in later life. *Br Med J* 322: 949–53.

Eriksson J, Forsen T, Tuomilehto J, Osmond C, and Barker D (2003). Early adiposity rebound in childhood and risk of type 2 diabetes in adult life. *Diabetologia* 46: 190–94.

Fall C (2011). Evidence for the intra-uterine programming of adiposity in later life. *Ann Human Biol* 38: 410–28.

Fraser A, Tilling K, Macdonald-Wallis C, et al. (2010). Association of maternal weight gain in pregnancy with offspring obesity and metabolic and vascular traits in childhood. *Circulation* 121: 2557–64.

Gillman M, Oakley H, Baghurst P, Volkmer R, Robinson J, and Crowther C (2010). Effect of treatment of gestational diabetes mellitus on obesity in the next generation. *Diabetes Care* 33: 964–86.

Godfrey K, Costello P, and Lillycrop K (2015). The developmental environment, epigenetic biomarkers and long-term health. *J Dev Orig Health Dis* 6: 399–406.

Horta B and Victora C (2013). *Long-term Effects of Breastfeeding: a Systematic Review*. World Health Organization: Geneva.

Li Y, Ley S, Tobias D, et al. (2015). Birth weight and later life adherence to unhealthy lifestyles in predicting type 2 diabetes. *BMJ* 351: h3672.

Oken E, Levitan E, and Gillman M (2008). Maternal smoking during pregnancy and child overweight: systematic review and meta-analysis. *Int J Obesity* 32: 201–10.

Potdar R, Sahariah S, Gandhi M, et al. (2014). Improving women's diet quality pre-conceptionally and during gestation: effects on birth weight and prevalence of LBW; a randomized controlled efficacy trial in India. *Am J Clin Nutr* 100: 1257–68.

Reynolds R, Allan K, Raja E, et al. (2013). Maternal obesity during pregnancy and premature mortality from cardiovascular events in adult offspring. *BMJ*: F4539.

Sahariah S, Potdar R, Gandhi M, et al. (2016). A daily snack containing leafy green vegetables, fruit, and milk before and during pregnancy prevents gestational diabetes. *J Nutr* 146(7): 1453S–60S.

Tanvig M, Vinter C, Jørgensen J, et al. (2015). Effects of lifestyle intervention in pregnancy and anthropometrics at birth on offspring metabolic profile at 2.8 years: results from the Lifestyle in Pregnancy and Offspring (LiPO) study. *J Clin Endocrinol Metab* 100: 175–83.

CHAPTER 8

Health workers and health systems

Kate Mandeville and Ingrid Wolfe

This chapter describes the role that health workers and strong health systems play in improving women's, children's, and adolescents' health.

Key points

- Strong health systems that are adequately financed and resourced are crucial for securing good health.

- There are many demonstrably effective and cost-effective interventions to strengthen health systems and improve health, including in resource-poor settings.

- Health workforces need to be aligned to a country's population and disease burden, with retention of health workers given as much priority as increased production.

- Universal health coverage is vital for ensuring equity and good health for all; however, both establishing and expanding such coverage is fraught with challenges, and countries can learn from the experiences of others further along in the process.

Background

Understanding health systems is vital for improving women's, children's, and adolescents' health. Health systems are defined as the people, institutions, and resources whose primary purpose is the production of health. The World Health Organization (WHO) defines six 'building blocks' for a health system:

- A robust financing mechanism
- Trained and motivated health workers
- Facilities and frameworks to deliver safe and high-quality services
- Strong leadership and governance
- Reliable and timely information for decision and policymaking
- Access to essential medicines and technologies

This framework has been criticised as being too simplistic to capture the complexity and interconnectedness of these elements. Indeed, it is difficult to set the boundaries of a health system: should this include industries such as pharmaceutical producers and sectors that are important for determining health, such as education? Perhaps it is easier to agree on what a strong health system should deliver: improved health and other social goals, including protection from financial ruin due to healthcare payments, equity of access, and responsive services. Delivering these goals relies on strengthening all parts of the health system, in the context of social, political, and historical factors.

Health system financing illustrates many of the challenges facing policymakers. There is substantial variation in financial means and efficiency between countries, as shown by the proportion of the public budget allocated to health. For example, in 2014 health accounted for 23.4% of government expenditure in New Zealand compared with 3.6% in Myanmar. Insufficient government spending on health necessitates out-of-pocket payments in the form of user fees or co-payments. This can discourage the appropriate use of health services, especially by women, children, and adolescents. Chronic or severe illnesses can lead to catastrophic or impoverishing health expenditures. Every year, around 100 million people are pushed into poverty through out-of-pocket payments. Universal health coverage is a means of assuring financial protection from catastrophic individual health expenditure.

Achieving universal health coverage requires sufficient health workers. Many poor countries do not have enough health workers to provide care for the population. For instance, Africa has the second highest proportion of the global burden of disease, but the fewest health workers and the least resources (Figure 8.1). Approximately 11,000 doctors are trained annually in the whole of sub-Saharan Africa, while the UK alone produces around 6,000 new doctors every year. In Malawi in 2012, there were just seventeen obstetricians for nearly seventeen million people. Health care is labour intensive, so insufficient or poorly distributed health workers inevitably constrains the equitable delivery of services. Low production of health workers is exacerbated by migration from poor to rich countries, and from rural to urban areas, usually in search of better job and living conditions. For example, one in every four doctors in England's National Health Service is of foreign nationality. There has been considerable debate over this 'brain drain', with recipient countries urged to implement ethical recruitment practices or compensate poorer countries for their training investment.

Targets and recommendations

Article 24 of the United Nations Convention on the Rights of the Child (UNCRC) states that every child has the right to the best possible health and health care. Richer countries must help poorer countries achieve this goal. In 2001, African Union countries agreed to allocate at least 15% of their national budget to health. By 2013, only six countries had met this target, known as the Abuja Declaration.

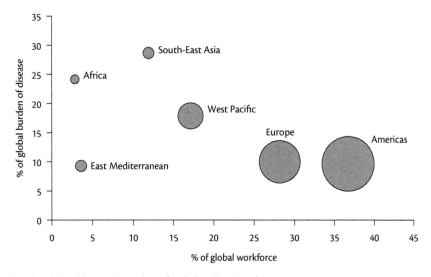

Figure 8.1 Distribution of health workers by health expenditure (size of circles) and burden of disease.
Reproduced with permission from World Health Organization. *The World Health Report 2006 - Working Together for Health.* WHO Document Production Services, Geneva, Switzerland. Copyright © 2006 World Health Organization.

Sustainable Development Goals (SDGs) Target 3c is to substantially increase health financing and the recruitment, development, training, and retention of the health workforce in developing countries. Many of the other SDGs are unachievable without adequate development of the health workforce and systems.

The 2016 global strategy on human resources for health (another term for the health workforce) suggests that, by 2030, all countries should be making progress towards halving inequalities in access to a health worker and halving their dependency on foreign-trained health professionals.

Training and retaining health workers

Increasing attention to human resources for health has led to a recent scaling up of health worker training in many countries. Based on several studies showing a significant relation between the number of health professionals per population and service delivery outcomes, the WHO identified a threshold of 2.28 health workers per 1000 people as necessary to achieve the Millennium Development Goals (MDGs). This is challenging, as, for example, some countries would have to devote more than 30% of their gross domestic product to health in order to achieve this threshold. However, the studies on which the WHO recommendation was made did not take into account the mitigating impact of mid-level or volunteer health workers who can provide effective and cost-effective care.

Measures used to retain health workers after qualification include compulsory service programmes, discouraging emigration, and incentive packages. Evidence from high-income countries shows that compulsory service programmes can improve health worker supply to underserved areas, but many participants do not complete their commitment. Voluntary codes discouraging active recruitment of health workers by rich countries have limited impact; however, changes to immigration rules can deliver more substantial changes. Finally, non-financial incentives such as training opportunities are as important as monetary incentives.

The path to universal health coverage

Universal health coverage is an intervention for delivering health equity. It allows the financial risks associated with the cost of health care to be pooled across the population, preventing people from being pushed into poverty due to ill health. Mechanisms of pooling funds to pay for health services include general taxation, social health insurance, community financing schemes, or private health insurance. In practice, most countries use a combination of financing mechanisms to maximise equity, risk pooling, and efficiency from their available income sources. Country experiences show that leveraging political, economic, or social changes (such as a financial crisis or post-conflict) and overcoming resistance from interest groups are crucial for achieving universal health coverage.

Challenges

Achieving sustainable scale-up of health workers is challenging. Salaries, benefits, and training absorb on average a third of public spending on health, so most governments have limited ability to substantially increase health worker supply. Task-shifting and the use of mid-level and community health workers can effectively ensure delivery of life-saving and cost-effective interventions, especially in remote and resource-poor settings (Case study 1). Transforming health professionals' education is important to ensure graduates are equipped to deliver health care for evolving and complex needs and provide equitable high-quality care for underserved communities.

Rolling out universal health coverage without bankrupting countries is another challenge. Once countries are on the path to universal health coverage, further expansion requires a delicate balance between who is covered, what services are covered, and at what cost (Figure 8.2). Expanding subsidised coverage to more vulnerable groups may cause resentment among those paying high premia or tax rates. Increasing the scope of covered services may run into political or social resistance (Case study 2). Reducing co-payments and user fees causes problems if there are insufficient pooled funds. Experiences of high-income countries highlight the importance of incremental expansion of coverage, judicious financing mechanisms, and leveraging purchasing power to improve efficiency. This is particularly the case with more expensive technologies and

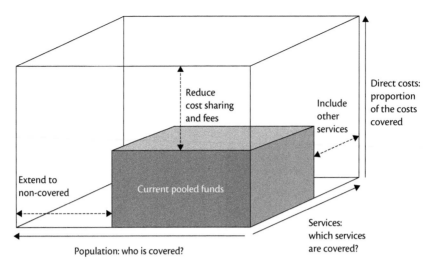

Three dimensions to consider when moving towards universal coverage

Figure 8.2 The UHC cube: dimensions to consider when moving towards universal health coverage.
Reproduced with permission from World Health Organization. *Health systems financing: the path to universal coverage. World Health Report 2010.* Geneva: World Health Organization. Copyright © 2010 World Health Organization.

medicines, and here the effective early implementation of prioritisation mechanisms, such as the use of essential medicines lists or health technology assessment, is vital.

Future priorities

- In high- and middle-income countries, rapidly ageing populations will lead to greater demand for health workers to provide clinical and long-term care that will fast outstrip supply.

- Health workers may migrate from poorer countries, leaving gaps in formal and informal care in their own countries.

- Increasing numbers of women with competing responsibilities are joining the labour force in low- and middle-income countries, requiring concomitant changes to cultural gender norms and policies for child and elder care.

- Further advances in medical technology, ever rising demand, and the ongoing epidemiological transition towards chronic illness will continue to put pressure on finite resources.

- Countries will have to find sustainable ways to secure the future health of mothers and children. Creative solutions will be needed, and countries may learn from each other's experiences.

Conclusions

There are many current and emerging challenges facing countries in their attempts to secure and improve the health of their populations. Strengthening health systems is an essential part of the global effort to safeguard health for women, children, and adolescents, now and in the future. There are many lessons to be learned from country experiences, including the vital importance of universal health coverage, which requires robust financing mechanisms and investment in human resources for health.

Case studies

Case study 1: mid-level providers delivering obstetric care in sub-Saharan Africa

Five African countries (Ethiopia, Ghana, Malawi, Mozambique, and Tanzania) allow mid-level providers to carry out Caesarean sections and other emergency obstetric surgery such as hysterectomies. These health workers often provide the majority of emergency obstetric care in rural and remote areas in these countries, where access to doctors is limited. This means that a larger proportion of maternal and child health needs are met than in countries where the role of mid-level providers is restricted. Studies comparing key outcomes between mid-level providers and doctors have found little difference in maternal or foetal mortality or major postoperative complications between these two groups.

Case study 2: contraception coverage in the US expanded by reforming healthcare insurance

The 2010 Affordable Care Act (also known as Obamacare) reformed health insurance in the US, where coverage has historically been low and costs high. Under the new legislation, private insurance companies are mandated to offer, without co-payments, at least one type of contraception to female clients. 'Male' contraception, including condoms and vasectomies, are not covered by the mandate. Reproductive health such as contraception can be controversial, and some religious organisations have launched legal challenges on the grounds that providing insurance to their employees, and thereby contraception, contravenes religious freedom.

Questions

1. What is a health system, and what should it deliver?

2. List the three dimensions that should be considered when expanding universal health coverage.

3. Describe three policies that could be implemented to strengthen the health workforce in a low-income country.

Key publications

Joint Learning Initiative (2004). Human resources for health: overcoming the crisis.
Global Health Initiative Harvard University: Washington, DC.
The first report to re-focus the global health community's attention on the importance of health workers to well-functioning health systems. It led to the 2006 World Health Report.

World Health Organization (2010). *The World Health Report 2010: health systems financing: the path to universal coverage.* World Health Organization: Geneva.
A report analysing the importance of health system financing in achieving universal health care.

Maeda A, Araujo E, Cashin C, et al. (2014). *Universal health coverage for inclusive and sustainable development: a synthesis of 11 country case studies.* Washington, DC: World Bank.
These publications outline the evidence for and country experiences of moving towards universal health coverage.

Balabanova D, McKee M, and Mills A (2011). '*Good health at low cost': 25 years on. What makes a successful health system?* London School of Hygiene and Tropical Medicine: London, UK.
A key report examining the factors supporting strong health systems in resource-poor countries

Bibliography

Bärnighausen T and Bloom D (2009). Financial incentives for return of service in underserved areas: a systematic review. *BMC Health Services Research* 9: 86.

Bossert T and Ono T (2010). Finding affordable health workforce targets in low-income nations. *Health Affairs* 29: 1376–82.

Crisp N, Gawanas B, and Sharp I (2008). Training the health workforce: scaling up, saving lives. *Lancet* 371: 689–91.

Frenk J, Chen L, Bhutta Z, et al. (2010). Health professionals for a new century: transforming education to strengthen health systems in an interdependent world. *Lancet* 376: 1923–58.

Hanson K and Smith R (2012). *Health Systems in Low- and Middle-Income Countries: an Economic and Policy Perspective.* Oxford University Press: Oxford, UK.

Hernandez-Pena P, Poullier J, Van Mosseveld C, et al. (2013). Health worker remuneration in WHO Member States. *Bull World Health Organ* 91: 808–815.

Mullan F, Frehywot S, Omaswa F, et al. (2011). Medical schools in sub-Saharan Africa. *Lancet* 377: 1113–21.

NHS workforce statistics (September 2013). The Health and Social Care Information Centre: London, UK.

Wilson A, Lissauer D, Thangaratinam S, Khan K, Macarthur C, and Coomarasamy A (2011). A comparison of clinical officers with medical doctors on outcomes of Caesarean section in the developing world: meta-analysis of controlled studies. *BMJ* 342: d2600.

World Bank (2015). *Universal Health Coverage for Inclusive and Sustainable Development: a Synthesis of 11 Country Case Studies.* World Bank: Washington, DC.

World Health Organization (2000). *World Health Report 2000.* World Health Organization: Geneva.

World Health Organization (2006). *World Health Report 2006: Working Together for Health.* World Health Organization: Geneva.

World Health Organization (2007). *Everybody's Business—Strengthening Health Systems to Improve Health Outcomes: WHO's Framework for Action.* World Health Organization: Geneva.

World Health Organization (2010). Global code of practice on the international recruitment of health personnel. World Health Organization: Geneva.

World Health Organization (2010). *Increasing Access to Health Workers in Remote and Rural Areas Through Improved Retention: Global Policy Recommendations.* World Health Organization: Geneva.

World Health Organization (2016). Global Health Observatory database. Available at: www.who.int/gho. World Health Organization: Geneva.

World Health Organization (2016). Global strategy on human resources for health: Workforce 2030. Draft for the 69th World Health Assembly. World Health Organization: Geneva.

CHAPTER 9

The environment and health

Nicholas Watts

This chapter explores the key environmental determinants that underpin good health in women, children, and adolescents, when these determinants are threatened, and the impacts of climate change on human health and wellbeing.

Key points

- Human and environmental systems are inextricably linked, and the environmental determinants of health—clean air, safe water, reliable shelter, nutritious food—are essential in maximising wellbeing.
- The health impacts of climate change are being felt today, are potentially catastrophic, and leave no country untouched.
- The effects of climate change and of environmental degradation are disproportionately felt by the most vulnerable in society, particularly women, children, and adolescents.

Background

'The Anthropocene' has been proposed as the new geological epoch to succeed the Holocene, which began some 11,700 years ago, and has encompassed almost all of human history to date, where, in the main, there has been relatively little geological change. Whilst the precise start date of the Anthropocene is debatable, what is not is that over recent decades, human activity has begun to have substantial, global, and irreversible impacts on Earth's ecosystems.

Social and environmental systems are inextricably linked. The World Health Organization (WHO) estimates that modifiable environmental factors are the root cause of almost one quarter (12.6 million) of all global deaths, every year. These risk factors work through a variety of pathways and interactions, and include the quality of household and outdoor ambient air quality; safe and reliable drinking water; the design and spatial infrastructure of cities and buildings; and many other aspects of human life. Climate change undermines many of these determinants, threatening a number of the essential prerequisites for a healthy society. These effects are being felt today, are disproportionately affecting women, children, and adolescents, and are projected to worsen substantially over the coming years.

Targets/recommendations

Sustainable Development Goal (SDG)

Goal 6 (Clean water and Sanitation)

- Available and sustainable management of water and sanitation for all.

Goal 7

- Ensure universal access to affordable, reliable, and modern energy services, by 2030.

Goal 11

- Provide access to safe, affordable, accessible, and sustainable transport systems for all, by 2030.

Goal 13

- Take urgent action to combat climate change and its impacts.

World Health Organization-United Nations Environment Programme (WHO-UNEP)

- Halve the number of deaths caused by air pollution, by 2030 WHO-UNEP.

United Nations Framework Convention on Climate Change (UNFCCC) Paris Agreement

- Limit global average temperature rise to 'well below 2ºC', requiring net-zero green house gas (GHG) emissions by the end of the century.

Air pollution

Combined, indoor and outdoor air pollution are responsible for approximately 6.5 million deaths every year, and represent the second largest risk factor for health, globally. In 2012 alone, ambient (outdoor) air pollution resulted in an additional three million premature deaths worldwide, with the vast majority of these deaths occurring in low- and middle-income countries (LMICs), and the West Pacific and South-East Asia experiencing the brunt of the burden. The types of air pollution and its sources vary from country to country, with motorised road transport and coal-fired power responsible for the majority of human exposure to outdoor ambient air pollution. On the other hand, exposure to household air pollution is found principally as a result of inefficient cooking, heating, and lighting from the combustion of solid fuels (such as wood or coal). Particulate matter smaller than 10 or 2.5 microns in diameter (PM_{10} and $PM_{2.5}$), as well as smaller gaseous emissions such as nitrogen oxides (NO_x) and sulphur dioxide, are among the most damaging to human health. Stroke and ischaemic heart disease are responsible for the vast majority of deaths from outdoor air pollution; however, chronic obstructive pulmonary disease, asthma, childhood pneumonia, and lung cancer are also common sequelae from high concentrations of dangerous particulates and emissions. Children and those with pre-existing cardiopulmonary conditions are among the worst affected, with new evidence also linking poor air quality to a range of in-utero disorders and reduced lung development in early life.

Transport and health

Ensuring affordable, accessible, and sustainable transport for all is a key target for SDG 11. A well-designed transport system can promote social inclusivity, stimulate local economic development, encourage physical activity, and form part of the mitigation efforts needed to tackle climate change (indeed, the transport sector is currently responsible for 27% of global greenhouse gas emissions). Too often urban transport networks are conceived with little consideration for human health. Globally, motor vehicle accidents are responsible for 1.2 million deaths and are the principle source of outdoor ambient air pollution in many countries. In many European countries, policies designed to tackle climate change by incentivising diesel motors had the perverse incentive of greatly exacerbating air pollution, with diesel producing four times as much $PM_{2.5}$ and 22 times as much NO_x.

Investing in active transport infrastructure (like cycle-lanes and pedestrian-friendly streets) and improved urban design not only reduces the health burden from motor vehicle accidents and noise and air pollution, but it also encourages physical activity, helping to tackle a range of non-communicable diseases such as diabetes, cancer, and cardiovascular disease. Indeed, projected scenarios for alternative, sustainable transport systems in Delhi, India, find a reduction in the number of years of life lost from ischaemic heart disease of 11–25% by 2030, as compared to a business-as-usual scenario. In rapidly developing cities, these active transport and air pollution considerations must be balanced with a desire for road safety, social inclusion, and the economic benefits of a locally and globally integrated community. Long-term policy objectives include a modal shift to active and public transport, and ultimately, electrification of the transport fleet, yielding impressive and immediate gains in public health, whilst also responding to climate change.

Water and sanitation

Ensuring the 'availability and sustainable management of water and sanitation for all' is the SDG 6. Whilst much progress has been made on improving access to potable water—between 1990 and 2015, coverage has risen from 76% to 91% of the global population—663 million people are still living without it. This, combined with a lack of basic infrastructure that leaves 2.4 billion people without access to basic sanitation services, leads to 760,000 premature deaths in children under the age of five every year, mostly due to infectious diarrhoea.

In LMICs, these issues extend in to healthcare facilities, which need reliable and safe sources of water. A recent assessment from the WHO and United Nations Children's Fund (UNICEF) concluded that 38% of healthcare facilities in LMICs do not have access to improved water.

Poor water management, growing demographic challenges, and mass urbanisation are increasing water consumption and demand. Simultaneously, climate change is exacerbating water scarcity, altering precipitation and temperature patterns, and increasing the duration and severity of drought in certain regions. Left unabated, projections suggest that some 3.9 billion people will be living in highly water-stressed areas, and water demand will have increased by 55%, by 2050.

In addition to infectious sources, environmental contamination of agriculture and water sources, either naturally or from human activity, from inorganic compounds, fertilisers, and industrial by-products also poses significant risks to health. Table 9.1 provides a brief summary of some contaminants and their impacts.

The health impacts of climate change

Climate change acts as a threat-multiplier, acting through the various environmental determinants of health, and exacerbating many of the major public health challenges faced today. The Intergovernmental Panel on Climate Change's (IPCC) 2014 Assessment Report definitively concluded that 'warming of the climate system is unequivocal' and 'human influence on the climate system is clear'.

Climate change brings a number of physical effects, including changes in patterns of precipitation and extreme weather events, sea-level rise and ocean acidification, raised average and extremes of temperature, and an exacerbation of existing air pollution. These effects have important social and demographic dimensions to them, with the greatest burden being experienced by the most vulnerable populations, particularly women, children, and adolescents. The health impacts of climate change are divided into direct and indirect (i.e. mediated through social or environmental systems), as shown in Figure 9.1. The WHO estimates that 99% of deaths related to climate change occur in low- and middle-income countries, and almost 80% of these in children. Whilst shocking, the underlying logic behind such inequalities is perhaps straightforward. Whilst the pathways from climate change to human health are many and varied, they can be easily conceptualised as the product of exposure to weather and climate phenomena, and the underlying health and social vulnerability of the affected population. As a result of these vulnerabilities (often disadvantaging marginalised populations and communities), climate change exacerbates existing health inequalities. Geography also plays a role here, with many of these already disadvantaged communities living in parts of the world worst affected by climate change, such as low-lying coastal zones and flood plains, mountainous regions, small island developing states, and water-scarce arid and semi-arid zones. Many of the direct and indirect effects combine into what is often described as a 'multi-hit scenario', where previously uncorrelated risks align as a result of a common driver (climate change), and erode the resilient capacity of a community or country.

Challenges

At its heart, the effects that the environment and climate change have on human health are the result of a siloed approach to policymaking that has proven poorly suited to capturing the health consequences of decisions in other sectors, such as transport, agriculture, or energy. In the case of climate change, its impacts are unfairly borne by low- and middle-income countries and by future generations, who had little to do with creating the problem. This poses the question: are today's national and global governance structures equipped to handle tomorrow's problems?

Future priorities

◆ Future research must expand on traditional health impact assessments to more successfully embed health considerations into local planning and infrastructure decisions. By considering the broader environmental and social consequences of agriculture or transport policies, decision makers can unlock important health benefits that often pay for the initial investment through reduced healthcare costs and increased productivity from a healthier workforce.

Table 9.1 Environmental contaminants and their potential health effects

Inorganic contaminant	Source	Potential health effects
Arsenic	Natural, industry, pesticides, smelting	Acute and chronic toxicity, liver and kidney damage, decreases blood haemoglobin, a carcinogen.
Beryllium	Natural, industry, mining, waste	Acute and chronic toxicity, can cause damage to lungs and bones. Possible carcinogen.
Cadmium	Natural, industry, mining, waste	Causes high blood pressure, liver and kidney damage, and anaemia. Destroys testicular tissue.
Chromium	Industry, mining, waste	Chromium VI causes liver and kidney damage, internal bleeding, respiratory damage, skin conditions.
Copper	Industry, mining, waste	Stomach and intestinal distress, liver and kidney damage, anaemia in high doses.
Cyanide	Industry, waste	Damages spleen, brain, and liver.
Lead	Industry, mining	Affects red blood cell chemistry; delays normal physical and mental development in babies and young children. Causes slight deficits in attention span, hearing, and learning in children. Can cause slight increase in blood pressure in some adults. Probable carcinogen.
Mercury	Electrical waste, industry, mining, pesticides, smelting	Acute and chronic toxicity. Affects the kidneys and can cause nervous system disorders.
Nitrate (as nitrogen)	Natural, fertiliser, sewage	Toxicity results from the body's natural breakdown of nitrate to nitrite. Causes 'blue baby disease,' by affecting the oxygen-carrying capacity of the blood.
Nitrite (combined nitrate/nitrite)	Fertiliser, sewage	
Volatile organic compounds	Used in plastics, dyes, rubbers, paints, disinfectants, pharmaceuticals, etc.	Can cause cancer and liver damage, anaemia, gastrointestinal disorders, skin irritation, blurred vision, exhaustion, weight loss, damage to the nervous system, and respiratory tract irritation.
Pesticides	Herbicides, insecticides, fungicides, rodenticides, and algicides.	Cause poisoning, headaches, dizziness, gastrointestinal disturbance, numbness, weakness, and cancer. Destroys nervous system, thyroid, reproductive system, liver, and kidneys.
Plasticisers, chlorinated solvents, benzo(a)pyrene, and dioxin	Improper waste disposal, leaching and industrial runoff	Cause cancer. Damages nervous and reproductive systems, kidney, stomach, and liver.

Source: data from The USGS Water Science School. Contaminants Found in Groundwater. Reston, USA: U.S. Department of the Interior. Copyright © 2017 U.S. Department of the Interior. Available at: https://water.usgs.gov/edu/groundwater-contaminants.html

◆ Through the same pathways that climate change undermines the environmental determinants of health, a robust response to climate change can yield substantial health co-benefits. Many policy responses require sensible, cost-effective public health interventions in their own right. This is in large part because a number of health challenges—for example poor air quality and physical inactivity—share a common driver climate change in the form of the combustion of fossil fuels. For example, urban spatial planning and active transport infrastructure that encourages a transition away from personal motorised transport will reduce GHG emissions, increase physical activity, and improve local air quality.

Conclusions

The alarming rate of environmental degradation and climate change experienced today demands an exceptional response. In 2015, the United Nations (UN) reached two land-mark agreements: the 2030 Agenda for Sustainable Development, and the Paris Agreement on climate change. Responsibility for their implementation now falls to everyone, with national and municipal governments, health systems, businesses, and local communities all having an important role to play. Women, children, and adolescents are particularly susceptible to the health impacts of climate change and environmental degradation, and also stand to gain the most from a comprehensive response. The complex interlinkages between environmental and social systems make it an essential component for consideration in the mind of any public health or development professional.

Case study: sustainable energy for health care in sub-Saharan Africa addressing an unmet need

Lack of access to modern energy services has long-hampered development efforts across sub-Saharan Africa. This is most apparent in Liberia, a country with a 2% electrification rate. A reliable source of electricity is essential for hospitals and clinics for a range of basic functions, including the maintenance of cold-chains and refrigeration, adequate washing and sterilisation, and lighting and indoor thermal regulation. Without this, running a functioning health system is difficult.

A WHO survey suggested that in sub-Saharan African countries studied, only 33% of hospitals had access to 'reliable electricity provision', and over a quarter of health facilities had no access to electricity at all. Here, solar photovoltaic energy is a preferable and often more cost-effective solution in the long-run, when compared to

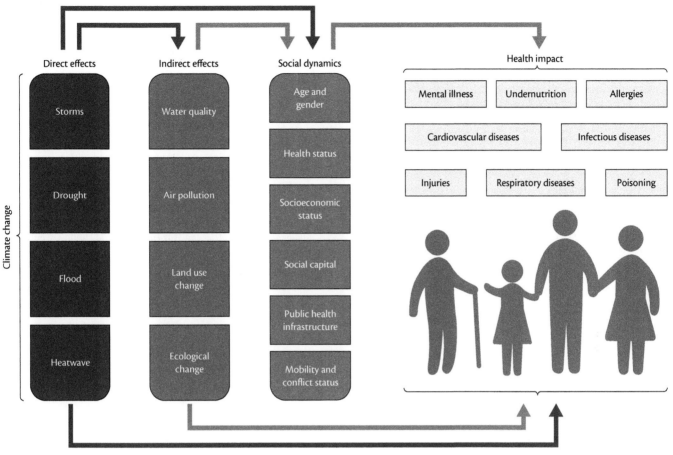

Figure 9.1 The direct and indirect health impacts of climate change.

diesel generators, which worsen local air quality. Decentralised renewable energy technology is particularly useful in countries such as Liberia or South Sudan, which lack a national grid and cannot hope for one in the near future. Investments in decentralised solar energy will not only strengthen the national health system and help tackle poverty, but it will also reduce deaths from air pollution and help mitigate climate change.

Questions

1. To what extent should healthcare professionals get involved in the discussions around climate change, and for what reason?

2. In what ways does climate change disproportionately affect the health of women, children, and adolescents?

3. How can we encourage more joined-up policymaking across disiplines, that considers the broader social and environmental implications of our actions, rather than operating in silos?

Key publications

Watts N, Adger W, Agnolucci P, et al. (2015). Lancet commission on health and climate change: policy responses to protect public health. *Lancet* 386(10006): 1861–914.

This provides an overview of the health impacts of climate change; and the health co-benefits of mitigation and adaptation.

Whitmee S, Haines A, Beyrer C, et al. (2015) Rockefeller Foundation-Lancet commission on planetary health: safeguarding human health in the Anthropocene epoch. *Lancet* 386(10007): 1973–2028.
This provides an overview of the relationship between public health and a broad range of planetary boundaries.

World Health Organization (2016). Preventing *Disease Through Healthy Environments: a Global Assessment of the Burden of Disease from Environmental Risks.* World Health Organization: Geneva.
This is the latest quantitative assessments of the burden of disease from environmental hazards

Further reading

Costello A, Abbas M, Allen A, et al. (2009). Managing the health effects of climate change. *Lancet* 373(9676): 1693–733.

Edenhofer O, Pichs-Madruga R, Sokona Y, et al. (2014). Technical summary. In: Edenhofer O, Pichs-Madruga R, Sokona Y, et al. (eds). *Mitigation of Climate Change: Contribution of Working Group III to the Fifth Assessment Report of the Intergovernmental Panel on Climate Change.* Cambridge University Press: Cambridge, UK and New York, US.

Holgate S, Grigg J, Agius R, et al. (2016) *Every Breath We Take: the Lifelong Impact of Air Pollution.* Royal College of Physicians & Royal College of Paediatrics and Child Health: London, UK.

Intergovernmental Panel on Climate Change (2014). Climate change 2014: synthesis report. In: Pachauri R and Meyer L (eds). *Contribution of Working Groups I, II and III to The Fifth Assessment Report of the IPCC*. Intergovernmental Panel on Climate Change: Geneva.

Lewis S and Maslin M (2015). Defining the Anthropocene. *Nature* 519(7542): 171–80.

Smith K, Woodward A, Campbell-Lendrum D, et al. (2014). Human health: impacts, adaptation, and co-benefits. In: Field C, Barros V, Dokken D, et al. (eds). *Climate Change 2014: Impacts, Adaptation, and Vulnerability Part A: Global and Sectoral Aspects Contribution of Working Group II to the Fifth Assessment Report of the Intergovernmental Panel of Climate Change*. Cambridge University Press: Cambridge, UK and New York, US. pp. 709–54.

United Nations (2014). *The Millennium Development Goals Report*. United Nations: Geneva.

Watts N, Adger N, Ayeb-Karlsson S, et al. (2016). The Lancet Countdown: tracking progress on health and climate change. *Lancet* 389(10074): 1151–64.

Woodcock J, Edwards P, Tonne C, et al. (2009). Public health benefits of strategies to reduce greenhouse-gas emissions: urban land transport. *Lancet* 374(9705): 1930–43.

World Health Organization (2009). *Global Health Risks*. World Health Organization: Geneva.

World Health Organization (2014). *Gender, Climate Change and Health*. World Health Organization: Geneva.

World Health Organization (2016). *Summary Results—Urban Ambient Air Pollution Database*. World Health Organization: Geneva.

World Health Organization and UN Children's Fund (2013). *Progress on Sanitation and Drinking Water: Joint Monitoring Programme Update 2013*. World Health Organization and UN Children's Fund: Geneva.

World Health Organization (2015). *Global Status Report on Road Safety 2015*. World Health Organization: Geneva.

World Health Organization and UN Children's Fund (2015). *Progress on Sanitation and Drinking Water: 2015 Update and MDG Assessment*. World Health Organization and UN Children's Fund: Geneva.

World Health Organization and UN Children's Fund (2015). *Water, Sanitation and Hygiene in Health Care Facilities: Status in Low- And Middle-income Countries and Way Forward* World Health Organization and UN Children's Fund: Geneva.

CHAPTER 10

Conflict, disasters, and humanitarian response

Miriam Orcutt, Clare Shortall, and Aula Abbara

This chapter will outline the main challenges for women's, children's, and adolescents' health in conflict and natural disasters, including existing frameworks for the provision of health care within these contexts.

Key points

◆ A growing number of people are affected by conflict, protracted humanitarian crises, and natural disasters worldwide.

◆ Armed conflict and natural disasters have direct and indirect impacts on public health; provision of health care to the most vulnerable within these populations is a priority.

◆ Early integration of sexual, reproductive, maternal, and child health into all humanitarian programmes is essential.

◆ The current provision of services in these contexts are insufficient in comparison with demonstrated need.

Background

From 1990 to 2013, almost 217 million people per year were affected by natural disasters (EM-DAT, 2016) and according to United Nations High Commissioner for Refugees (UNHCR) by 2017, at least 68.5 million people had been forcibly displaced as a result of persecution, conflict or violence. Around half of all forcefully displaced populations are women, children, and adolescents under the age of 18 made up 52% of the world's refugees in 2017. Addressing global women's, children's, and adolescents' health within conflict and disasters caused by natural hazards involves considering a complex interplay between wider determinants of health, population movement, and shifting patterns of health and disease.

During and after conflict and disaster there is often a collapse of healthcare infrastructure, in addition to other factors such as loss of shelter, access to water, hygiene, and sanitation, and food insecurity. Key needs in these settings include: protection, communicable disease prevention, treatment of non-communicable diseases, treatment of physical injury, treatment of mental health trauma, and addressing nutritional needs. The impact of natural disasters and conflict on child health extends from the period of pregnancy and childbirth to adolescence, through a myriad of direct and indirect effects encompassing loss of life, separation from family, physical trauma, psychological distress, and multiple human rights abuses including torture, forced recruitment, and sexual and gender-based violence.

Of the ten countries with the highest maternal mortality ratios worldwide, eight are experiencing or have experienced recent conflict, demonstrating the direct impact of conflict on health outcomes. Fifteen per cent of pregnant women who are displaced encounter a life-threatening obstetric emergency, such as obstructed labour, eclampsia, haemorrhage, or sepsis, increasing the need for improved access to effective antenatal and delivery services in these situations. Although some frameworks exist for addressing maternal and reproductive health, there is a need for greater emphasis on inclusion of these areas in the formation of all stages of response, from emergency humanitarian response to longer term development response. Given the increasingly protracted nature of the majority of armed conflicts there is also an urgent need to bridge the gap between the humanitarian and development approaches when dealing with women, children and adolescents. Additionally, the Sustainable Development Goals (SDGs) have set the aim to: 'Significantly reduce all forms of violence and related death rates everywhere', which highlights the importance of this topic on the global policy agenda.

Public health in humanitarian crises

Armed conflict and disasters caused by natural hazards create morbidity and mortality spikes, with children under five particularly affected. Both share certain impacts on health; however, there are also important differences. For example, during natural disasters, particularly in previously functioning states experiencing a single event, the immediate relief needs may be for a shorter duration. However, in poorer nations, or those with multiple events, such as earthquakes, there may be a requirement for ongoing needs. Both stressors have the capacity to create a large number of dead and wounded with most deaths from disasters occurring in conflict-affected states. Violence can lead to injuries from small arms or larger weaponry, resulting in greater destruction; chemical weapons, cluster bombs, landmines, and barrel bombs take a particularly high toll on civilians. The use of these can result in fatal injuries or disabilities which can leave both women, children, and adolescents more susceptible to further health issues. It is notable that despite attempts to curtail the deaths amongst civilians by International Human Rights Law, the ratio of civilian to military deaths is increasing, with a rising toll on children.

Health infrastructure

Floods, droughts, cyclones, and armed conflict may lead to population displacement and a breakdown of health infrastructure. This, in turn, can result in both a rise in communicable diseases and greater morbidity and mortality from non-communicable diseases.

Civilians will move to areas of safety: either internally or across country borders as migrants or refugees, temporarily or permanently. In recent conflicts, there has been a rise in the number of urban refugees rather than those resident in refugee camps; this complicates access to services, such as distribution of food and health care, and hinders vaccination campaigns. Refugee camps, particularly those with poor infrastructure, which are overcrowded and exist in areas otherwise unfit for habitation, may lack water and sanitation or be subject to extremes of temperature. Breakdown of vaccination programmes, lack of sanitation, malnutrition, and overcrowded conditions can lead to outbreaks of communicable diseases. The majority of child deaths in these settings are caused by diarrhoeal disease, respiratory infections, measles, malaria, and malnutrition. Disrupted food supplies can occur in both armed conflict and after disasters, leaving those most vulnerable prone to severe malnutrition, resulting in higher mortality and increased risk of disease.

Health systems

Health systems can be disrupted, directly or indirectly, during conflict and disaster. Once destabilised, this results in increased morbidity and mortality amongst the affected population and an increased strain on the remaining structures. Direct disruption of the health system can result from deliberate or coincidental attacks on healthcare facilities during conflict. Increasingly, deliberate attacks are being seen on hospitals and health workers, leading to a reduced health workforce, which may suffer ongoing trauma or become refugees. Indirect effects on health systems, such as interruption of already inadequate health information systems, makes outbreaks more challenging to detect. Additionally, the lack of security in the aftermath of a disaster or during conflict can result in the looting of medical supplies and equipment; and health financing, leadership, and governance may break down, leading to increased costs of healthcare delivery, but without regulation or accountability. These impacts result in limited and inadequate possibilities for health service delivery with reduced access and poor coverage.

Psychological trauma

Conflict presents a particular type of trauma exposure and forced migrants may present with varying responses to the trauma of conflict and the additional trauma of their flight from the conflict-affected area. If their movement is abruptly stopped, either by borders or by being interned in camps, this presents a series of traumas, acute or chronic in nature and impacting on the individual at many levels. Psychological trauma after a disaster or from conflict or ongoing displacement can be significant, compounded by the disintegration of social structures, including family units, the lack of educational opportunities, greater likelihood of poverty, and the death of peers or relatives. This is particularly the case for child soldiers who are abducted and forced into combat with physical threats and drugs. In recent conflicts, there have been deliberate attacks on schools, further disrupting education and resulting in trauma to children. Symptoms of psychological trauma can range from anxiety to depression to post-traumatic stress disorder. For both maternal and child health, the consequences of armed conflict or disaster last for years and can also affect the next generation.

Emergency humanitarian response

Emergency humanitarian response to conflict and natural disasters needs to cover important issues as diverse as child health, child protection (including from violence, abuse, exploitation), pregnancy and childbirth, the provision of emergency obstetric care, and prevention of unwanted pregnancies and unsafe abortions. In addition, the prevention of sexually transmitted infections, including human immunodeficiency virus and acquired immune deficiency syndrome (HIV/AIDS), discouragement of harmful practices such as female genital mutilation, and the protection of women from sexual and gender-based violence (SGBV), are important. Reproductive health outcomes and SGBV have been shown to worsen substantially during conflict and displacement, and women are often particularly vulnerable in these situations. Various guidelines have been developed to integrate reproductive health into humanitarian response. Guidelines most commonly used in emergency humanitarian response situations include the World Health Organization (WHO) Guidance, Sphere, the Inter-Agency Working Group (IAWG) Field Manual, and the Minimum Initial Service Package for Reproductive Health in Crises (MISP). MISP outlines how to integrate comprehensive reproductive health services in the areas of family planning, prevention of gender-based and sexual violence, prevention of maternal and infant mortality, and HIV prevention and treatment. These guidelines should be implemented at the start of humanitarian emergencies to reduce morbidity and mortality among women, children, and adolescents.

Future priorities

- ◆ There is a lack of evidence-based practice used in humanitarian emergencies. Further research and data collection, increased development, implementation, and monitoring and evaluation of maternal and child health interventions, is necessary.

- ◆ Attention must be paid to the potential broader sociocultural and education barriers in the provision of reproductive and child health care. In these settings, community involvement and sustainable access to reproductive and child health care is necessary.

Conclusions

With growing numbers of people affected by conflict and protracted humanitarian crises worldwide and the increasing frequency of disasters caused by natural hazards, provision of health care to those experiencing vulnerabilities, especially women, children and adolescents, remains a priority. The current provision of services in these situations is insufficient in comparison with demonstrated need. Overcoming political and operational hurdles, including difficulties accessing these populations, as well as addressing resource constraints, is essential to provide effective health provision in each phase of the humanitarian response for these populations.

Case study: measles outbreak in an informal refugee camp

In 2015, migrants and refugees fleeing protracted conflicts and poverty became stranded in informal camps across Europe, such as the Calais Camp. Between 5 January and 11 February 2015, a total of 13 clinical measles cases associated with the Calais settlement were detected in a population of 3500 refugees. The impossibility of implementing contact tracing and the risk of further outbreak led to the regional and national public health authorities agreeing to a mass measles immunisation programme for all those aged six months to thirty-five, with vitamin A for children. This outbreak was not entirely unexpected as a previous rapid risk assessment concluded that while the risk of introduction of communicable diseases into Europe from the refugee population is extremely low; poor living conditions overcrowding, inadequate water, sanitation, hygiene and shelter and unknown vaccination status make this population vulnerable. Measles has long been seen as a priority in refugee health due to its highly infectious nature, association with poor nutrition, ability to lead to significant morbidity and mortality (particularly in children under five and pregnant women) and its preventable nature.

Questions

1. Explain the ways in which health systems can be destabilised during a conflict or natural disaster.

2. Outline some of the psychological impacts which might be seen secondary to traumatic exposures during conflict or natural disasters.

3. Describe three important areas emergency humanitarian response must cover to effectively address the health needs of women, children, and adolescents.

Key publications

Sphere Project (2011). *Sphere Handbook: Humanitarian Charter and Minimum Standards in Disaster Response*. Available at: http://www.refworld.org/docid/4ed8ae592.html.
The aim of the handbook is to improve the quality of humanitarian response in situations of disaster and conflict, and to enhance the accountability of the humanitarian system to disaster-affected people.

Kuruvilla S, Bustreo F, Kuo T, et al. (2016). The Global Strategy for Women's, Children's and Adolescents' Health (2016–2030): A Roadmap Based on Evidence and Country Experience. *Bull World Health Organ* 94: 398–400.
Provides a roadmap for ending preventable deaths of women, children, and adolescents. The global strategy has three objectives: survive, thrive, and transform.

WHO Reproductive health during conflict and displacement: A guide for programme managers, 2000.
(http://www.who.int/reproductivehealth/publications/maternal_perinatal_health/RHR_00_13/en/).
This manual provides a tool for developing practical and appropriately focused sexual and reproductive health programmes during each phase of conflict and displacement—pre-conflict, conflict, stabilisation, and post-conflict.

Inter-agency Working Group (2010). *Inter-agency Working Group on Reproductive Health in Crisis. Inter-agency Field Manual on Reproductive Health in Humanitarian Settings, 2010 Revision for Field Review*. IAWG: New York, US.
Serves as a tool to facilitate implementation, monitoring, and evaluation of reproductive health interventions, based on refugee needs.

Child Protection Working Group (2012). Minimum standards for child protection in humanitarian action. Child Protection Working Group (2012). (http://cpwg.net/?get=006914%7C2014/03/CP-Minimum-Standards-English-2013.pdf)
Inter-agency minimum standards for child protection from violence, exploitation, abuse, and neglect in humanitarian situations.

Further reading

Black B, Bouanchaud P, Bignall J, Simpson E, and Gupta M (2014). Reproductive health during conflict. *The Obstetrician & Gynaecologist*.

Centre for Research on the Epidemiology of Disasters (CRED). *EM-DAT: The OFDA/CRED International Disaster Database*. Brussels, Belgium: Catholic University of Leuven.

Fazel M and Stein A (2002). The mental health of refugee children. *Arch Dis Child* 87(5): 366–70.

Leaning J and Guha-Sapir D (2013). Natural disasters, armed conflict, and public health. *N Eng J Med* 369(19): 1836–42.

Levenson R and Sharma A (1999). *The Health of Refugee Children: Guidelines for Paediatricians*. King's Fund and Royal College of Paediatrics and Child Health: London, UK.

Machel G (1996). *Impact of Armed Conflict on Children: Report of the Expert of the Secretary-General, Ms. Graça Machel, Submitted Pursuant to General Assembly Resolution 48/157*. United Nations and UNICEF: New York, US.

Rieder M (2012). Armed conflict and child health. *Arch Dis Child* 97(1): 59–62.

Thomas S and Thomas S (2004). Displacement and health. *Br Med Bull* 69:115–27.

United Nations High Commissioner for Refugees (1992). *Handbook on Procedures and Criteria for Determining Refugee Status: Under the 1951 Convention and the 1967 Protocol Relating to the Status of Refugees*. UNHCR: Geneva.

United Nations High Commissioner for Refugees (2015). *UNHCR Mid-year Trends 2015*. UNHCR: Geneva. p. 3.

United Nations Office for the Coordination of Humanitarian Affairs (2016). *Global Humanitarian Overview 2016*. United Nations OCHA: New York, US. p. 3.

United Nations (2015). *Transforming our World: The 2030 Agenda for Sustainable Development*. https://sustainabledevelopment.un.org/content/documents/21252030 Agenda for Sustainable Development web.pdf.

Women's Refugee Commission (2011). *Minimum Initial Service Package (MISP) for Reproductive Health in Crisis Situations: A Distance Learning Model*. Women's Refugee Commission: New York, US, Geneva. p. 58.

World Health Organization, UNFPA (2011). Trends in maternal mortality: 1990–2008; estimates developed by the WHO, UNICEF, UNFPA, and the World Bank.

SECTION 4

Adolescent health

CHAPTER 11

Introduction to adolescent health

Susan M Sawyer, Suraya Abdul-Razak, and George C Patton

This chapter highlights the significance of health and wellbeing in adolescents and young adults and the importance of this time period within the lifecourse. The most effective actions for adolescent health are intersectoral, multi-component, and multi-level.

Key points

- Investment in building adolescent capabilities yields a triple dividend by improving the health of adolescents, reducing the burden of disease in adults, and improving the health and development of the next generation.

- Beyond early childhood influences, brain maturation and social-role transitions that accompany puberty affect the health of adolescents, shaped by social determinants of health.

- Adolescent health profiles differ greatly between and within countries reflecting different social, educational, economic, cultural, and technological opportunities and risks.

- Different platforms can deliver preventive and treatment-oriented health actions. These include structural actions (e.g. laws, taxation), media (e.g. health promotion), community-based actions (e.g. positive youth development programmes), online and social media, school-based actions and clinical services.

Background

This generation of 10–24-year-olds is the largest in human history. With a population of 1.8 billion, adolescents and young adults constitute a quarter of the world's population. Unparalleled global forces shape their health and wellbeing, including economic development, unemployment, family instability, global communications, and population displacement. Adolescence is a critical life phase for achieving human potential. How young people traverse these years in terms of the capabilities they develop and the behaviours they adopt will influence their future health as individuals, as well as their countries' economic and social prospects. Adolescence itself is a highly dynamic period of human development. Unique maturational windows open with puberty (e.g. brain development, sexual maturation) within which interactions with physical, educational, social, emotional, and cultural environments powerfully influence adolescent behaviours and capabilities that play out across the lifecourse. Early childhood development influences the health and capabilities of children as they enter adolescence, and the health of adolescents is key to achieving a healthy start to life for the next generation.

Reducing mortality is the focus of many global health investments. Road traffic accidents, self-harm, and human immunodeficiency virus and acquired immune deficiency syndrome (HIV/AIDS) are the major causes of death in adolescents and young adults. These are all preventable, but require interventions well beyond the health sector (Table 11.1).

However, the scope of prevention extends beyond mortality, with adolescent health needs and actions defined at three levels (Figure 11.1): (1) current health problems (including mortality); (2) health risks for health problems in adolescence, adulthood, and the next generation; and (3) important structural and proximal social determinants of health. The most important actions for adolescent health and wellbeing are intersectoral, multi-level, and multi-component.

Young people have high unmet needs for health services, which have historically neglected this age group. Most health professionals who work with young people receive little training, and most health services are not well oriented to the needs of the young. Establishing systems for training, mentoring, and for the participation of youth health advocates has the potential to transform traditional models of healthcare delivery to create more adolescent-responsive health systems. The Global Strategy for Women's, Children's and Adolescents' Health (2016-2030) in 2016 included adolescents for the first time, in an appreciation that the Sustainable Development Goals (SDGs) could not be achieved without greater attention to this group.

Global targets

Sustainable Development Goals (2015)

Goal 2 (Zero hunger)

- Address the nutritional needs of adolescent girls.

Goal 3 (Health)

- By 2020, halve the number of global deaths and injuries from road traffic injuries.

- By 2030, reduce by one third premature mortality from non-communicable diseases through prevention and treatment and promote mental health and wellbeing.

- Strengthen the prevention and treatment of substance abuse, including narcotic drug abuse and harmful use of alcohol.

Goal 4 (Education)

- Ensure that all girls and boys complete free, equitable, and quality primary and secondary education leading to relevant and effective learning outcomes.

Goal 5 (Gender equality)

- End all forms of discrimination against all women and girls everywhere.

Table 11.1 Leading causes of death, risk factors, and years lived with disability, by age and sex (2016)

	10–14 years		15–19 years		20–24 years	
	Boys	**Girls**	**Boys**	**Girls**	**Boys**	**Girls**
Leading causes of death, by age group and sex	Road injuries	HIV/AIDS	Road injuries	Self-harm	Road injuries	Self-harm
	Drowning	Intestinal infections	Interpersonal violence	HIV/AIDS	Self-harm	HIV/AIDS
	HIV/AIDS	Malaria	Self-harm	Road injuries	Interpersonal violence	Road injuries
	Intestinal infections	Road injuries	HIV/AIDS	Diarrhoeal diseases	Tuberculosis	Tuberculosis
	Malaria	Diarrhoeal diseases	Drowning	Tuberculosis	Conflict and terror	Maternal haemorrhage
Leading risk factors for death, by age and sex	Unsafe water	Unsafe sex	Unsafe sex	Unsafe sex	Alcohol use	Unsafe sex
	Unsafe sex	Unsafe water	Occupational injury	Unsafe water	Occupational injury	Unsafe water
	Unsafe sanitation	Unsafe sanitation	Alcohol use	Unsafe sanitation	Unsafe sex	Unsafe sanitation
	Handwashing	Handwashing	Unsafe water	Handwashing	Drug use	Alcohol use
	Household air pollution	Household air pollution	Unsafe sanitation	Alcohol use	High BMI	High BMI
Leading causes of years lived with disability, by age and sex	Skin diseases	Skin diseases	Skin diseases	Skin diseases	Skin diseases	Skin diseases
	Conduct disorder	Iron deficiency anaemia	Migraine	Migraine	Low back and neck pain	Migraine
	Iron deficiency anaemia	Migraine	Conduct disorder	Depressive disorders	Migraine	Depressive disorders
	Migraine	Anxiety disorders	Depressive disorders	Iron deficiency anaemia	Depressive disorders	Iron deficiency anaemia
	Anxiety disorders	Conduct disorder	Low back and neck pain	Anxiety disorders	Drug use disorders	Low back and neck pain

Source: data from Institute for Health Metrics and Evaluation (IHME). *Global Burden of Disease Study 2016.* Seattle, USA: Institute for Health Metrics and Evaluation. Copyright © 2016 Institute for Health Metrics and Evaluation.

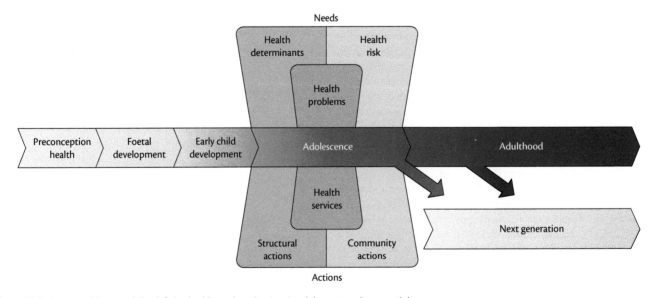

Figure 11.1 Conceptual framework for defining health needs and actions in adolescents and young adults.
Reproduced with permission from Patton, G. et al. Our future: a Lancet commission on adolescent health and wellbeing. *The Lancet.* 387(10036), 2423–78. Copyright © 2016 Elsevier Limited. All rights reserved.

Why adolescent health and wellbeing?

Interest in adolescents and their health is higher than ever, for many reasons. First, the period of the Millenium Development Goals (MDGs) oversaw great reductions in the mortality of under fives. Survival of young children has resulted in a population bulge such that a quarter of the world's population is 10–24 years old. While the health of adolescents and young adults has also improved over this period, it has not occurred to the same extent. In many countries, the mortality rate of older adolescent males is now higher than in 1–4 year old males. Investments made to improve the health of young children will not be sustained without new investments during adolescence.

Second, the significance of adolescence within the lifecourse is better understood. The capabilities achieved during adolescence yield a triple dividend of improved health in adolescence itself, in adulthood and for the next generation. Improved health and nutrition have led to a reduction in the age of onset of puberty, and in most parts of the world, upward extension in the age of adoption of adult roles and responsibilities (e.g. later transition to employment, financial independence, and the formation of life partnerships). Adolescence now constitutes a greater proportion of the lifecourse. Young people are biologically primed to engage. Whether they do so in socially acceptable ways or in more antisocial and dangerous ways reflects the extent to which the young can be engaged by civil society in structures and processes that are meaningful and rewarding for them.

Third, attention is shifting to adolescence due to the adult burden of disease being disproportionately related to non-communicable diseases (NCDs). Primary prevention of NCDs means attending to adolescent health, as many risk factors for adult NCDs have their origin in behaviours and states that commence in adolescence, such as tobacco smoking and other drug use; obesity, poor diet and physical inactivity; and mental health conditions. The lifecourse approach also shows us that health of adolescents now has important implications for future generations.

Finally, young people are at the forefront of global megatrends, such as technology and social media, that profoundly influence health. Young people are also disproportionately affected by population displacement, whether from economic migration, conflict, or climate change. While young people have much to gain from these megatrends, they also have most to lose.

The effect of economic development on adolescent health

The demographic transition describes a country's shift from a high birth rate and high mortality rate to lower fertility, lower mortality, and longer life expectancy. This is accompanied by an epidemiological transition, or shift in the burden of disease. These processes occur because of economic development.

The Lancet Commission on Adolescent Health and Wellbeing grouped the Disability Adjusted Life Years (DALYs) of nine conditions into three categories (diseases of poverty, injuries, and NCDs) that were used to define three groups of countries (multi-burden, injury excess, and NCD predominant). The epidemiological transition is typically accompanied by reductions of communicable diseases, lower maternal mortality, and greater survival of children into adolescence. During adolescence, diseases of poverty are conditions that are prominent prior to a country passing through the epidemiological transition and include undernutrition, major sexual and reproductive health problems (e.g. maternal deaths, high rates of sexually transmitted infections), and infectious diseases.

Just over half of the world's adolescents are growing up in multi-burden countries (n = 68) which are characterised by all three categories of health problems (Figure 11.2). Many such countries are in southern and eastern sub-Saharan Africa where HIV has been a growing contributor to the adolescent disease burden. Others are in South-East Asia and Oceania. These countries have made some progress in the past 15 years in reducing infectious diseases other than HIV, sexual and reproductive health, and nutritional deficiencies (Figure 11.3).

One in eight adolescents is growing up in injury excess countries (n = 28), which are characterised by high levels of unintentional injury or violence and high adolescent birth rates. The majority of these countries have made little progress in reducing the burden of adolescent disease since 2000. Only six countries have made good progress in reducing unintentional injuries and to a lesser extent violence, including Russia, Thailand, Colombia, and Bolivia.

Just over a third of adolescents are growing up in countries that can be classified as NCD predominant (n = 92), where the major burden lies in chronic physical and mental disorders, and substance use disorders. These countries have made substantial progress in reducing the burden of communicable diseases and of injuries and violence, but little progress in chronic physical conditions, mental health, and substance use disorders.

Within any country, there are major differences in health between different regions and within different groups of adolescents. Poverty, gender, and social marginalisation are important determinants of adolescent health. Young people from ethnic and sexual minorities, and who are displaced, homeless, disabled, or in detention face additional health risks.

Actions for health

Investments in adolescent health extend from actions directed towards conspicuous health problems (e.g. conditions such as asthma or anxiety) to the health risks that emerge during this phase of life (e.g. behaviours such as tobacco smoking), and to the broader social determinants of health (e.g. participation in quality schooling, avoidance of child marriage). The most effective actions for adolescent health are intersectoral, multi-component, and multi-level.

Challenges

Adolescents have been missing in the middle, quietly invisible within the health system and social and health policies that have emerged in response to the burden of women's, children's, and adolescents' health and infectious diseases. There are also risks that the growing cost to health budgets from NCDs and the elderly will derail the necessary investments in the developmental years of 0–24, even though they provide the foundation for future health.

The SDGs and the new Global Strategy for Women's, Children's and Adolescents' Health (2016–2030) provide a global framework for investing in adolescents' health and wellbeing, with a promised triple dividend. However, in comparison to women's and child health, which has had decades of technical investments (e.g. data monitoring systems, research, health systems, professional education, and

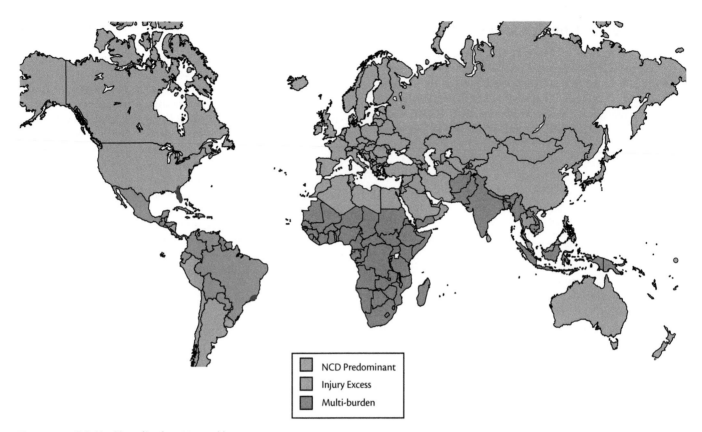

Figure 11.2 Global health profile of 10–24-year-olds.

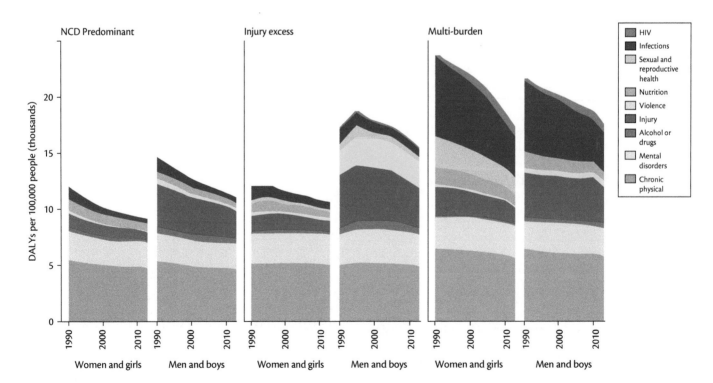

Figure 11.3 Changes in disease burden in 10–24-year-olds between 1990 and 2013.

policy), the technical underpinnings of adolescent health are much more limited. Knowledge of effective programmes and policies lags well behind the urgent need for action; investments will need to be made without the usual surety of evidence. This places greater reliance on the need for co-investment in robust evaluation.

The strength of the SDGs is that they require investments beyond the vertical or disease silos that have so characterised the MDGs. The requirement for intersectoral, multi-component and multi-level actions fits squarely within the SDG remit. Finding ways of working more smartly across sectors, especially the health and education sectors, will greatly benefit adolescents; quality secondary education is arguably the smartest investment in adolescent health. Disaggregating the various SDG targets by age (10–14, 15–19, and 20–24 years) would be helpful in making adolescent health more visible.

We also need better monitoring and accountability systems. One explanation of why adolescent health has been neglected for so long is the lack of visibility that has accrued from a failure of data systems to be sufficiently inclusive of adolescents. This must change. We need to both extend and achieve greater harmonisation of data collection systems for the range of conditions that affect adolescents and young adults, not just sexual and reproductive health.

Achieving universal health coverage for adolescents will require unprecedented coordination across sectors. Substantial investments are required in healthcare systems and preventive strategies to address the growing dominance of NCDs in adolescents, including mental and substance use disorders. Realigning service systems to ensure equity of access for socially and economically marginalised adolescents is required. This will be most effective when adolescents and young adults are themselves engaged as active partners in their own health.

Future priorities

◆ More research is required: about the effectiveness (and cost-effectiveness) of interventions in adolescents and young adults.

◆ Research needs to particularly focus on those from low- and middle-income countries with different cultures, beliefs, lifestyles, and health systems.

Conclusions

As the United Nations (UN) Secretary General Ban Ki-moon stated, 'Young people are the world's greatest resource'. Whether we make smarter investments to optimise the health of future adolescents will depend more on what we wish to do than what we think we can afford to do. Different actions are required by each of the three country groups to address their excess adolescent health burden.

NCD predominant: physical disorders, mental disorders, substance use disorders.

Injury excess: unintentional injuries, violence.

Multi-burden: infectious and vaccine preventable diseases, undernutrition, HIV, sexual and reproductive health

Case study: complex picture of adolescent health in Nigeria

Nigeria is a multi-burden country with a high disease burden related to maternal health and major differences across states. Adolescent pregnancy rates in the northern states of Nigeria are more than four times higher than in the south. There is a lower age of marriage in rural compared to urban areas. Nigeria has an emerging HIV epidemic, particularly in the north-central region, with high rates of unsafe sexual activity. High rates of other infectious diseases include malaria and neglected tropical diseases. Diseases of poverty are priorities to address, as are road traffic injuries and sexual violence, which are prominent. Chronic physical illness (including anaemia from haemoglobinopathies) and obesity are on the rise. Retention in secondary school is increasing, but fewer than 50% of adolescents and young adults receive a basic level of education (ten years).

Responses to Nigeria's adolescent health profile include scaling up school attendance and health service coverage for maternal health care, greater contraceptive coverage, treatment of HIV and other infectious diseases, and responding to chronic physical illness. Emerging priorities of road traffic injury and obesity warrant specific policy and legislative responses.

Questions

1. Why is adolescent health no longer neglected in low- and middle-income countries?

2. What are the factors that can affect health and wellbeing during adolescence?

3. Why are there such differences in the adolescent burden of disease across countries?

Key publications

Patton G, Sawyer S, Santelli J, et al. (2016). Our future: a Lancet commission on adolescent health and wellbeing. *Lancet* 387: 2423–78.
With global interest in adolescent health at unprecedented levels, the Lancet Commission outlines the next steps to advance from advocacy to action. There are also two previous Lancet series on adolescent health (2012 and 2007).

Mokdad A, Forouzanfar M, Daoud F, et al. (2013). Global burden of diseases, injuries, and risk factors for young people's health during 1990–2013: a systematic analysis for the Global Burden of Disease Study 2013. *Lancet* 387: 2383–401.
This paper details the global burden of disease, including injuries and risk factors for 10–24-year-olds.

Bibliography

Ki-moon B, (2016). Sustainability—engaging future generations now. *Lancet* 387: 2356–8.

Kyu H, Pinho C, Wagner J, et al. (2016). Global and national burden of diseases and injuries among children and adolescents between 1990 and 2013: findings from the Global Burden of Disease 2013 Study. *JAMA Pediatrics* 170(3): 267–87.

Viner R, Coffey C, Mathers C, et al. (2011). Fifty-year mortality trends in children and young people: a study of 50 low-income, middle-income, and high-income countries. *Lancet* 377: 1162–74.

World Health Organization (2001). *The Second Decade: Improving Adolescent Health and Development*. WHO: Geneva.

World Health Organization (2009). *Global Health Risks: Mortality and Burden of Disease Attributable to Selected Major Risks*. WHO: Geneva.

CHAPTER 12

Adolescent sexual and reproductive health

Saiqa Mullick, Melanie Pleaner, Mopo Radebe, and Chelsea Morroni

This chapter provides an overview of key sexual and reproductive health (SRH) issues affecting adolescents, with insight into the multiple SRH needs of adolescents and the challenges and barriers to access. It should be read in conjunction with Chapter 15 (HIV and infection in adolescents) and Chapter 19 (Sexual and Reproductive Health).

Key points

◆ This chapter is framed by an integrated definition of SRH and rights which defines SRH as a state of physical, emotional, mental, and social wellbeing in relation to all aspects of sexuality and reproduction, not merely the absence of disease, dysfunction, or infirmity. It embraces a positive approach to sexuality and reproduction, the right of individuals to make decisions governing their bodies and to access services that support these rights.

◆ Adolescents have the poorest level of universal health coverage of any age group and experience disproportionately high rates of preventable sexual behaviour morbidities, including unintended pregnancy, sexually transmitted infections (STIs), and human immunodeficiency virus (HIV).

◆ Adolescents face many barriers in accessing their SRH and rights, which include the right to receive accurate information and confidential services tailored to their specific needs and provided in a non-discriminatory manner.

Background

Adolescents in developing countries or living in economically disadvantaged settings experience disproportionately high rates of preventable morbidities related to sexual behaviour, including teenage pregnancy (resulting in poor pregnancy outcomes and higher risk of maternal mortality) STIs, and HIV. Inadequate policies, lack of resources, poor knowledge about how and where to obtain SRH services, negative provider attitudes, and high risk of sexual coercion and gender-based violence are some of the reasons why adolescents are especially vulnerable. Other contributing factors include sexual exploitation, transactional sex, peer pressure, alcohol and substance abuse, and age-disparate sex. It is important to note that adolescents are not a homogenous group and that adolescents may have very different SRH needs depending on their age, maturation, and experience. Additionally, there are groups of adolescents that may be more vulnerable than others depending on factors such as whether they are orphaned, in school, or in a rural or an urban setting.

Targets

Sustainable Development Goals (SDGs) (2015)

Goal 3 (Health)

◆ By 2030, ensure universal access to SRH services, including family planning, information and education, and the integration of reproductive health into national strategies and programmes.

Goal 5 (Gender equality)

◆ End all forms of discrimination against all women and girls everywhere.

◆ Eliminate all forms of violence against all women and girls.

◆ Ensure universal access to sexual and reproductive health and reproductive rights.

Goal 4 (Inclusive and quality education)

◆ By 2030, eliminate gender disparities in education and ensure equal access to all levels of education and vocational training.

Issues in adolescent SRH

The following sub-sections highlight some of the most common SRH outcomes of concern amongst adolescents.

Sexually transmitted infections

Globally, adolescents and young adults under 25 have the highest rates of curable STIs. Each year, one in every 20 adolescents and young adults will develop a new STI. Comprehensive age and sex-specific data on STIs other than HIV infection are currently lacking. Younger adolescent girls face an even greater risk than older adolescents of acquiring STIs including HIV as, biologically, their immature reproductive and immune systems result in increased susceptibility. Untreated STIs can result in serious health problems including infertility, pelvic pain, and increased risk of HIV co-infection.

Gender-based violence

Extreme violence, including sexual assault and rape, affects at least one-third of all females, 29% of women aged 15–19 and a high proportion of girls younger than 15 years (Figure 12.1). Sexual assault also affects adolescent males, but it remains highly stigmatised and is largely a hidden problem. The most common form of violence that women experience is from an intimate partner (IPV) and includes physical, sexual, or emotional abuse. Sexual assault is also common, with a high proportion of young women under the age of 18 reporting sexual assault (Figure 12.1), which includes their first sexual encounter being forced. Adolescents are at high risk for IPV and their young age and relative inexperience can increase vulnerability through limiting their power in relationships, particularly for young women involved with older men. Furthermore, traumatic experiences and fear of such abuse undermine gender equity for adolescent women, both by conveying the notion that they are not valued and by constraining their engagement in education, employment, and general mobility in society, based on fears for safety.

Female genital mutilation/cutting (FGM/C)

There are four types of FGM/C: clitoridectomy, excision, infibulations, and all other harmful procedures to the female genitalia. FGM/C is a form of gender-based violence that may be performed to preserve the dignity of the family, guarantee of virginity and fidelity to the husband, to dampen or remove a woman's sexual pleasure, prevent sexual deviance, or enhance male pleasure, or for other cultural and traditional beliefs.

FGM/C can potentially affect a woman's physical and mental health throughout her life, from the moment of cutting as a child or adolescent, to sexuality and childbirth in adulthood. The complications of FGM/C include severe pain, excessive bleeding, shock, infections, urination problems, impaired wound healing, and death. It is associated with prolonged or obstructed labour, obstetric lacerations, obstetric haemorrhage and difficult delivery. Women can also experience psychological problems, including fear of having sexual intercourse, anxiety, and depression.

Early marriage

Around the world, 15 million girls marry each year before 18 years; in developing countries, one in nine girls marry before 15 years, and a third of girls are married before 18 years. Child marriage is most common in South Asia and sub-Saharan Africa. A combination of economic, cultural, traditional, and religious reasons are used to justify early marriage. Early marriage often results in adolescent pregnancy, increasing the risk of complications in pregnancy or childbirth, as well as having a negative effect on education, economic security, rights, and wellbeing.

Early and unintended pregnancy

Approximately 16 million girls aged 15–19 give birth each year, accounting for roughly 11% of all births worldwide; 95% of these births occur in developing countries. Factors contributing to teenage pregnancy include early marriage, sexual coercion, lack of information, poor access to contraceptive services and social pressure. Adolescents are less likely to be able to obtain legal and safe abortions, or obtain skilled antenatal, childbirth, and postnatal care.

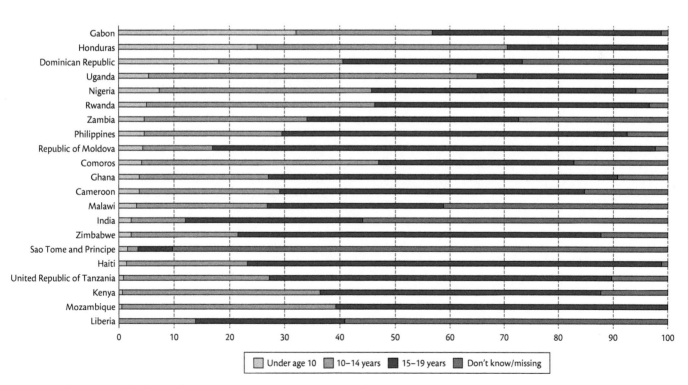

Figure 12.1 The percentage distribution of girls aged 15–19 years who have experienced forced sexual intercourse or any other forced sexual acts, by age at first incident of the violence.

Note: Data for Comoros are based on 25–49 unweighted cases.

Reproduced with permission from Unite for Childen, UNICEF. Hidden in Plain Sight – A statistical analysis of violence against children. UNICEF, New York, 2017, https://data.unicef.org/wp-content/uploads/2015/12/VR-full-report_Final-LR-3_2_15_189.pdf; and source: data from UNICEF global databases, 2014, based on DHS, 2005-2013.

Childbirth at an early age is associated with greater health risks for both the mother and her baby as many adolescents enter pregnancy with incomplete body growth or in poor health. Pregnant adolescent girls are more likely to experience health problems, such as anaemia, HIV and other STIs, postpartum haemorrhage and mental disorders, and their babies are at greater risk of pre-term birth, low birthweight, and asphyxia, all of which increase the chance of death and of future health complications for the baby. The risk of maternal death about a third higher among 15–19-year-olds than among 20–24-year-olds.

The prevention of adolescent pregnancies, and the provision of support to pregnant adolescents are key strategies in improving maternal and child outcomes. Barriers to effective use of contraception include poor understanding of pregnancy risks, concerns about the effect of contraceptives on health or fertility, lack of knowledge of services, community stigma about sexual activity, and disapproving attitudes from providers.

Abortion

A large proportion of adolescent pregnancies are unintended, and over a third of these end in abortion (Table 12.1). An estimated 3.2 million unsafe abortions occur annually in adolescent girls, contributing to maternal mortality and health problems which are often long lasting and affect future SRH. Adolescents girls are more likely to present in the second trimester and are more likely to use unregulated providers. As such, younger women experience a higher risk of abortion-related deaths than women over 25 years.

Interventions

Research studies and programmatic experiences over the last 20 years have improved our knowledge and understanding of adolescent programmes and interventions (Table 12.2). Although there are still many gaps, there is a much better understanding of what works and what does not, in responding to the SRH needs of adolescents. The SRH and rights of adolescents is affected by a country's cultural, religious, legal, political, and economic contexts, and as such, actions must take account of these contexts. Actions are needed at each level, from structural, through to community settings, including schools, and health services. The most effective programmes are typically multi-component, targeting one or more of these settings.

Challenges

Although nearly all countries have signed and ratified the United Nations Convention on the Rights of the Child, profound differences in the legal frameworks underpinning adolescent SRH across countries still exist. Even where national legal frameworks exist, customary or religious laws often take precedence, leaving the right of adolescents to health neglected and undermined. Age of consent, age of marriage and age at which adolescents can access SRH services are inconsistent, particularly in developing country settings. Although evidence-based interventions are required to feed into policy and practice, adolescents are often excluded from research due to ethical restrictions and the need for parental/guardian's consent.

Future priorities

◆ More research on effective interventions and better age-disagreggated data from existing programmes is needed to monitor, evaluate, and plan for effective programmes.

◆ Inequalities in health and wellbeing are evident in socially and economically marginalised adolescents, including ethnic minorities and refugees; health service systems need to be restructured to ensure engagement of adolescents and equity of access regardless of sex, ethnic, or socioeconomic status.

◆ A concerted effort needs to be made to address specific needs of younger adolescents aged 10–14 years. While this age group is less likely to be sexually active and thus in need of SRH services than older adolescents, those in need of services are likely to be underserved by providers and neglected by national policies.

◆ Research is needed to identify aspects that will contribute to the elimination and prevention of FGM/C and how to better care for girls and women who have been subjected to the practice.

Conclusions

Adolescents are at risk of adverse SRH outcomes. However, they are a diverse group and risk of adverse outcomes may be higher in some groups than others. It is a well-documented fact that adolescents face structural, cultural, legal, and health system barriers to obtaining reproductive health information and services. These barriers operate at the individual, family, community, and sometimes policy levels. Addressing these barriers is crucial for enabling

Table 12.1 Adolescent abortion in five developing countries

Country (and year)	No. of abortions to women aged 15–19	Rate per 1000 women 15–19	Percentage of pregnancies to women 15–19 that end in abortion
Burkina Faso (2008)	23,630	30	16
Ethiopia (2008)	46,860	11	9
Kenya (2012)	76,760	38	22
Malawi (2009)	14,040	21	14
Mexico (2009)	230,180	44	34

Source: data from Sedgh G et al., Adolescent pregnancy, birth and abortion rates across countries: levels and recent trends. *Journal of Adolescent Health*. 56(2), 223–230. Copyright © 2015 Elsevier Inc. All rights reserved.

Table 12.2 Evidence of effectiveness of sexual and reproductive health interventions among adolescents

Intervention	Key findings/evidence	Recommendations
School-based interventions		
Comprehensive sexuality education; a curriculum-based approach that aims to provide young people with the knowledge, attitudes, and skills to make informed decisions about their sexuality and sexual and reproductive health.	Greater benefit with the intervention that involve contraception and programmes combining education and contraceptive promotions.	Ensure that all adolescent rights to essential health information are met, including comprehensive sexuality education. More efforts and action needed to convince governments and other stakeholders to invest resources in this area.
Abstinence-only education.	Ineffective in preventing HIV, incidence of STIs adolescent pregnancy.	Abstinence-only education is not recommended.
School-based health services ranging from permanent medical staff to nurse clinics a few hours per week.	Significant impact on safe sex behaviours and pregnancy if contraceptives are offered on site.	Provision of essential resources for health in schools and easy access to adolescent health services including condoms and modern contraception.
Community based interventions		
Generating community support: for interventions in schools and health services through social marketing, public hearings, and dialogues.	Evidence of reduction in STI incidence and pregnancy. Integrated programmes that focus on empowerment and incentives shown to be effective in delaying marriage.	Play a role in the success of interventions within other settings and should feature in multi-component interventions.
Positive youth development (PYD) programmes which aim to address the cause of sexual health risks and early pregnancy.	Have an impact on knowledge and attitudes and safe-sex behaviours (contraceptive use, delayed sexual initiation, and number of sexual partners).	Promising intervention and warrants further research.
Youth-friendly venues in which young people access information and services that address sexual and reproductive health needs.	Moderate quality evidence of mixed impact on uptake of services; ineffective in changing safe-sex behaviours, HIV, or sexually transmitted infection prevalence or incidence, and adolescent pregnancy.	Not recommended in current form.
Cash transfers (in LMICs) may be unconditional, with payments going to individuals who are not required to do anything to receive these, or conditional, with payments tied to behaviours such as staying in school.	Evidence of impact on safe sex behaviours with both unconditional and conditional transfers. Interventions also shown to have an impact reducing unintended pregnancies and delaying marriage.	Promising intervention, further research needed.
Peer education (education delivered by young people to their peers).	Positive impact on safe sex behaviours within programmes that include provision of contraception.	Promising interventions in low- and middle-income countries; further research needed.
Family-based interventions		
Interventions to improve parent-child communication about sexual health and sexuality.	Evidence of effect on parent-child communication, improved contra-ception and condom use.	Should feature in multi-component interventions; more research into science-driven, skills-based programmes to support parent and child.
Promoting universal health coverage		
Health service interventions which include the provision of information and counselling, including preconception advice, contraception, antenatal and postnatal care and delivery, abortion services, treatment and prevention of STIs/HIV, and care of sexual and gender-based violence.	Evidence shows that making services more adolescent friendly increases service utilisation.	Health services should provide all essential healthcare responses, including modern contraception and, when necessary, safe abortion regardless of age, marital, and socioeconomic status.

adolescents to exercise their right to sexual and reproductive health information and services.

Case study: using school-based interventions in Rwanda to optimise adolescent health

School-aged children in Rwanda face many challenges related to poor health, poverty, and environmental hazards, such as inadequate water and sanitation facilities (which can particularly impact on menstruating girls), limited school infrastructure, communicable and non-communicable diseases, and gender-based violence. Other important health issues relate to sexuality, SRH, HIV prevention, trauma, violence, substance abuse, and mental health problems. These factors impact on attendance at schools and on learners' abilities to concentrate on school lessons, leading to poor retention rates.

In order to overcome such barriers, the Government of Rwanda has developed a comprehensive national school health policy as an integrated set of planned and sequential efforts designed to promote the students' physical, social, psychological, and educational development.

The school health policy recommends policy actions in eight key areas:

- Health promotion and disease prevention and control
- HIV, acquired immune deficiency syndrome (AIDS), and other STIs
- Sexual and reproductive health and rights
- Environmental health including sanitation
- School nutrition
- Physical education
- Mental health and related needs
- Gender and gender-based violence (GBV) issues

The policy takes a whole-school approach, with interventions directed at improving the school curriculum, physical infrastructure, access to school-based health services, school ethos, school policies, and linkages with the community. It recommends a school health 'minimum package', including health promotion and education, referral and follow-up of minor health issues, safe water and sanitation provision, deworming, and school nutrition. Nine ministries implement the policy, each with its specific areas of responsibility. This has allowed for early, preventative intervention to optimise child health at an early age.

Questions

1. Describe key components of a holistic, youth-friendly healthcare package of services that could improve adolescent SRH in developing country settings.

2. Describe the barriers to SRH information and care faced by young people in low- and middle-income countries (LMICs), and consider how and why these barriers may or may not differ from barriers faced by adults in the same settings.

3. Outline the short and long-term impacts of adolescent childbearing for individuals, families, and societies.

4. Explain the multi-level (individual, relationship, cultural, and social) and multi-factorial reasons why adolescent girls may not practice safer sex.

Key publications

Salam R, Faqqah A, Sajjad N, et al. (2016). Improving adolescent sexual and reproductive health: a systematic review of potential interventions. *J Adolesc Health* 59(4 Suppl): S11–S28.
  This systematic review assesses the effectiveness of different interventions, with a focus on key issues such as the prevention of adolescent pregnancy, FGM/C, and gender-based violence.

Chandra Mouli V, Lane C, and Wong S (2015). What does not work in adolescent sexual and reproductive health: a review of evidence on interventions commonly accepted as best practices. *Glob Health Sci Pract* 3(333): 40.
  This paper questions the value of ineffective interventions that waste human and financial resources, and fail to demonstrate results. There are useful recommendations that highlight the importance of adapting

evidence-based prevention science approaches that address both risk and protective factors for adolescents in LMICs.

Chandra-Mouli V, Lane C, and Wong S (2014). Contraception for adolescents in low and middle income countries: needs, barriers, and access. *Reprod Health* 11(1): 1.
  A review of research and programmatic experiences on the needs, barriers, and effective strategies to improve access to and use of contraception by adolescents in LMICs.

McCarthy K, Brady M, and Hallman K, et al. (2016). *Investing When it Counts: Reviewing the Evidence and Charting a Course of Research and Action for Very Young Adolescents*. Population Council: New York.
  This paper focuses on younger adolescents specifically, looking at why it is imperative to invest in this younger age group, the social and contextual influences on younger adolescents' health, and ways to improve both research and programmes to respond more effectively to this vulnerable age group.

Bibliography

Ahman E and Shah I (2011). New estimates and trends regarding unsafe abortion mortality. *Int J Gynaecol Obstet* 115: 121–6.

Banwari G (2013). Adolescent male peer sexual abuse: an issue often neglected. *Indian J Psychol Med* 35: 394–6.

Bearinger L, Sieving R, Ferguson J, and Sharma V (2007). Global perspectives on the sexual and reproductive health of adolescents: patterns, prevention, and potential. *Lancet* 369: 1220–31.

Blanc A, Tsui A, Croft T, and Trevitt J (2009). Patterns and trends in adolescents' contraceptive use and discontinuation in developing countries and comparisons with adult women. *Int Perspect Sex Reprod Health* 35: 63–71.

Christiansen C, Gibbs S, and Chandra-Mouli V (2013). Preventing early pregnancy and pregnancy-related mortality and morbidity in adolescents in developing countries: the place of interventions in the prepregnancy period. *J Pregnancy* 257546.

Decker M, Peitzmeier S, Olumide A, et al. (2014). Prevalence and health impact of intimate partner violence and non-partner sexual violence among female adolescents aged 15–19 years in vulnerable urban environments: a multi-country study. *J Adolesc Health* 55: S58–67.

Dehne K and Riedner G (2001). Sexually transmitted infections among adolescents: the need for adequate health services. *Reprod Health Matters* 9: 170–83.

Nour N (2009). Child marriage: a silent health and human rights issue. *Rev Obstet Gynecol* 2: 51–6.

Patton GC, Sawyer SM, Santelli JS, et al. (2016). Our future: a Lancet commission on adolescent health and wellbeing. *The Lancet* 387(10036): 2423–78.

Nove A, Matthews Z, Neal S, and Camacho A (2014). Maternal mortality in adolescents compared with women of other ages: evidence from 144 countries. *Lancet Global Health* 2: e155–64.

Starrs AM, Ezeh AC, Barker G, et al. (2018). Accelerate progress—sexual and reproductive health and rights for all: report of the Guttmacher–Lancet Commission. *The Lancet Commissions* 391(10140): 2642–92.

Sedgh G, Finer L, Bankole A, et al. (2015). Adolescent pregnancy, birth and abortion rates across countries: levels and recent trends, *J Adolesc Health* 56(2): 223–30.

Wellings K, Collumbien M, Slaymaker E, et al. (2006). Sexual behaviour in context: a global perspective. *Lancet* 368: 1706–28.

World Health Organization (2013). *Global and Regional Estimates of Violence Against Women: Prevalence and Health Effects of Intimate Partner Violence and Non-partner Sexual Violence*. WHO: Geneva.

World Health Organization (2013). *Safe Abortion: Technical and Policy Guidance for Health Systems*, second edition. WHO, Department of Reproductive Health and Research: Geneva.

World Health Organization (2014). *Adolescent Pregnancy*. WHO: Geneva.

Woog V, Singh S, Browne M, and Philbin J (2015). *Adolescent Women's Need for and Use of Sexual and Reproductive Health Services in Developing Countries*. Guttmacher Institute: New York.

CHAPTER 13

Adolescent non-communicable diseases

Jacqueline Pitchforth and Dougal Hargreaves

This chapter will explore key non-communicable diseases (NCDs) and risk factors, focusing on their prevalence and impact on current adolescent health as well as future population health. Mental health (Chapter 14), injuries (Chapter 16), and adolescent sexual and reproductive health (Chapter 12) contribute to adolescent NCDs but are covered elsewhere. This chapter should also be read in conjunction with Chapter 39 (NCDs in children).

Key points

◆ NCDs are responsible for 63% of deaths worldwide and a significant cause of mortality in adolescents. It encompasses a broad range of pathologies with varied aetiologies.

◆ The main risk factors for NCDs, including smoking, unhealthy diet, physical inactivity, and harmful use of alcohol, are established or influenced by behaviours in adolescence.

◆ Interventions are heavily linked to behavioural modification, especially related to advertising and health promotion campaigns.

Background

Non-communicable diseases, including mental health problems, injuries, cancer, asthma, diabetes, epilepsy, and sickle cell disease are major causes of morbidity and mortality during adolescence. In addition, adolescence is a formative period when lifelong patterns of health behaviours, such as tobacco use, are often established. The same is also true for unhealthy diet, physical inactivity, and harmful use of alcohol. For example, globally 100,000 young people start smoking each day and over 90% of adults who smoke started during childhood or adolescence. Thus, risk factors acquired in adolescence account for a significant proportion of deaths from cardiovascular disease, cancer, diabetes, and chronic respiratory conditions in adulthood.

In 2013 the World Health Organization (WHO) adopted nine Voluntary Global targets for reducing deaths from NCDs by 2025. These contained four adolescent-specific indicators: the prevalence of heavy drinking amongst adolescents, alcohol related morbidity and mortality among adolescents, prevalence of insufficiently physically active adolescents, and prevalence of tobacco use among adolescents.

Global targets

Sustainable Development Goals (SDGs) (2015)

Goal 3 (Health)

◆ By 2030, reduce by one third, premature mortality from NCDs through prevention and treatment and promote mental health and wellbeing.

WHO Global Action Plan for the prevention of NCDs (2013)

◆ A 25% relative reduction in the risk of premature death from cardiovascular disease, cancer, diabetes, or chronic respiratory disease by 2020.

◆ A 10% relative reduction in the prevalence of insufficient physical activity by 2020.

◆ A 30% relative reduction in prevalence of current tobacco use by persons aged 15+ by 2020.

Why are NCDs important?

Most NCDs are considered preventable because they are caused by common modifiable risk factors which include: tobacco use, unhealthy diet, physical inactivity, and harmful use of alcohol. NCDs in adolescents are similar to those in adults, with diabetes, asthma, and cancer (especially leukaemia, lymphoma, and solid tumors) being the most common. There are also chronic childhood conditions such as rheumatic heart disease, congenital heart disease, and epilepsy. Over half of the new 36 million NCDs in adults every year are associated with behaviours that begin or were reinforced in adolescence and 1.2 million youth under age 20 died of NCDs in 2002. The NCD-predominant country categorisation (see Chapter 11) accounted for 92 of 188 countries in the 2013 adolescent burden of disease.

NCDs account for a significant proportion of mortality and disease burden in adolescence. Globally, eight of the top twenty-five leading causes of death in 10–19-year-olds are due to NCDs (including leukaemia, ischaemic heart disease, and epilepsy), with a higher proportion in high-income countries (HICs) than low-income countries (LICs). However, the majority (>70%) of global adolescent deaths occur in LICs. The relative importance of different NCDs in specific countries is described in Figure 13.1. Although there is significant variation between countries, NCDs result in a

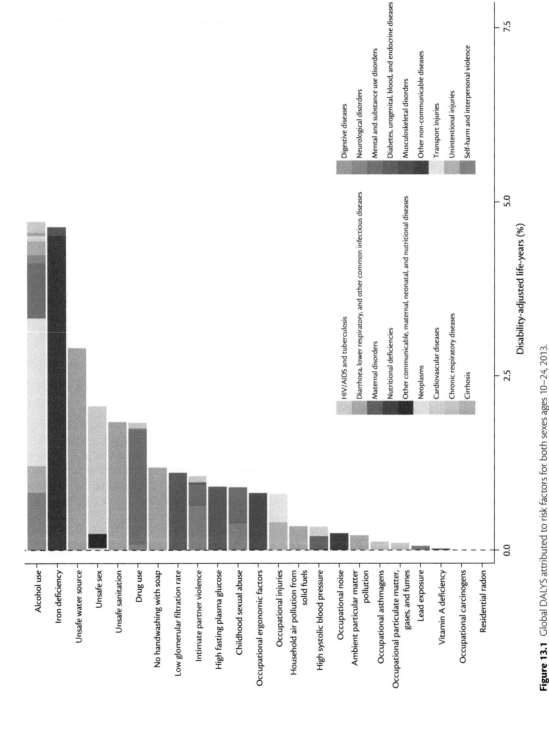

Figure 13.1 Global DALYS attributed to risk factors for both sexes ages 10–24, 2013.

significant disease burden and are the leading cause of years lived with disability (YLDs) worldwide.

Relevance of adolescence to NCDs

Adolescence has traditionally been thought of as a time of relative health. Mortality rates have decreased more rapidly among young children than adolescents from 1955–2004, reflecting a transition from communicable diseases to NCDs and injury-related deaths. Adolescents are uniquely vulnerable by virtue of their low social-economic, legal, and political status and increased exposure to risk factors. Adolescence can be a time of increased risk-taking behaviour. Maturation of the neural systems underpinning emotional processes might be one reason for higher risk of mental and substance abuse disorders in adolescence. Although family influences are less dominant in adolescence, family connectedness, parental involvement, and supportive peer relationships are associated with improved mental health outcomes.

The primary causes of mortality and morbidity in adolescents worldwide are due to NCDs. The leading global risk factor for death is unsafe water for young people aged 10–14 years and unsafe sex for those aged 15–19 years. In addition, the greatest cause of Disability Adjusted Life Years (DALYs) in 10–14 years and for 15–19 years were skin diseases (see Table 11.1).

Specific adolescent NCDs

Diabetes

Type 1 diabetes is the most common autoimmune disorder in childhood and adolescence, affecting 490,000 (0–14 years) worldwide, with 70,000 new cases each year. Adolescents with diabetes experience a deterioration in metabolic control during this period, often attributable to erratic meal and exercise patterns, poor adherence to treatment regimens, hazardous and risk-taking behaviours, eating disorders, and endocrine changes associated with puberty. Overweight or obesity are the single most important predictors of type 2 diabetes (T2DM). As a result of increasing global rates of adolescent obesity, T2DM accounts for a growing proportion of diabetes cases in children and young people (<10% of the total in most countries but estimated to be 60–80% in Japan).

Cancer

Data from the American Cancer Society shows that in the US, the annual incidence rate of all cancers is 186.6 per 1 million children and adolescents (0–19 years). Approximately 175,000 new cases of cancer are diagnosed each year in children younger than 15 years worldwide, and fewer than 40% are adequately diagnosed and treated, mostly in HICs. In the US, 1 in 285 children will be diagnosed with cancer before age 20 and, despite increased survival rates for many childhood cancers, the disease is still the second leading cause of death (following accidents) in children aged 5–14 and the most common cause of death from disease in 1–19 years. The most common cancers among adolescents aged 15–19 are Hodgkin's lymphoma (15%), thyroid carcinoma (11%), and brain and central nervous system cancers (10%). Survival rates for Hodgkin's lymphoma have improved from 87% in 1975–1979 to 97% in 2003–2009 in the US. However, the reduction in mortality has not been without cost, and the long-term side effects of treatment include pulmonary and cardiac diseases, thyroid abnormalities, infertility, and secondary cancers.

Asthma

Asthma has a low mortality rate but high prevalence rate in adolescents with a significant burden of disease. Mortality is highest among the youngest children, lower during school age, and then increases from puberty to adulthood. In 2012, asthma was the fourth highest global cause of YLDs in 10–14-year-olds and in 2014 it was ranked the ninth leading cause of illness and disability in all adolescents (10–19 years). Asthma morbidity is a major burden for the child, their family, and community. In England, 69% of parents or partners of parents of asthmatic children reported taking time off work because of the child's asthma, while 13% had given up their jobs completely. A US study of 17,000 families by Taylor and Newacheck reported 10.1 million days' absence from schools due to asthma in one year.

Epilepsy

Epilepsy was ranked the ninth leading cause of death amongst adolescents worldwide in 2014 and is the most common neurological disease in adolescents. Hauser showed that the incidence of epilepsy (recurrent unprovoked seizures) in children and adolescents seems relatively consistent across all populations studied, ranging from 50 to 100/100,000.

Nearly 80% of people with epilepsy live in low- and middle-income countries (LMICs) and 75% of these do not get the treatment they need. In many parts of the world, people with epilepsy and their families suffer from stigma and discrimination. Children and adolescents with seizures are socially and economically disadvantaged, more likely to have concurrent health conditions, and more likely to face barriers to care. Cui et al. (2015) found that children and adolescents with seizures missed six or more school days associated with any illness or injury than did children and adolescents without seizures (41.9% compared with 14.3%).

Future effect: population health and later life determinants of health

Adolescence is a sensitive period for determining lifelong trajectories in health and wellbeing. While exploratory behaviour is normal during adolescence, attitudes and habits acquired at this age can determine lifelong health risks. The 2010 Global Burden of Disease study identified ten risk factors which were responsible for the highest burden of disability and premature death (Figure 13.2). Of these, two (smoking and drinking alcohol) are largely initiated during adolescence, while others such as diet, overweight/obesity, and physical inactivity are strongly determined by behaviours and attitudes acquired during adolescence.

Risk factors

Tobacco use

Smoking is a common and significant risk factor for NCDs. Approximately 80% of lifetime smokers initiate the habit as adolescents. One fifth of 13–15-year-olds smoke, and 50% of those who commence smoking in adolescence continue for more than 15 years. Half of 150 million adolescents who continue smoking for more than 15 years will die from tobacco-related causes.

Smoking is also a risk factor for other adverse health behaviours as smokers are three times more likely to use alcohol regularly and eight times more likely to use cannabis. Tobacco smoke also causes asthma, and ear and respiratory infections in children

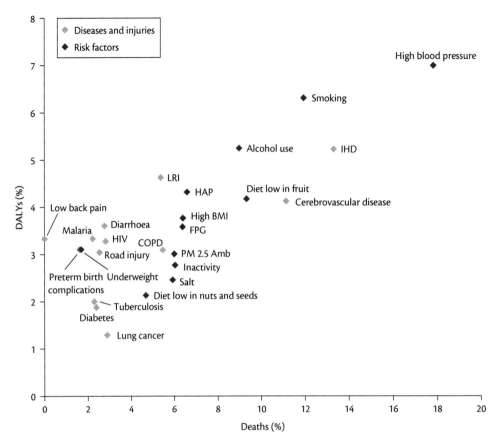

Figure 13.2 Comparison of the magnitude of the ten leading diseases and injuries and the ten leading risk factors based on the percentages of global deaths and percentage of global DALYs.

DALYs = disability-adjusted life years, IHD = ischaemic heart disease, LRI = lower respiratory infections, COPD = chronic obstructive pulmonary disease, HAP = household air pollution from solid fuels, BMI = body-mass index, FPG = fasting plasma glucose, PM2.5 Amb = ambient particulate matter pollution.

Reproduced with permission from Murray, CLJ. et al. GBD 2010: design, definitions, and metrics. *The Lancet.* 380(9859), 2063-2066. Copyright © 2012 Elsevier Ltd. All rights reserved.

and young people. Female adolescents have lower rates of tobacco use globally.

Unhealthy diet

Perhaps the most striking change in health risks has been the shift from undernutrition and stunting to increasing rates of obesity. First in HICs and now in LMICs there has been a dietary switch toward greater consumption of foods high in added sugars, salt, and unhealthy fats, and low in important micronutrients. Combined with decreases in physical activity, these patterns have fueled the global obesity epidemic. Ng et al. (2013) found that overweight and obesity prevalence has now reached more than 20% in some developed countries, with more than 25% of obese adolescents having signs of diabetes or impaired glucose tolerance by age 15. Eighty per cent of US adolescents who are obese at the age of eighteen will remain obese throughout their lives.

As described by Mokdad et al. (2016), unhealthy diets are not just associated with overnutrition but also undernutrition, with iron deficiency anaemia being the leading global risk factor for DALYS in 10–14-year-olds. This has led to a dual burden of unhealthy diet in some LMICs.

Physical inactivity

The WHO recommends that children and youth aged 5–17 years should do at least 60 minutes of moderate to vigorous-intensity physical activity daily, but 84% of girls and 78% of boys do not meet

these requirements. The prevalence of physical inactivity is highest in HICs, where it is almost double that of LICs.

Harmful use of alcohol

Alcohol and drug use in young people aged 10–24 years accounted for 3% of DALYS in 1990 and 6% in 2013. Adolescents are more vulnerable than older adults to alcohol-related harm from a given volume of alcohol, partially related to an increased propensity to reckless behaviour when intoxicated. Some of the increased risks are related to the greater proportion of alcohol consumed by adolescents during heavy drinking episodes as adolescents tend to drink on fewer occasions per month but are more likely to binge drink than older adults. Early initiation of alcohol use (before 14 years of age) is also associated with increased risk for alcohol dependence and abuse at later ages, and increased alcohol-related motor vehicle and other unintentional injuries.

Interventions

The WHO Global Action Plan for Prevention and Control of NCD's 2013–2020 is a comprehensive strategy to achieve the nine global NCD targets, including a 25% relative reduction in premature mortality from NCDs by 2025. This intervention plan primarily works through implementing policy change especially relating to advertising and health promotion, as well as using the WHO tools to monitor NCDs globally. This plan is not adolescent specific.

Challenges

Adolescence is often viewed as the healthiest time of one's life, and consequentially can be neglected by health policymakers. As data are often not available in appropriate age bands (e.g. 10–19 or 10–14, 15–19, 20–24), it is hard to study trends and evaluate the impact of interventions in adolescence. Adolescents can be perceived by healthcare workers as a difficult group to engage and work with, with patchy coverage of interventions to address this, such as the WHO adolescent friendly services initiative. Young people are less likely to vote than older adults, and the full health benefits of investment may only be realised over long time periods, so they may not be prioritised by politicians and other decision makers looking for short-term wins.

Future priorities

◆ In 2015 the WHO report: *Non-communicable Diseases Progress Monitor*, demonstrated that not only were many targets not being met, but there was minimal attention placed on adolescent NCDs.

◆ Surveillance and monitoring of NCD progress especially in low-income countries is likely to be challenging but is essential to reduce morbidity.

Conclusions

NCDs are an important and increasing global health issue for adolescents and the future. Early intervention targeting risk factors and increased prioritisation of adolescent health is key to reducing this growing disease burden.

Case study: developing evidence for school-based interventions to improve adolescent health in the US

A US school-based randomised trial by Peterson et al. (2009) of smoking cessation, used motivational interviewing and cognitive behavioural skills counseling via telephone for 2151 smokers aged 16–18. They demonstrated a 4% increase in six-month smoking abstinence. A Cochrane review and meta-analysis by Lindson-Hawley et al. (2015) showed that this type of motivation-based intervention can also be effective in other contexts.

Evidence from a wide variety of countries and contexts shows that school-based prevention programmes and family-based intensive interventions, which typically focus on improving family functioning, can be effective in reducing smoking among adolescents. Sustained mass media campaigns can also be effective. Similarly, as described by Das et al. (2016), school-based prevention programmes can be effective in reducing the use of alcohol, cannabis, and other drugs, while family-based interventions reduce rates of alcohol misuse, although the effect size is often small.

Questions

1. Why do you think the rate of increase in NCDs is higher in low-income countries?

2. What strategy would you employ to specifically target adolescent NCDs and how would you measure its effectiveness?

3. Do you think there should be a global or country specific response to tackling adolescent NCDs?

Key publications

Neinstein L (2016). *Neinstein's Adolescent and Young Adult Health Care: a Practical Guide*, sixth edition. Wolters Kluwer.
This highlights the importance of adolescent behaviours in determining lifelong health patterns of behaviour.

World Health Organization (2013). *Global Action Plan For Prevention and Control of NCDs 2013–2020*. WHO: Geneva.
This outlines the current global strategy to address the issue of increasing NCDs.

Proimos J and Klein J (2012). Noncommunicable diseases in children and adolescents. *Pediatrics* 130(3): 379–81.
This paper details the role of NCDs specifically in adolescence and provides unique adolescent data.

Global Burden of Disease Pediatrics Collaboration (2016). Global and national burden of diseases and injuries among children and adolescents between 1990 and 2013: findings from the global burden of disease 2013 study. *JAMA Pediatrics* 170: 267–87.
This article provides the data on the disease burden of NCDs globally.

Bibliography

American Cancer Society (2014). *Cancer Facts and Figures 13.s 2014*. Special section: childhood and adolescent cancers. ACS: Atlanta, US.

Cui W, Kobau R, Zack M, Helmers S, and Yeargin-Allsopp M (2015). Seizures in children and adolescents aged 6–17 years—United States, 2010–2014 *CDC—Morbidity and Mortality Weekly Report (MMWR)* 64: 1209–14.

Das J, Salam R, Arshad A, Finkelstein Y, and Bhutta Z (2016). Interventions for adolescent substance abuse: an overview of systematic reviews. *J Adolesc Health* 59: S61–S75.

European Respiratory Society (2013). *European Lung White Book: the Burden of Lung Disease*. ERS: Sheffield, UK.

Hauser W (1994). The prevalence and incidence of convulsive disorders in children. *Epilepsia* 35: S1–6.

International Diabetes Federation/International Society for Paediatrics and Adolescence (2011). *Global IDF/ISPAD Guideline for Diabetes in Childhood and Adolescence*. IDF/ISPAD: Berlin, Germany.

Lindson-Hawley N, Thompson TP, Begh R (2015). Motivational interviewing for smoking cessation. *Cochrane Database of Systematic Reviews* 3. Art. No.: CD006936.

Mokdad A, Forouzanfar M, Daoud F, Mokdad A, El Bcheraoui C, Moradi-Lakeh M, et al. (2016). Global burden of diseases, injuries, and risk factors for young people's health during 1990–2013: a systematic analysis for the Global Burden of Disease Study 2013. *Lancet* 387: 2383–401.

Murray C, Ezzati M, Flaxman A, et al. (2012). GBD 2010: design, definitions, and metrics. *Lancet* 380: 2063–6.

Ng M, Fleming T, Robinson M, et al. (2013). Global, regional, and national prevalence of overweight and obesity in children and adults during 1980–2013: a systematic analysis for the Global Burden of Disease Study 2013. *Lancet* 384: 766–81.

Peterson AV Jr, Kealey KA, Mann SL, et al. (2009). Group-randomized trial of a proactive, personalized telephone counseling intervention for adolescent smoking cessation. *Journal of the National Cancer Institute* 101: 1378–92.

Patton G, Sawyer , Santelli J, et al. (2016). Our future: a Lancet commission on adolescent health and wellbeing. *Lancet* 387: 2423–78.

Proimos J and Klein J (2012). Noncommunicable diseases in children and adolescents. *Pediatrics* 130(3): 379–81.

United Nations Children's Fund (UNICEF) (2011). The state of the world's children 2011. www.unicef.org/sowc2011/.

William RT and Newacheck PW. (1992). Impact of Childhood Asthma on Health. *Pediatrics*, 90(5).

World Health Organization (2014). *Health for the world's adolescents: a second chance in the second decade*. WHO: Geneva.

World Health Organization (2016). *Global Report on Diabetes*. WHO: Geneva.

CHAPTER 14

Adolescent mental health

Kelly Clarke, Sílvia Shikanai Yasuda, and Atif Rahman

This chapter explains how adolescent mental health relates to other areas of health and has relevance across the lifecourse. Particular attention is paid to preventative and treatment interventions in low- and middle-income countries (LMICs), and how these have been adapted for adolescents. It should be read in conjunction with Chapter 25 (Maternal mental health).

Key points

◆ Adolescent mental health disorders are a major cause of morbidity and mortality, and can have devastating health and socioeconomic effects in adolescence and adulthood.

◆ Adolescent mental health and wellbeing is a neglected area of public health, and there has been a global lack of research and investment in mental health interventions.

◆ Physical and mental health are intimately linked. Mental health preventive and treatment approaches must involve coordination across multiple health sectors.

Background

More than 70% of all mental health disorders begin before the age of 25. Depression, self-harm, anxiety, and conduct disorders constitute four of the top ten causes of disbality adjusted life-years (DALYs) among girls and boys aged 15–19 years (Table 14.1) and suicide is a leading cause of adolescent mortality. Risk factors for mental disorders include genetic pre-disposition, deficiencies in psychosocial or educational environments, alcohol and drug misuse, and unresolved family, peer, or school problems. Some risk factors are age-specific and may have reciprocal relationships with mental ill health (Figure 14.1). Mental disorders have serious health and socioeconomic costs, which may persist into adulthood and have intergenerational effects (Figure 14.1).

The lives of adolescents around the world are rapidly changing through armed conflict, urbanisation, and use of digital devices. Gang violence, cyberbullying, and negative online peer influences pose new and important threats to adolescent mental health.

More nuanced definitions of mental health incorporate resilience, that is, an individual's ability to cope with stress, and to realise his or her own potential despite adversity. Resilience relies on psychosocial and interpersonal 'life skills', as well as social and community-level resources, such as parental support and neighbourhood and school connectedness. For adolescents living in war-affected and other humanitarian settings, psychological resilience is central to their long-term health and wellbeing.

Global targets

Sustainable Development Goals (SDGs) (2015)

Goal 3 (Health)

◆ By 2030, reduce by one third premature mortality from non-communicable diseases (NCDs) through prevention and treatment and promote mental health and wellbeing.

◆ Strengthen the prevention and treatment of substance abuse, including narcotic drug abuse and harmful use of alcohol.

The World Health Organization's (WHO's) Mental Health Action Plan 2013–2020

◆ Strengthen effective leadership and governance for mental health.

◆ Provide comprehensive, integrated, and responsive mental health and social care services in community-based settings.

◆ Implement strategies for promotion and prevention in mental health.

◆ Strengthen information systems, evidence, and research for mental health.

Interventions

Globally there is a deficit of mental health resources for young people, including specialised personnel, facilities, and training schemes, and many LMICs lack adequate mental health policies and laws. General principles to address the resource deficit include: (1) shifting mental health interventions from specialist services and hospitals in urban areas to community-based settings such as primary care centres and schools; (2) building the capacity of non-specialised health workers (e.g. general physicians, nurses and health volunteers); and (3) integrating mental health into existing adolescent health and social programmes. In high-income countries, computer-based 'e-therapies' are helping to reduce pressure on existing services.

Mental health interventions can be broadly categorised as preventive (universal, selective, and indicated strategies) or treatment. Universal preventive strategies target all adolescents in a population. Examples include taxation and legislation on selling addictive substances, and community or school-based interventions with direct or indirect benefits for mental health, including life skills education and physical fitness programmes. Life skills education enables young people to develop critical thinking, decision-making, problem-solving, interpersonal communication, and coping skills, and can have positive effects on self-esteem, self-efficacy, and motivation. The United Nations Children's Fund (UNICEF) has

Table 14.1 DALYs due to mental health and behaviour disorders among adolescents aged 10–19 years in 2012

Disorder	DALYs in 1000s females (% of DALYs)	DALYs in 1000s males (% of DALYs)	Management*
All causes for ages 10–19 years	84,315	96,746	—
Mental and behavioural disorders	14,411 (100.0)	15,706 (100.0)	—
Depressive disorders Anxiety disorders	7382 (51.2)** 3456 (24.0)	4800 (30.6)** 1972 (12.6)	◆ Family psychoeducation and carer support ◆ Address psychosocial stressors, strengthen social support and link with other community resources ◆ Liaise with the child/adolescent's school ◆ Consider Cognitive Behavioural Therapy (CBT), behavioural activation, interpersonal psychotherapy, family therapy, and parent skills training ◆ Do not use pharmacotherapy as first-line intervention and do not prescribe for under 12s ◆ If partial/no response to psychosocial intervention, consult a specialist for antidepressants ◆ Monitor closely and assess for suicidal thoughts, especially after starting antidepressants
Behavioural disorders	1090 (7.6)	2828 (18.0)	◆ Family psychoeducation ◆ Address psychosocial stressors ◆ Consider parent skills training ◆ Liaise with the child/adolescent's school ◆ Consider psychosocial interventions including CBT and social skills training ◆ Support the family to manage behavioural problems ◆ Assess impact of behavioural disorders on the carer and offer support ◆ For ADHD: consult a specialist regarding psychostimulant medication if the above fail
Alcohol use disorders Drug use disorders	556 (3.9) 460 (3.2)	2972 (18.9) 783 (5.0)	◆ Motivational interviewing (brief psychotherapeutic intervention to motivate change) ◆ Prevention and harm reduction of blood-borne/sexually transmitted infections and unwanted pregnancy ◆ Consider pharmacotherapy by specialist team with caution since evidence is limited and licensing age varies (continuous 24-hour monitoring is necessary).
Self-harm	Not available	Not available	◆ Restrict access to means (firearms, medication, pesticide) ◆ Treat any injuries/comorbidities ◆ Family psychoeducation ◆ Risk and needs assessment (including mental/physical health, social and financial circumstances) ◆ No clear evidence of effectiveness of psychosocial interventions

*Based on Mental Health GAP Intervention Guide (WHO), National Institute for Health and Care Excellence and British Association of Psychopharmacology guidelines.

**For unipolar depressive disorder.

Source: data from World Health Organization (WHO). Global Health Estimates 2013. Geneva, Switzerland: WHO. Copyright © 2013 WHO; Gilvarry, E. et al. Guidance for the pharmacological management of substance misuse among young people. National Treatment Agency for Substance Misuse, National Treatment Agency. Copyright © 2009 Crown; and Hawton K et al. Interventions for self-harm in children and adolescents. Cochrane Database of Systematic Reviews. 2015 Dec 21;(12):CD012013.

recommended incorporating life skills education into the core school curriculum, with adaptations to local culture and needs. Selective and indicated preventive strategies target adolescents at high risk (e.g. acquired immune deficiency syndrome (AIDS)-orphaned and out-of-school adolescents) and with subclinical presentations of mental disorders, respectively. Strategies include peer support groups, microfinance schemes, and parental training.

Treatment strategies for adolescent mental disorders are outlined in Table 14.1. Psychosocial interventions (e.g. cognitive behaviour therapy (CBT) and other talking therapies) are usually the

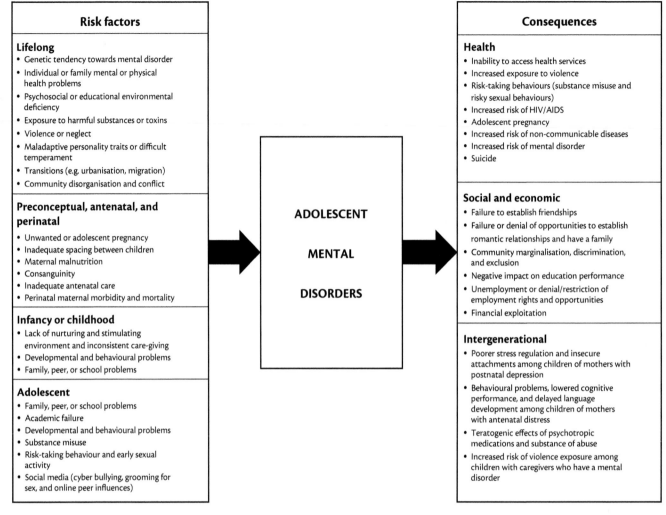

Figure 14.1 Risk factors for and consequences of adolescent mental disorders.

first-line approach. Pharmacotherapy must be considered carefully due to special issues in this age group, such as capacity to consent, diagnostic uncertainty, co-morbidity, drug licensing, and pharmacokinetics (faster metabolism). The WHO developed the Mental Health Gap Action Programme Intervention Guide, which provides guidelines for treating mental, neurological and substance use disorders in adults, children, and adolescents. The guidelines are aimed at non-specialist healthcare providers, especially in LMICs.

Challenges

Conflict and humanitarian settings pose a threat to youth mental health. Violence, lack of security, and unmet basic needs, combined with disruptions in individual, family, and community relations put adolescents at risk of mental disorders. Group psychotherapy (especially CBT), school-based interventions and other psychosocial support can reduce symptoms of depression, anxiety, and post-traumatic stress disorder (PTSD). However, further research is needed to identify the optimum content, duration, and target age-range of such interventions.

Future priorities

◆ Large-scale and sustainable improvements in adolescent mental health require government commitment, strong leadership, and involvement of stakeholders to influence resource allocation, and to develop mental health policies and evidence-based interventions.

◆ Liaison with the education, youth affairs, criminal justice, and humanitarian aid agencies is needed to improve access to mental health care, especially for vulnerable adolescents (e.g. with learning disabilities, young offenders, and trafficked and immigrant adolescents).

◆ Research priorities include: (1) epidemiological data to help plan services, especially in LMICs; (2) validation of tools for screening and referral, suitable for use by non-specialist workers in diverse community settings; (3) translational research to adapt existing mental health interventions for different cultural contexts and low-resource settings, including exploring the use of technology to make such care more accessible.

Conclusions

Adolescent mental health and wellbeing presents an important public health opportunity to improve the health of today's adolescents and tomorrow's adults. Addressing the gap between the burden of mental disorders and allocated resources is an essential first step. Adopting a broader approach to mental health promotion by engaging both health and non-health sectors, and by fostering youth resilience and channelling negative behaviours will help more young people reach their full potential and lead healthy happy lives. Engaging adolescents, either in the development or delivery of mental health interventions, could lead to more appropriate and relevant interventions, and help to empower adolescents to take responsibility for their own mental health.

Case study: low-resource, high-impact intervention to improve both mental and physical health in India

Research among young people in Goa, India, indicated strong associations between sexual and reproductive health (SRH), substance abuse, depression and exposure to violence, with urban youths at greater risk of depression compared to their rural peers. The *Yuva Mitr* ('Friend of Youth') intervention was designed to address these health problems concurrently, in urban and rural communities. The intervention comprised three parts: (1) peer education involving group sessions and street plays; (2) teacher training on teaching methods, improving teacher-student relations, managing common problems faced by students, and counselling; and (3) distribution of health information materials to youth. The intervention was associated with significant positive effects on depression, prevalence of violence perpetrated, and knowledge and attitudes about SRH. Benefits in rural communities included fewer reported menstrual problems and increased knowledge and attitudes about emotional health and substance use. In urban communities, substance use, suicidal behaviour, sexual abuse, and SRH complaints were significantly lower. This case study highlights a low-resource approach to incorporating mental health into a population-level adolescent health promotion programme.

Questions

1. Increasingly, adolescents are using social media—can you list some of the advantages and disadvantages of this for their mental health?

2. What are the main economic arguments for addressing adolescent mental health?

3. Adolescent mental health interventions are commonly based in schools—why might this be beneficial, and what are the challenges of school-based intervention?

Key publications

Kieling C, Baker-Henningham H, Belfer M, et al. (2011). Child and adolescent mental health worldwide: evidence for action. *Lancet* 378(9801): 1515–25.
Review of the global literature on prevalence, risk and protective factors, and interventions for child and adolescent mental health problems.

Barry M, Clarke A, Jenkins R, and Patel V (2013). A systematic review of the effectiveness of mental health promotion interventions for young people in low and middle income countries. *BMC Public Health* 13: 835.
Reviews evidence for interventions to promote mental health among young people in school and community settings

World Health Organization (2016). Mental health gap action programme (mhGAP) Intervention Guide for mental, neurological, and substance use disorders in non-specialized health settings—Version 2.0. WHO: Geneva.
Aimed at doctors, nurses, other health workers, and health planners and managers, this guide presents clinical decision-making algorithms for key mental neurological and substance use disorders

Bibliography

Balaji M, Andrews T, Andrew G, and Patel V (2011). The acceptability, feasibility and effectiveness of a population-based intervention to promote youth health: an exploratory study in Goa, India. *J Adolesc Health* 48: 453–60.

Betancourt T and Khan K (2008). The mental health of children affected by armed conflict: protective processes and pathways to resilience. *International Review of Psychiatry* 20: 317–28.

Drew N, Funk M, Tang S, et al. (2011). Human rights violations of people with mental and psychosocial disabilities: an unresolved global crisis. *Lancet* 378: 1664–75.

Fergus S and Zimmerman M (2005). Adolescent resilience: a framework for understanding healthy development in the face of risk. *Annual Review of Public Health* 26.

Gordon R (1983). An operational classification of disease prevention. *Public Health Reports* 98: 107–9.

Kessler R, Berglund P, Demler O, Jin R, Merikangas K, and Walters E (2005). Lifetime prevalence of and age-of-onset distributions of DSM-IV disorders in the national comorbidity survey replication. *Archives of General Psychiatry* 62: 593–603.

Lewis A, Galbally M, Gannon T, and Symeonides C (2014). Early life programming as a target for prevention of child and adolescent mental disorders. *BMC Medicine* 12: 33.

Mokdad A, Forouzanfar M, Daoud F, et al. (2016). Global burden of diseases, injuries, and risk factors for young people's health during 1990–2013: a systematic analysis for the Global Burden of Disease Study 2013. *Lancet* 387(10036): 2383–401.

National Collaborating Centre for Mental Health (2014.) *E-therapies Systematic Review for Children and Young People with Mental Health Problems*. National Collaborating Centre for Mental Health: UK.

Panter-Brick C, Eggerman M, Gonzalez V, and Safdar S (2009). Violence, suffering, and mental health in Afghanistan: a school-based survey. *Lancet* 374: 807–816.

Patel V, Flisher A, Hetrick S, and Mcgorry P (2007). Mental health of young people: a global public health challenge. *Lancet* 369: 1302–1313.

Tyrer R and Fazel M (2014). School and community-based interventions for refugee and asylum seeking children: a systematic review. *PLoS ONE* 9: e89359.

United Nations Children's Fund (2012). *Global Evaluation of Life Skills Education Programmes*. UNICEF: New York, US.

World Health Organization (2014). *Health for the world's adolescents—a second chance in the second decade*. WHO: Geneva.

World Health Organization (2014). *Mental Health: a State of Wellbeing*. WHO: Geneva.

CHAPTER 15

Adolescent HIV and infection

Rashida Ferrand

This chapter describes the burden of human immunodeficiency virus (HIV) and other major infections in adolescents. It should be read in conjunction with adolescent sexual and reproductive health (Chapter 12), neonatal (Chapter 31), maternal (Chapter 21 and 22), and child (Chapter 36) infections.

Key points

- Infectious diseases remain a leading cause of morbidity and mortality among adolescents, despite the improvements in public health over the past five decades.

- Many infections have long-term chronic complications that result in disability in adulthood.

- While effective interventions to prevent and treat many of the common and serious infectious diseases exist, the main challenge is how to make these accessible to adolescents, an age group that is under-reached by public health programmes.

Background

Infectious diseases remain among the leading causes of death in adolescents, despite the epidemiological transition taking place globally. While non-communicable diseases account for the largest percentage of disability adjusted life-years (DALYs), infectious diseases continue to make a significant contribution, particularly in 10–14-year-olds, where they were responsible for 24% of total DALYs lost in 2012. The largest burden of infections in this age group is due to HIV/AIDS (acquired immune deficiency syndrome), intestinal infections, lower respiratory tract infections (LRTI), diarrhoeal disease, malaria, and tuberculosis.

Overall, the mortality rates for these infections have been slowly declining, with a bigger decline in countries in whom all-cause mortality has also fallen. A notable exception is HIV/AIDS. HIV-related deaths have more than tripled since 2000, making it the second biggest cause of mortality and the fourth leading cause of DALYs lost among adolescents worldwide (Figure 15.1). In 2000, HIV was not even among the top ten causes of death or lost DALYs in adolescents; importantly, adolescents are the only age group in whom HIV-related mortality is rising. This is because adolescents are less likely to access HIV testing and care, and, among those who do get started on treatment, adherence is poorer than in other age groups. The increase in global HIV-related deaths among adolescents results primarily from high mortality in sub-Saharan Africa, where it ranks as the number one cause of death.

As with HIV, there are large regional and between-country differences in the burden of other infections in adolescents. Lower respiratory tract infections rank among the top five causes of adolescent deaths in all regions except for high-income countries and the West Pacific Region, with more deaths occurring among younger adolescents. Half of the world's diarrhoeal deaths in adolescents occur in just five countries (India, Pakistan, Nigeria, Ethiopia, Democratic Republic of Congo).

The regional differences in the prevalence of infections are partly explained by the biological (e.g. prevalence of organisms and vectors) and physical environment (e.g. sanitation and pollution). In addition, the age-related risk of certain infections reflects the biological changes and the social and behavioural context of adolescence. These may have differing effects on adolescent boys and girls. HIV incidence is extremely low in young adolescents, but escalates rapidly after they become sexually active, especially in girls and young women. The difference is mainly due to young women tending to have older male sexual partners and their increased biological susceptibility. The increased incidence of certain infectious diseases in adolescents, for example schistosomiasis, may result from more frequent contact with contaminated water for work or for play, compared to younger children. Similarly, the risk of *Mycobacterium tuberculosis* infection and progression to active disease increases in adolescence. It is important to note that some infections may result in long-term complications and consequent disability (Table 15.1).

Global targets

Sustainable Development Goals (2015)

Goal 3 (Health)

- Ensuring healthy lives and promoting wellbeing for all ages includes reduction in incidence of major infectious diseases as one of the targets.

UNAIDS 90-90-90 (2014)

- By 2020, 90% of all people living with HIV will know their HIV status, 90% of all people with diagnosed HIV infection will receive sustained antiretroviral therapy (ART), and 90% of all people receiving ART will have adequate viral suppression.

Interventions

Effective methods to prevent, treat, and control the spread of most common infections exist (Table 15.1). The Integrated Management of Adolescent and Adult Illness (IMAI) is a standardised World Health Organization (WHO) guideline providing a syndromic approach to managing febrile illness and HIV infection, targeted at first-level health facility workers. At a public health level, prevention and eradication campaigns for common endemic diseases

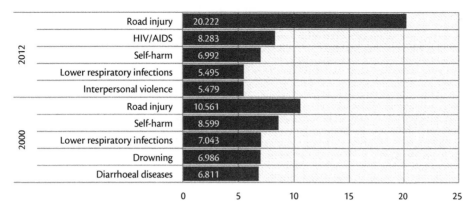

Figure 15.1 Top five causes of mortality (per 100,000 10–19-year-olds), 2000 and 2012.
Source: data from World Health Organization. *Global Health Estimates*. Geneva: World Health Organization. Copyright © 2017 World Health Organization.

have been underway, focusing on vector control, promoting water, sanitation, and hygiene (WASH), and age-targeted mass treatment programmes. School children and schools are a natural target because of the existing school infrastructure and the larger numbers of schools and teachers compared to health facilities and healthcare providers.

For HIV, the choice of interventions should depend on the type of epidemic, that is, whether low-level (prevalence of HIV infection is less than or equal to 1% in the general population or less than 5% in any subpopulation), concentrated (HIV prevalence is over 5% in at least one subpopulation but is less than 1% in the general population), or generalised (HIV prevalence is greater than 1% in the general population), and the specific local context. Interventions for key affected populations, such as young sex workers, men who have sex with men, and people who inject drugs will require different approaches from those in generalised epidemics where population-wide interventions assume increased importance. Experience has shown that interventions combining prevention, treatment, and care and a multi-sectoral approach are most effective.

Challenges

In many, but not all, countries, the burden of infectious diseases is slowly falling, but for some infections the drop in incidence has been much lower in adolescents. The main challenges are:

♦ Access

Adolescents are a difficult age group to reach for provision of interventions. They often seek care late or not at all, due to factors such as poverty, low social status, and lack of awareness. This can be exacerbated by health facilities that are often not set up to cater for their needs, for example confidentiality, non-judgemental attitudes when dealing with sensitive issues (e.g. HIV), and age-appropriate communication. In addition, the requirement for parental consent can be a barrier for adolescents to access health services such as HIV testing.

♦ Adherence

Adherence to interventions drops during adolescence. In a study from Uganda, adolescents frequently did not use bed nets, resulting in an increased risk of malaria (Figure 15.2). This is particularly problematic in HIV, given that lifelong treatment is required and poor adherence increases the risk of onward sexual transmission and the emergence of resistance to drugs used for treatment.

♦ Coverage and impact

Despite the substantial burden in adolescents, helminth infections have received much less attention than HIV, tuberculosis, and malaria. These 'neglected tropical diseases' have longer incubation periods and the clinical manifestations are not immediately obvious. Furthermore, available control interventions do not achieve optimal coverage and impact is achieved slowly over decades.

Future priorities

♦ Improving the evidence base for interventions (e.g. adherence to HIV treatment and school-based malaria treatment programmes) will lead to better choice of interventions.

♦ Innovative strategies should be utilised to improve uptake of and delivery of interventions (e.g. intermittent preventive therapy for malaria, bed nets, and HIV testing).

♦ Improving surveillance data on disease burden should be implemented to inform programming.

Conclusions

Infectious diseases cause a considerable burden among adolescents despite improvements in public health. The developmental, social, and behavioural context of adolescence impacts on risk of infection and treatment outcomes. Effective interventions do exist but how to deliver and reach broader coverage remain to be elucidated.

Case study: poor uptake of routine HIV testing in Zimbabwe among adolescents

Routine HIV testing of all attendees to healthcare facilities (termed provider-initiated HIV testing and counselling or PITC) is recommended by the WHO in high HIV prevalence countries. Guardian consent is required for those under 16 years to access HIV testing in Zimbabwe. In an evaluation of HIV testing practices in seven public sector primary healthcare clinics in Harare, Zimbabwe, only around 50% of adolescents who attended the clinics underwent HIV testing. Those who were sick and attended with female caregivers were more likely to be offered testing. The main reasons for the low coverage of testing were healthcare providers not offering HIV testing because they perceived the accompanying caregiver to

Table 15.1 Common infections in adolescence

Infection	Causative agent(s)	Transmission	Long-term complications	Treatment	Prevention and control
HIV/AIDS	Human immune-deficiency virus (HIV)	Mother to child Intravenous drug use Sexual Blood transfusion	Mainly perinatally-infected adolescents: Stunting and pubertal delay Heart, lung, and bone disease Neurocognitive disease Opportunistic infection	Lifelong antiretroviral therapy (ART)	HIV testing with linkage to prevention and care Voluntary male medical circumcision Prevention of mother-to-child transmission Condoms Post-exposure prophylaxis Pre-exposure prophylaxis Health education Integrated sexual and reproductive health services Needle exchange programmes
Tuberculosis	*Mycobacterium tuberculosis*	Airborne	Chronic lung disease	Anti-TB drugs	Isoniazid preventive therapy BCG (variable efficacy) Contact tracing
Respiratory tract infection	Bacteria Viruses	Airborne	Poor lung function	Antibiotics	Influenza vaccine Pollution control Reduce exposure to biomass fuels
Diarrhoea	Bacteria Viruses Parasites	Faecal-oral	Malabsorption and stunting if recurrent or chronic diarrhoea	Hydration Antibiotics	Water and sanitation Health education
Malaria	*Plasmodium falciparum* (responsible for >90% of malaria in Africa) Others: *Vivax, ovale, malariae, and knowlesi*	Bite of female anopheles mosquito	Complications in pregnancy: High levels of parasitaemia, maternal death, anaemias, low birthweight, miscarriage, and stillbirth	Antimalarials	Intermittent preventive treatment in pregnancy Insecticide treated bed nets
Schistosomiasis	*Schistosoma. haematobium* (bladder and kidney) and *Schistosoma. mansoni* (intestinal) Others: *Japonicum, mekongi, intercalatum* (intestinal)	Contact with water infected with cercariae from specific snail species	Growth restriction Impaired cognition Anaemia *S. haematobium:* Bladder cancer Kidney failure Genital schistosomiasis (leads to ectopic pregnancy, infertility, irregular menstruation, cervical lesions and risk of HIV acquisition) *S. mansoni* Liver fibrosis and failure Portal hypertension	Antischistosomal drugs	Snail control Water and sanitation Health education
Soil-transmitted helminths (STH)	Hookworm Trichuris Ascaris	Faecal-oral Direct penetration of skin (hookworm)	Growth retardation Anaemia	Anti-helminthic drugs Iron supplementation	Improved sanitation Health education Treatment for schoolchildren

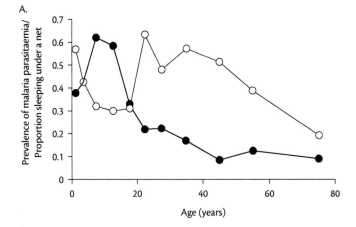

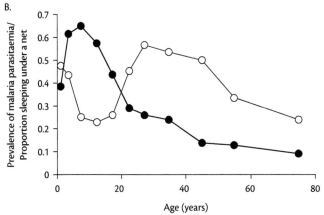

Figure 15.2 Age patterns in the prevalence of malaria parasitaemia (solid circles) and proportion reporting sleeping under a bed net the previous night (open circles) for females (A) and males (B) (Uganda). 0.6 refers to 60% of population sleeping under a net/60% of population have malaria parasitaemia.

Pullan, R. et al. Plasmodium infection and its risk factors in eastern Uganda. *Malaria Journal.* 9(2). https://doi.org/10.1186/1475-2875-9-2. Copyright © 2010 Pullan, R. et al; licensee BioMed Central Ltd.

be unsuitable to provide consent, and because of the lack of staff and HIV testing kits, indicating that PITC in children is not optimally practiced.

Questions

1. Why has HIV-related mortality increased when mortality from other infectious diseases is generally declining?

2. What specific barriers are adolescents likely to encounter in accessing prevention and treatment of infections?

3. What can be done on a public health level to reduce the incidence of infectious diseases in the adolescent age group?

Key publications

Das J, Salam, R, Arshad A, et al. (2016) Systematic review and meta-analysis of interventions to improve access and coverage of adolescent immunizations. *J Adolesc Health,* Suppl 9: S40–48.

Discusses coverage and impact of vaccines and how to improve vaccine coverage in adolescents

Global Burden of Disease Pediatrics Collaboration (2013). Global and national burden of diseases and injuries among children and adolescents between 1990 and 2013: findings From the Global Burden of Disease 2013 Study. *JAMA Pediatrics* 170: 267–87.

Reports leading causes of and trends in mortality among adolescents globally and demonstrates that infection remains a leading cause of death in this age group

Mavedzenge S, Luecke E, and Ross D (2014). Effective approaches for programming to reduce adolescent vulnerability to HIV infection, HIV risk, and HIV-related morbidity and mortality: a systematic review of systematic reviews. *J Acquir Immune Defic Syndr* 66(Suppl 2): S154–69.

A comprehensive review of the programmatic strategies to reduce the risk of HIV infection in adolescents and the risk of morbidity and mortality among adolescents living with HIV.

World Health Organization (2013). *World Health Organization Informal Consultation on Fever Management in Peripheral Health Care Settings: a Global Review of Evidence and Practice.* WHO: Geneva.

Provides an understanding of how infection is managed in peripheral health facilities globally.

Bibliography

Bernays S, Jarrett P, Kranzer K, and Ferrand R (2014). Children growing up with HIV infection: the responsibility of success. *Lancet* 383: 1355–7.

Butterworth A, Dalton P, Dunne D, et al. (1984). Immunity after treatment of human schistosomiasis mansoni. I. Study design, pretreatment observations and the results of treatment. *Trans R Soc Trop Med Hyg* 78: 108–23.

Chandiwana S and Woolhouse M (1991). Heterogeneities in water contact patterns and the epidemiology of Schistosoma haematobium. *Parasitology* 103(Pt 3): 363–70.

Garner P and Gulmezoglu A (2006). Drugs for preventing malaria in pregnant women. *Cochrane Database Systematic Reviews* CD000169.

Gore F, Bloem P, Patton G, et al. (2011). Global burden of disease in young people aged 10–24 years: a systematic analysis. *Lancet* 377: 2093–102.

Granja A, Machungo F, Gomes A, and Bergstrom S (2001). Adolescent maternal mortality in Mozambique. *J Adolesc Health* 28: 303–6.

Kappagoda S and Ioannidis J (2014). Prevention and control of neglected tropical diseases: overview of randomized trials, systematic reviews and meta-analyses. *Bull World Health Organ* 92: 356–366C.

Kranzer K, Meghji J, Bandason T, et al. (2014). Barriers to provider-initiated testing and counselling for children in a high HIV prevalence setting: a mixed methods study. *PLoS Med* 11: e1001649.

Lowenthal E, Bakeera-Kitaka S, Marukutira T, Chapman J, Goldrath K, and Ferrand R (2014). Perinatally acquired HIV infection in adolescents from sub-Saharan Africa: a review of emerging challenges. *Lancet Infect Dis* 14: 627–39.

Pasha O, Del Rosso J, Mukaka M, and Marsh D (2003). The effect of providing fansidar (sulfadoxine-pyrimethamine) in schools on mortality in school-age children in Malawi. *Lancet* 361: 577–8.

Pullan R, Bukirwa H, Staedke S, Snow, R, and Brooker S (2010). Plasmodium infection and its risk factors in eastern Uganda. *Malar J* 9: 2.

World Health Organization (2007). *Global Plan to Combat Neglected Tropical Diseases 2008–2015.* WHO: Geneva.

World Health Organization (2014). *Health for the World's Adolescents: a Second Chance in the Second Decade.* WHO: Geneva.

CHAPTER 16

Adolescent injuries

Qingfeng Li and Adnan A Hyder

This chapter focuses on unintentional injuries in the 10–19-years-old age group, with brief mention of intentional injuries. Information specific to injuries among younger children is included in Chapter 41.

Key points

♦ Injuries are the leading cause of death and disability in children 10–19 years old, accounting for 37% of all deaths in this age group.

♦ Road traffic crashes, drowning, and burns are the most common types of unintentional injuries; these three main causes respectively account for 46%, 20%, and 7% of all deaths caused by unintentional injuries.

♦ Low- and middle-income countries (LMICs) bear a burden of injuries disproportional to their population, vehicle possession, and economic activities.

Background

An injury can be characterised as either intentional or unintentional. According the *International Classification of Disease* tenth edition (ICD-10), unintentional injuries include road injuries, drowning, falls, fire/burns, poisoning, suffocation, bites, and natural disasters. Intentional injuries include self-harm, interpersonal violence, and collective violence. Self-harm is a common type of intentional injury, but its actual burden is poorly understood due to the sensitivity of suicides globally and the illegality of suicide in some countries. According to the World Health Organization (WHO), quality vital registration data on suicide are only available in sixty WHO member states because suicide registration requires a complicated, multi-sectoral effort that includes both medical and legal concerns.

Injuries have been traditionally known as 'accidents', suggesting they are random or even unavoidable events. Studies and interventions in recent decades dramatically improved our understanding of the nature, mechanism, and determinants of injuries. Abundant evidence from a variety of settings has proven that injuries are not 'accidents', but predictable and preventable events. Consequently, many in the field now use the term injury exclusively in preference to the term accident.

Adolescents have a growing curiosity and wish to experiment; however, this is not always matched by their capacity to understand or respond to danger. Consequently, they face elevated risk for all types of injuries. They may also fall victim to intentional injuries, such as sexual assaults, neglect, abandonment, other maltreatment, and collective violence.

In 2013, about 350,000 children 10–19 years of age died due to injuries, around the world. As shown in Figure 16.1, 72% of these deaths were unintentional. Road traffic injuries caused 33% (115,065) of these deaths; drowning was ranked second and other major causes included fire, falls, and poisoning.

The incidence of fatal injuries varies greatly across regions, (Figure 16.2). Latin America and the Caribbean (LAC) have the highest injury death rate, followed by South Asia; their injury death rate is more than twice that in high-income countries. This may be due to the inverted U-shaped relationship between road traffic deaths and economic development. Previous studies have found this relationship in many countries and proposed a few explanations, such as competing risks, vehicle mix, externalities (i.e. unintended and uncompensated effects of policies), and medical technology. For example, LAC tends to be economically more developed than sub-Saharan African, but it has not reached the turning point for reversing the trend. The huge disparity between countries indicates opportunities for high-risk regions and countries to catch up by learning from best practices in the better performing countries.

Child injury is related to poverty; poor children tend to live in unsafe environments and consequently face heightened risk of injuries. Their limited access to resources to overcome these risks and lack of access to affordable medical treatment after injuries occur, make them particularly vulnerable. Such economic disparity is true not only between poor and rich countries but also between poor and rich households within a country. For example, according to the Global Status Report on Road Safety 2015, LMICs account for 54% of the world's registered vehicles and 82% of the world's population, but have 90% of the world's road traffic deaths. Vulnerable road users (e.g. pedestrians, cyclists, and motorcyclists) make up more than half of these fatalities. In fact, in most countries, children in rural areas experience a higher risk for road traffic injuries, pesticide poisoning, and drowning than their urban counterparts.

Death, although the most notable, is not the only outcome of injury. A report from five countries in South and East Asia showed that for each death among children under eighteen years old, there were twelve hospitalised or permanently disabled children and thirty-four children who needed medical treatment or missed school or work because of an injury. Non-fatal injuries may cause severe disability and long-term need for medical treatment, which also leads to tremendous loss of economic productivity. For any injury intervention policy and programme, the design and evaluation plans should always consider both fatal and non-fatal injuries.

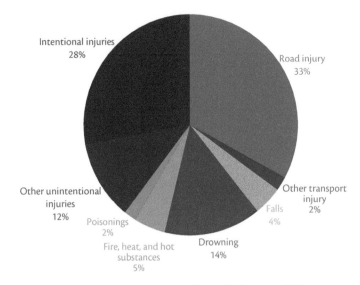

Figure 16.1 Global distribution of causes of injury deaths among children 10–19 years of age in 2013.

Source: data from Institute for Health Metrics and Evaluation. *GBD 2013: Global Burden of Diseases, Injuries, and Risk Factors Study Protocol.* Copyright © 2013 University of Washington.

Targets

Sustainable Development Goals (SDGs) (2015)

Goal 3 (Health)

♦ By 2020, halve the number of global deaths and injuries from road traffic injuries.

Interventions

Several effective and cost-effective interventions are available to prevent child injuries. This chapter takes a matrix approach to introduce a wide range of prevention strategies for child injury in relation to each cause of injury. The first axis is by type of prevention on a time scale:

♦ Primary prevention: preventing incidence of new injuries.

♦ Secondary prevention: reducing the severity of injuries once they have occurred.

♦ Tertiary prevention: decreasing the frequency and severity of disability after an injury.

The second axis is by location of the injury event:

♦ Home environment.

♦ Schools and playgrounds.

♦ Communities including roads.

Evidence-based and well-enforced legislation is a highly effective tool in preventing injuries. Disaggregated by type of environment, these interventions include roads (child restraints, seatbelts, bicycle/motorcycle helmets), homes (smoke alarm, child-resistant containers), and leisure environment (isolation of swimming pools). However, despite the widely available evidence, passing and enforcing legislation is still difficult in many countries. More evidence for the immediate and long-term health and economic benefits of injury prevention programmes is urgently needed to convince policymakers to take action, especially in LMICs. Rigorous studies and innovative approaches to conveying preventive messages to the public is also key to confronting the burden of injuries.

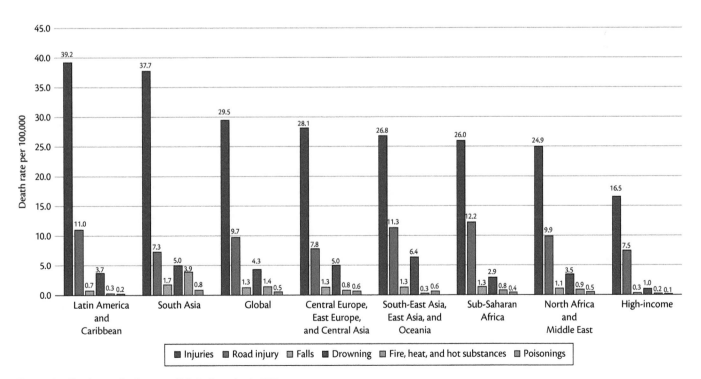

Figure 16.2 Death rate of major type of injuries by region in 2013.

Source: data from Institute for Health Metrics and Evaluation. *GBD 2013: Global Burden of Diseases, Injuries, and Risk Factors Study Protocol.* Copyright © 2013 University of Washington.

Table 16.1 Intervention approaches to prevent child injuries

Key approaches	Traffic	Drowning	Burns	Falls	Poisoning
Legislation, regulation and enforcement	Speed limits; comprehensive drink-driving laws; child restraints	Four-sided pool fencing	Hot water tap temperature legislation; smoke alarms	Playground equipment standards	Manufacture, storage and distribution of harmful substances requiring safe packaging
Product modification	Vehicle-front modification; child restraint system	Person floatation devices	Non-tip lanterns and candle holders	Baby walker modification; safety glass	Medication packaging; child restraint closures
Environmental modification	Child friendly infrastructure; safer routes to school; safer play spaces	Barriers, such as well covering and fencing	Separation of cooking area from living area	Window guards on tall buildings; non-climbable banisters	Safe storage of potentially harmful substances
Education and skills development	Helmet wearing; using child restraints	Swimming training and supervision	First aid, cool the burn	Supportive home visitation to identify fall hazards	Immediate first aid
Emergency medical care	Child-sized equipment; child-friendly environment	Immediate resuscitation	Burns centres	Appropriate paediatric acute care	Poison control centres

Source: data from Peden, M. et al (eds). World Report on Child Injury Prevention 2008. Geneva, Switzerland: World Health Organization. Copyright © 2008 World Health Organization.

Unlike communicable and vaccine-preventable diseases, injuries require a multi-sectoral approach. For example, road traffic injuries require actions from police, transportation, education, vehicle manufacturers, and infrastructure sectors; and drowning requires actions from water, education, and environment sectors (Table 16.1). The health sector needs to play a key role in advocating for actions across governmental agencies. Additionally, the health sector has to incorporate the prevention and treatment of injuries and support of community-based interventions, and pay particular attention to targeting socioeconomic disparities. Innovative theories, such as systems science (e.g. using computer simulation to study the dynamics of a transportation system), could be used to plan and monitor such interventions.

Challenges

A major challenge is the lack of quality data to support evidence-based intervention design, particularly in LMICs where most child injuries occur. Despite the progress in collecting data around the world, the availability and quality of data on incidence and consequences of injuries vary greatly between countries. Even in developed countries, where surveillance systems are relatively complete, important information is often missing for injuries, such as location, intent, circumstances, treatment, and outcome.

Future priorities

◆ In sharp contrast to the heavy burden of injuries, very few studies have estimated the economic cost of injuries, particularly the costs caused by the long-term or even permanent need for health care and loss of productivity. This cost information is critically important for evaluation and prioritisation of injury prevention strategies.

◆ Injury interventions are mostly based on evidence collected in high-income countries, therefore, large-scale and rigorous evaluations of interventions are urgently needed in LMICs.

◆ In recognition of the multi-sectoral approach for injury, a system-based framework is needed to scientifically address the problem. Given the complexity of these factors and interacting relationship, a classical linear approach may not be sufficient or effective in investigating and eliminating the burden of injuries.

Conclusions

Injures cause high mortality and morbidity among children, yet are nearly entirely preventable. Evidence-based interventions are available to prevent common causes of injuries, including road traffic injuries, drowning, and burns. Therefore, any comprehensive approach to child health and development must include injury prevention, especially in LMICs.

Case study: implementing graduated driver's licences reduces crashes amongst 16-year-olds by 23%

Rapid increase in motorisation is occurring all around the world and comes at the cost of increasing risk for traffic collisions. Young and novice drivers especially lack experience and skills in driving and in recognising possible dangers and dealing with unexpected situations.

To protect young drivers and other road users, a few high-income countries, such as New Zealand and the US, developed Graduated Driver Licensing (GDL). Generally, the programme divides obtaining a driver licence into three steps. The applicant first enters an extended period as a learner driver, to increase the amount of supervised driving experience. Then the applicant is given a provisional or intermediate licence that requires temporary provisions, restrictions on unsupervised driving, late-night driving, and driving with young passengers. Finally, a full licence is issued upon successful completion of the first two steps. A typical GDL scheme covers areas such as speed, seatbelt use, alcohol restrictions, passenger restrictions, and mobile phone use.

Studies from the US found GDL programme led to a 23% reduction in crashes over a decade among 16-year-olds. Similar programmes in other places are also shown to be effective in reducing crashes and fatalities, though the exact estimate of effectiveness varies due to differences in the programmes, drivers' age, and evaluation methodology.

Questions

1. Why is it misleading to refer to injuries as 'accidents'?

2. Why are children from LMICs and from poor households in high-income countries exposed to an elevated risk for injuries?

3. What are the evidence-based interventions to prevent childhood drowning?

Key publications

World Health Organization (2008). *World Report on Child Injury Prevention*. WHO: Geneva.
The joint effort of the WHO and UNICEF brings together all knowledges available about the five major types of child injuries (road traffic injuries, drowning, burns, falls, and poisonings), their risk factors, and proven prevention strategies.

World Health Organization (2015). *Global Status Report on Road Safety*. WHO: Geneva.
Based on inputs from 180 countries, this report is the most updated and comprehensive source of global, regional, and country-level road crash data and measures of the 'Decade of Action for Global Road Safety 2011–2020'.

World Health Organization (2014). *Global Report on Drowning: Preventing a Leading Killer*. WHO: Geneva.
The WHO's first global report dedicated exclusively to drowning systemically presents the global burden, risk factors, and prevention strategies.

Li Q, Alonge O, and Hyder AA (2016). 'Children and road traffic injuries: can't the world do better?' *Arch Dis Child* 101(11): 1063–1070.
Based on a triangulation of multiple data sources and an extensive literature review, this study provides an updated assessment of the burden of child injuries and a strategic roadmap to improve road safety for children.

Hyder AA, Sugerman D, Puvanachandra P, et al. (2009). Global childhood unintentional injury surveillance in four cities in developing countries: a pilot study. *Bull World Health Organ* 87(5): 345–52.

One of the first multi-country, emergency department-based injury surveillance systems for children in the developing world. This study illustrates the feasibility of documenting the burden of childhood injuries on health systems in LMICs and undertaking standardised child injury surveillance.

Bibliography

Alonge O and Hyder AA (2014). Reducing the global burden of childhood unintentional injuries. *Arch Dis Child* 99(1): 62–9.

Alonge O, Khan U, and Hyder AA (2016). Our shrinking globe: implications for child unintentional injuries. *Pediatric Clinics North Am* 63(1): 167–81.

Arbogast K, Durbin D, Cornejo R, Kallan M, and Winston F (2004). An evaluation of the effectiveness of forward facing child restraint systems. *Accident Analysis and Prevention* 36(4): 585–9.

Bartlett S (2002). The problem of children's injuries in low-income countries: a review. *Health Policy Plan* 17(1): 1–13.

Bishai D, Quresh A, James P, and Ghaffar A (2006). National road casualties and economic development. *Health Econ* 15(1): 65–81.

Brussoni M, Brunelle S, Pike I, et al. (2015). Can child injury prevention include healthy risk promotion? *Injury Prevention* 21(5): 344–7.

Haddon W Jr (1980). Advances in the epidemiology of injuries as a basis for public policy. *Public Health Rep* 95(5): 411–21.

Harvey A, Towner E, Peden M, Soori H, and Bartolomeos K (2009). Injury prevention and the attainment of child and adolescent health. *Bull World Health Organ* 87(5): 390–4.

He S, Lunnen J, Puvanachandra P, Amar S, Zia N, and Hyder AA (2014). Global childhood unintentional injury study: multisite surveillance data. *Am J Public Health* 104(3): e79–84.

Hyder AA, Alonge O, He S, et al. (2014). Saving of children's lives from drowning project in Bangladesh. *Am J Prev Med* 47(6): 842–5.

Hyder AA, Tran N, Bachani A, Bishai D, and Peden M (2012). Saving 1000 children a day: the potential of child and adolescent injury prevention. *International Journal of Child and Adolescent Health* 5(3): 267.

Langley J, Wagenaar A, and Begg D (1996). An evaluation of the New Zealand graduated driver licensing system. *Accid Anal Prev* 28(2): 139–46.

Miller T, Romano E, and Spicer R (2000). The cost of childhood unintentional injuries and the value of prevention. *Future Child* 10(1): 137–63.

Runyan C (2003). Introduction: back to the future—revisiting Haddon's conceptualization of injury epidemiology and prevention. *Epidemiol Rev* 25: 60–64.

United Nations Children's Fund (2011). *The State of the World's Children 2011—Executive Summary: Adolescence an Age of Opportunity*. UNICEF: New York, US.

CHAPTER 17

Strategies to improve adolescent health

Samantha Sadoo and David A Ross

This chapter discusses key priorities and strategies to improve adolescent health and wellbeing worldwide. We will take a broad view, looking at the various ecological levels that influence adolescent development, as well as ongoing challenges.

Key points

- Adolescents have previously been neglected on the global health agenda. Recent progress has been made with the inclusion of adolescents in the World Health Organization (WHO) *Global Strategy for Women's, Children's, and Adolescents' Health* (2016–2030), and the establishment of the Lancet Standing Commission on Adolescent Health and Wellbeing.

- Investing in adolescent programmes yields a triple return; improving the health and wellbeing of the adolescent, of their future selves as adults, and then of their children.

- The most powerful actions for adolescent health and wellbeing are intersectoral, multi-level, and multi-component.

- Adolescents must be engaged with and involved in developing and implementing programmes that respond to their particular health-related needs in order to maximise the likelihood of success.

Background

Only recently has adolescence been recognised as a key time period within the lifecourse, requiring targeted interventions in order to achieve goals for women's, children's, and adolescents' health, among others. Investment in the health of adolescents has the potential to provide a triple return through improving the health of the adolescent, their future selves as adults, and then of their children. The importance of adolescent health on the global agenda was highlighted by the explicit inclusion of adolescent health within the WHO *Global Strategy for Women's, Children's and Adolescents' Health (2016–2030)*. The Global Accelerated Action for the Health of Adolescents (AA-HA!) guidance supports implementation of the Global Strategy by providing technical guidance for countries as they decide what needs to be done to improve the health of adolescents, and how to do it.

Interventions

Figure 17.1 provides a summary of key evidence-based interventions related to prevention or treatment of specific adolescent diseases, as set out in the AA-HA! guidance. It is also important to keep in mind the continuum of care across the lifecourse when considering interventions to improve adolescent health; improving the health of women before and during pregnancy will improve the health of newborns, leading to better health status of children, and therefore of adolescents (Figure 17.2).

As the main determinants of adolescent health are outside the specific remit of the health sector, interventions must be delivered by multiple sectors, including education, social protection, roads and infrastructure, and employment, and be targeted more widely at various levels of influence. These include the individual and family, community, school, media and technology, environment, and legal and policy frameworks. Each of these levels acts as an important platform for action against major causes of morbidity and mortality, including smoking and alcohol, road traffic injury, violence, obesity, and sexual and reproductive health. Taking a comprehensive and intersectoral approach requires coordination between all levels of health care, the public and private sectors, governments, professional associations, development partners, donors, civil society, and adolescents themselves.

Individuals, families, and communities

Adolescent participation in the design, implementation, monitoring, and evaluation of programmes has multiple benefits; it allows policymakers to understand their needs and offer more effective solutions, as well as encouraging adolescents to engage with services, and it empowers them by enhancing their confidence, and social and leadership skills. Working with families and communities is important due to their potential positive influence on the behaviours and values of adolescents. Parents should be supported to promote stable and positive relationships with their children, for example encouraging them to spend time with their adolescent in enjoyable activities, enabling them to anticipate life changes such as puberty, and to provide support for regular sleep, a healthy diet, and physical activity. Community interventions such as encouraging sporting activities for girls can improve physical health, fitness, and social skills, as well as empowering girls through challenging traditional gender norms.

School

School is a key setting for interventions as it provides the opportunity for intensive long-term, large-scale programmes to be implemented, alongside the fact that education itself is a major determinant of health and wellbeing across the lifecourse. Providing

Positive development	Unintentional injury	Violence	Sexual and reproductive health, including HIV
• Adolescent-friendly health services • Health-promoting schools • Improving hygiene and nutrition • Child online protection • e-health and m-health interventions for health education and the involvement of adolescents in their own care • Parenting interventions • Adolescent participation and interventions to promote competence, confidence, connection, character, and caring	• Laws on drinking age, blood alcohol concentration, seat-belt, and helmet wearing, graduated driver licencing • Traffic calming and safety measures • Pre-hospital and hospital care • Community campaigns and individual interventions to promote behavioural change related to safe driving and good laws to encourage behavioural change • Population, community-based and individual level drowning prevention measures • Assessment and management of adolescents who present with unintentional injury, including alcohol-related injury • Infrastructure design and improvement • Vehicle safety standards	• INSPIRE strategies to preventing and responding to all forms of violence against children and adolescents: • Implementation and enforcement of laws: banning violent punishment, criminalising sexual abuse, and exploitation of children, prevent alcohol misuse, limit youth access to firearms and other weapons • Norms and values: changing adherence to restrictive and harmful gender and social norms, community mobilisation programmes, bystander interventions • Safe environments: addressing 'hotspots', interrupting the spread of violence, improving the built environment • Parent and caregiver support through home visits, community approaches, and comprehensive programmes • Income and economic strengthening: cash transfers, group saving and loans, microfinance • Response and support services: screening and interventions, counselling and therapeutic approaches, programmes for juvenile offenders, foster care interventions • Education and life skills: increasing school enrolment, safe and enabling school environment, life and social skills training	• Comprehensive sexuality education • Information, counselling, and services for comprehensive sexual and reproductive health, including contraception • Prevention of, and response to, harmful practices, such as female genital mutilation and early and forced marriage • Preconception, antenatal, birth, postnatal, abortion (where legal), and post-abortion care, as relevant to adolescents • Prevention, detection, and treatment of sexually transmitted and reproductive tract infections, including HIV and syphilis • Voluntary medical male circumcision (VMMC) in countries with generalised HIV epidemics • Comprehensive care of children (including adolescents) living with, or exposed to HIV

Communicable diseases	Noncommunicable diseases, nutrition and physical activity	Mental health, substance abuse and self-harm	Conditions with particularly high priority in humanitarian and fragile settings
• Prevention, detection, and treatment of communicable diseases, including tuberculosis • Routine vaccinations, e.g. human papillomavirus, hepatitis B, diphtheria-tetanus, rubella, measles • Prevention and management of childhood illness, including malaria, pneumonia, meningitis, and diarrhoea • Case management of meningitis	• Structural, environmental, organisational, community, interpersonal, and individual level interventions to promote healthy behaviour (e.g. nutrition; physical activity; no tobacco, alcohol, or drugs) • Prevention, detection, and treatment of noncommunicable diseases • Prevention, detection, and management of anaemia, especially for adolescent girls; iron supplementation where appropriate • Treatment and rehabilitation of children with congenital abnormalities and disabilities	• Care for children with developmental delays • Responsive caregiving and stimulation • Psychosocial support and related services for adolescent mental health and wellbeing • Parent skills training, as appropriate, for managing behavioural disorders in adolescents • Structural environment, organisational, community, interpersonal, and individual level interventions to prevent substance abuse • Detection and management of hazardous and harmful substance use • Structural, environmental, organisational, community, interpersonal, and individual level interventions to prevent adolescent suicide • Management of self-harm and suicide risks	• Assess conditions and ensure adequate nutrition for adolescent population groups according to age, gender, weight, physical activity levels, and other key factors • Ensure core health services to support adolescents with disabilities in an emergency • Medical screening of former child soldiers, and clinical management and community-based psychosocial support for survivors of sexual and/or gender-based violence • Implement a minimal initial sexual and reproductive health service package • Ensure safe access to and use and maintenance of toilets; materials and facilities for menstrual hygiene management and other interventions to improve water, sanitation, and hygiene • Promote mental health through recreational activities for adolescents, formal or informal education, and involvement in concrete, purposeful activities • Provide psychological first aid and first-line management of adolescent mental, neurological and substance-use conditions

Figure 17.1 Key evidence-based interventions related to prevention or treatment of specific adolescent diseases.
Reproduced with permission from the WHO, UNAIDS, UNESCO, UNFPA, UNICEF, UN Women, World Bank, PMNCH, EWEC. 2017. *Global accelerated action for the health of adolescents (AA-HA!): guidance to support country implementation. Summary.* Geneva: World Health Organization. Copyright © 2017 World Health Organization.

access to free, good-quality secondary education for adolescents, particularly for girls in low- and middle-income countries (LMICs), can yield some of the greatest returns on investment for their wellbeing. National school health programmes should be established and all schools should be 'health promoting'. Health-promoting schools have the capability to promote healthy behaviours and lifestyles, mental health, sexual and reproductive health, enhance cognitive abilities, reduce the risk of non-communicable diseases (NCDs) in later life, and increase productivity in the future workforce. Good nutrition can be encouraged by providing healthy meals, snacks, and drinks, and healthy dietary advice.

Reducing barriers to school attendance is vital. The United Nations Educational, Scientific and Cultural Organisation (UNESCO) has referred to menstruation as one of the biggest barriers to school attendance and performance; appropriate materials for menstrual hygiene should be accessible to all girls, as well as suitable water and sanitation facilities. Cost is a significant barrier, not just the direct cost of education but also the indirect cost to families due to the loss of adolescent labour, particularly in rural areas. Conditional and unconditional cash transfers, scholarships, free education or school fee reduction, free uniforms, equipment, and meals can be beneficial. Early marriage and pregnancy account for

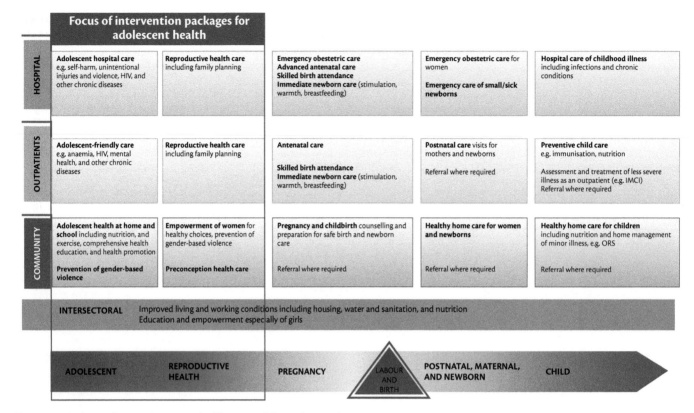

Figure 17.2 Packages of interventions across the lifecourse and the continuum of care.

higher dropout rates of girls in many LMICs; strategies to address this include programmes to change social norms, comprehensive sexuality education and providing access to contraception. There are significant equity gaps that need addressing; disadvantaged groups include girls, those affected by armed conflict, those who speak a different language at home to that in school, and students with disabilities. There is also a need for flexible learning schemes for those who are not able to stay in mainstream education, such as child labourers or married adolescents.

Health services

Adolescents have different health care needs to adults and younger children; however, only recently have programmes been specifically targeted to this age group to try to meet their unique needs. Demand barriers include a lack of knowledge about how to access care, and greater concern about confidentiality. Healthcare providers should be trained to provide adolescent-friendly services, responding to the needs of adolescents in a non-judgemental way that fosters engagement with the individual and the community. In particular, sexual and reproductive health services must be acceptable and confidential; usage is low in many settings and this is often at least partly due to a lack of respect for adolescents from health workers. Integrating the delivery of services can improve efficiency and access to care, for example using the HEADSS assessment opportunistically (Home, Education, Activities/employment, Drugs, Suicidality, Sex), at any contact with the health system and providing advice and implementing preventive interventions alongside management of the initial presentation.

Environment

Interventions targeted at the environment can have a significant impact on adolescent health and wellbeing. Targeting the physical environment includes improving water and sanitation facilities which can particularly benefit menstruating girls, promoting road-safety measures particularly around schools or other places where adolescents gather, and supporting access to safe fuel and safe cooking stoves within homes.

Media and technology

Advances in technology and media are transforming adolescents' social environments and networks and have the potential to substantially benefit multiple areas affecting their development, including education and health care. Mobile phones are now accessible to the majority of young people, even in LMICs. Educational materials can increase individual knowledge, careseeking behaviours, and in some countries has changed social norms around challenging issues such as domestic violence and human immunodeficiency virus and acquired immune deficiency syndrome (HIV/AIDS). Adolescents can be empowered and autonomy encouraged, independently of their parents and peers. Social media can be harnessed to reach and engage more marginalised groups. Interventions can be delivered through a range of technologies including the Internet, video games, text messages, radio, and mobile phone apps. However, there is also an increased risk of harm, such as the promotion of unhealthy lifestyles and commodities through mass media, which can negatively affect health, and online safety concerns, including cyberbullying. A national strategy for online child protection is necessary, including reporting mechanisms, education, resources for awareness generation, and legislation. More evidence is required regarding effective strategies that utilise technology and media.

Policy and legal frameworks

Policies and laws can affect adolescent wellbeing in multiple ways; they can protect adolescents from harm (such as preventing child marriage, or placing health warnings and taxation on harmful commodities such as tobacco), and they can promote health (such as increasing access to contraception, providing incentives to attend school). Supporting social protection strategies is paramount, for example regarding adolescent victims who may need temporary protection and care. Legal frameworks relating to adolescent health vary significantly between countries, and in many settings customary or religious laws take precedence. In order for changes in laws to impact adolescents positively, cooperation of the police and judiciary system is required in supporting their implementation.

Challenges

Strategies must focus on addressing inequalities, specifically targeting socially and economically marginalised adolescents who often have the greatest health needs; these include ethnic minorities, refugees, young offenders, those with disabilities, or who are homeless. Increased efforts to engage and understand their needs are required. The WHO's Innov8 approach provides guidance on upholding rights and equity in programmes, including adolescent health programming.

Non-communicable diseases are increasingly of importance everywhere and among all social strata; addressing risk factors will require significant investment in health systems, coordination across sectors, and innovative approaches to prevention.

Programmes need to be better evaluated in order to assess outcomes and monitor progress towards the Sustainable Development Goals (SDGs). The Global Strategy for Women's, Children's, and Adolescents' Health (2016–2030) proposes sixty indicators, of which forty-three are either adolescent-specific, such as the adolescent mortality rate, or are relevant to adolescents, such as measures of sexual violence. At least the sixteen key indicators should be monitored (of which twelve are relevant to adolescents) in order to ensure effectiveness and sustainability of programmes.

Future priorities

◆ Research is needed to strengthen the evidence base for adolescent-specific interventions. However, contrary to popular belief, many interventions do have evidence, are recommended by the WHO, and are ready for implementation now.

Conclusions

The needs of adolescents have been overlooked in the global agenda until recently. As a result, there are gaps in our understanding of their health requirements, in the evidence base for strategies, in civil society structures for advocacy, and in systems for intersectoral action. Government leadership is vital, as is the participation of adolescents themselves. With improved child health and nutrition, access to education, delays in marriage and pregnancy, and the emergence of new technologies and social media, we have an unprecedented opportunity to greatly impact the health and wellbeing of adolescents worldwide.

Case study: the AA-HA! guidance to support country implementation: creating an international reference document to improve adolescent health

The AA-HA! guidance is a landmark document. It was published in 2017 in response to the 'coming of age' of adolescent health on the global health agenda. It has been designed as a reference document to support country implementation, with detailed guidance on planning, implementation, monitoring, and the evaluation of programmes. It is targeted at policymakers, healthcare professionals, researchers, donors, and governments, and aims to assist countries in translating the Global Strategy for women's, Children's and Adolescents' Health (2016-2030) into action for adolescents.

This document also contributes to a paradigm shift in how adolescent health is regarded:

1. It views adolescents as potentially powerful and autonomous assets to society, and shows how this potential can be harnessed through their engagement and participation in strategies. The development of the guidance itself included important contributions from adolescents and young adults themselves.

2. It highlights the significant potential triple return from investing in adolescent health. Historically, adolescent health programmes have had to look for 'entry points' such as the opportunities created by HIV-prevention programmes. This guidance argues that the evidence is strong enough to argue that adolescent health should be included in all policies and programmes, and in a variety of sectors including education, urban planning, and the criminal justice system.

3. It recognises that adolescents in humanitarian and fragile settings are particularly vulnerable, and has specific guidance for targeting this subpopulation. They will usually be harder to reach, and at greater risk of physical and mental health problems, and violence, than in more stable settings.

4. It celebrates what is already being done with regards to adolescent health programmes worldwide, with over 75 case studies demonstrating success in implementation in a variety of settings and sectors.

This case study demonstrates how even though strategies have to be selected to be appropriate to the local context, an international guidance document can help countries to prioritise and can support their implementation of evidence-based adolescent health interventions.

Questions

1. Why should adolescents be targeted specifically within national health programmes?

2. What sectors are important in influencing adolescent health, other than the health sector?

3. What is the AA-HA! guidance and how can it be used to support transformation of adolescent health care globally?

Key publications

WHO, UNAIDS, UNESCO, UNFPA, UNICEF, UN Women, World Bank, PMNCH, EWEC (2017). *Global Accelerated Action for the Health of Adolescents (AA-HA!): Guidance to Support Country Implementation.* World Health Organization: Geneva.
Recent publication outlining a strategy on how to improve adolescent health on a country level.

Patton G, Sawyer S, Santelli J, et al. (2016). Our future: a Lancet commission on adolescent health and wellbeing. *Lancet* 387: 2423–78.
Comprehensive narrative and plan to improve global adolescent health.

Bibliography

Crone E and Dahl R (2012). Understanding adolescence as a period of social-affective engagement and goal flexibility. *Nat Rev Neuroscience* 13(9): 636–50.

Dick B and Ferguson B (2015). Health for the world's adolescents: a second chance in the second decade. *J Adolesc Health* 56: 3–6.

Sawyer S, Afifi R, Bearinger L, et al. (2012). Adolescence: a foundation for future health. *Lancet* 379: 1630–40.

Viner R, Ozer E, Denny S, et al. (2012). Adolescence and the social determinants of health. *Lancet* 379: 1641–52.

United Nations Children's Fund (2011). *State of the World's Children—Adolescence: an Age of Opportunity.* http://www.unicef.org/sowc2011/pdfs/SOWC-2011-Main-Report_EN_02092011.pdf

World Bank (2007). *World Development Report 2007: Development and the Next Generation.* World Bank: Washington, DC.

World Health Organization (2015). *The Global Strategy for Women's, Children's, and Adolescents' Health (2016–2030). Every Woman, Every Child.* http://www.who.int/life-course/publications/global-strategy-2016-2030/en/

SECTION 5

Women's reproductive and maternal health

CHAPTER 18

Introduction to maternal and reproductive health

Martha Kamanga, Jennifer Hall, and Address Malata

This chapter focuses on the public health importance of maternal health, from preconception, through pregnancy, childbirth, and the postnatal period.

Key points

- Every day, approximately 830 women die from preventable causes related to pregnancy and childbirth.

- Improving maternal and newborn health remains an important priority and a basic human right. There is a strong link between maternal, newborn, and child health.

- A woman's chance of dying or becoming disabled during pregnancy and childbirth is closely connected to her social and economic status, the norms and values of her culture, and the geographic remoteness of her home.

- Women value good communication, high-quality information, having a sense of control, and the ability to participate in their care and make choices. Optimising women's health before and between pregnancies is an ongoing process that requires access to and the full participation of the healthcare system, as well as supportive policies across the broader determinants of health.

Background

Pregnancy and childbirth have a huge impact on the physical, mental, emotional, and socioeconomic health of women and their families. Physical and psychological problems are common, and may have a significant negative and long-term impact on women's wellbeing and daily functioning. 'Safe motherhood' aims to ensure that all women receive the care they need to be safe and healthy before, during, and after pregnancy and childbirth.

Safe motherhood begins before conception with good nutrition, a healthy weight and lifestyle, and the planning of pregnancy. It continues with appropriate antenatal care, preventing problems before they arise. The ideal result is a full-term pregnancy without unnecessary interventions, giving birth to a healthy baby, and experiencing a healthy postnatal period in a positive environment that supports the physical and emotional needs of the mother, baby, and family.

While motherhood offers a rewarding experience, for too many women it is associated with suffering, ill health, and even death. Many women, including adolescents, die from preventable causes related to pregnancy and childbirth. The poorer and more marginalised a woman is, the greater her risk of death. High maternal mortality ratios reflect disparities between wealthy and poor countries more than any other measure of health and are a marker of the state of health services. Despite women living longer than men, their lives are not necessarily healthy. Women's ill health and its consequences are poorly defined.

In many societies, women and girls are disadvantaged by discrimination rooted in sociocultural and structural factors including:

- Unequal power relationships between men and women.

- Social norms, such as early marriage or restricted mobility, that decrease education and paid employment opportunities.

- Lack of equal opportunities to realise rights recognised by law, such as property or land ownership.

- Low value placed on women's education.

- An exclusive focus on women's reproductive roles.

- Potential or actual experience of physical, sexual, and emotional violence, including female genital mutilation and so-called 'honour' killings.

Policy history of maternal and reproductive health

The health of the mother during pregnancy and childbirth was not a focus for policymaking, research, and programming until 1985, when Alan Rosenfield and Deborah Maine published a provocative paper titled 'Maternal health—a neglected tragedy: Where is the M in MCH (maternal and child health)?' They argued that, while the global policy and programmatic focus on child health was essential and worthy, the health of the mother had been neglected in the implementation of women's, children's, and adolescents' health services. They called on the United Nations to prioritise maternity care to reduce maternal morbidity and mortality.

In 1987, the first international Safe Motherhood Conference convened in Kenya. The conference raised global awareness of the devastating maternal mortality rates in developing nations and formally established the Safe Motherhood Initiative. The goal was to reduce maternal mortality by 50% by the year 2000. Initially efforts focused on two strategies to reduce maternal mortality: increasing antenatal care and training for traditional birth attendants. By the year 2000, the goal was far from realised. The global community reaffirmed its commitment to maternal health in 2000, with Millennium Development Goal (MDG) 5 targeting a reduction of the maternal mortality ratio (MMR) of 75% by 2015. A separate target on reproductive health was not included until 2007. While significant progress was made, MDG 5 was also not met. Much more work needs to be done to sustain the gains made whilst pursuing the post-2015 Sustainable Development Goals (SDGs). As described in Chapter 1, many of the SDGs are relevant to maternal health, given their focus on the determinants of health such as poverty, nutrition, and education. The SDGs specifically linked to maternal health are listed below.

Global targets

Sustainable Development Goals (2015)

Goal 3 (Health)

◆ Ensure universal access to sexual and reproductive health (SRH) services, including family planning, information and education, and the integration of reproductive health into national strategies and programmes by 2030.

◆ By 2030, reduce the global maternal mortality ratio to less than 70 maternal deaths per 100,000 live births.

Goal 5 (Gender equality)

◆ Ensure universal access to SRH and reproductive rights as agreed in accordance with the plan of action of the International Conference on Population and Development (ICPD).

◆ End all forms of discrimination against women and girls everywhere.

◆ Eliminate all forms of violence against women and girls.

Maternal mortality: classification, trends, and distribution

Classification of maternal mortality

The WHO definition of a maternal death is the death of a woman while pregnant, or within 42 days of the termination of pregnancy, irrespective of the duration and site of the pregnancy, from any cause related to or aggravated by the pregnancy or its management but not from accidental or incidental causes. Maternal deaths are classified as direct or indirect. Direct causes are those related to obstetric complications of pregnancy, labour, delivery, and the postnatal period, such as haemorrhage or infection. Indirect causes are those relating to pre-existing medical conditions that may be aggravated by the physiologic demands of pregnancy, such as human immunodeficiency virus (HIV) infection, malaria, cardiovascular disease, mental illness, and diabetes. To date, indirect deaths have been overlooked in key policies and strategies, with the exception of HIV.

The Obstetric Transition Model (Table 18.1) is a proposed theoretical framework to examine the dynamic process of maternal mortality reduction. As countries pass through the obstetric transition, indirect deaths become more important. This model allows identification of a country's current obstetric stage, which in turn indicates which strategies a country can use to make further improvements, providing guidance to public health decision makers on implementation of appropriate, dynamic, and efficient programmes at the global, regional, and national levels.

Trends in maternal mortality

By 2015, the number of maternal deaths had fallen globally by almost half (44%) since 1990, from about 532,000 to an estimated 303,000 per year. This equates to an estimated global MMR of 216 maternal deaths per 100,000 live births, down from 385 in 1990 (Table 18.2). This improvement is thought to be due to increases in skilled attendance at delivery; globally, coverage of skilled attendants during childbirth increased from 62% in 2000 to 73% in 2013. Women in the richest quartile are almost three times as likely to deliver with a skilled health attendant as those in the poorest quartile, an inequity that has not changed in fifteen years.

Table 18.1 Stages of the obstetric transition

Stages of the obstetric transition	Fertility level	Causes of death	Access to services
Stage I Maternal mortality ratio > 1000 maternal deaths/100,000 live births	Very high	Direct causes, particularly communicable diseases, e.g. malaria	Majority do not receive professional obstetric care or have access to affordable and quality health facilities.
Stage II Maternal mortality ratio: 300–999 maternal deaths/100,000 live births	Very high	Similar to stage I	Increase in proportion seeking and receiving care in health units.
Stage III Maternal mortality ratio: 50–299 maternal death/100,000 live births	High (variable)	Direct causes still predominate, although indirect causes increase proportionately	Improving care, but with access issues remaining a problem for a large part of the population.
Stage IV MMR < 50 maternal deaths/100,000 live births	Low	Indirect causes of maternal mortality, in particular non-communicable diseases, gain increasing importance	Access to care improving further, but with a threat to quality and outcomes from over medicalisation of pregnancy in select cases.
Stage V All avoidable maternal deaths are actually prevented; maternal mortality ratio < 5 maternal deaths/100,000 live births	Low/very low	Indirect causes become predominant	Majority receive high quality obstetric care, with awareness of issues surrounding over medicalisation of pregnancy.

Source: data from Souza, JP. et al. Obstetric transition: the pathway towards ending preventable maternal deaths. BJOG: An International Journal of Obstetrics & Gynaecology. 121(s1), 1–4. Copyright © 2014 Wiley Online Library.

Table 18.2 Global and regional estimates of maternal mortality by MDG region

	Maternal mortality ratio				Number of maternal deaths		Lifetime risk of maternal death			
	1990 ratio (80%UI)	2015 ratio (80%UI)	% change 1990–2015	Average annual % change	1990	2015	1990	2015	Absolute change	Relative change
World	385 (359–427)	216 (207–249)	44	2.3 (1.7–2.7)	532,000	303,000	73	180	107	2.47
HICs	23 (22–25)	12 (11–14)	48	2.6 (2.1–3.0)	3500	1700	2400	4900	2500	2.04
LMICs	430	239	44	2.4	—	302,000	—	150	—	—
Sub-Saharan Africa	987 (898–1120)	546 (511–652)	45	2.4 (1.6–2.8)	223,000	201,000	16	36	20	2.25
Northern Africa	171 (145–204)	70 (56–92)	59	3.6 (2.4–4.5)	6400	3100	130	450	320	3.46
East Asia	95 (79–114)	27 (23–33)	72	5.0 (4.0–6.0)	26,000	4800	370	2300	1930	6.22
East Asia excluding China	51	43	16	0.7	—	—	—	—	—	—
South Asia	538 (457–641)	176 (153–216)	67	4.5 (3.5–5.2)	210,000	66,000	40	210	170	5.25
South-East Asia	320 (277–376)	110 (95–142)	66	4.3 (3.1–5.0)	39,000	13,000	87	380	93	2.07
West Asia	160 (132–199)	91 (73–125)	43	2.2 (0.8–3.4)	6700	4700	130	360	230	2.77
Caucasus and central Asia	69 (65–73)	33 (27–45)	52	3 (1.7–3.8)	1300	610	360	1100	740	3.06
Latin American and the Caribbean	135	60	50	2.8	14,000	6000	220	760	540	3.45
Oceania	391 (242–673)	187 (95–381)	52	3.0 (1.1–4.9)	780	500	54	150	96	2.78

Source: data from Graham, W. et al. Diversity and divergence: the dynamic burden of poor maternal health. *The Lancet*. 388(10056), 2164–2175. Copyright © 2016 Elsevier. All rights reserved.

Distribution of maternal mortality

The distribution of maternal deaths is unequal between regions (Table 18.2). In 2015, 99% (302,000) of estimated global maternal deaths were in developing regions, with 66% (201,000) occurring in sub-Saharan Africa (SSA) followed by South Asia (66,000) (Table 18.2). The global lifetime risk of maternal mortality is 1 in 180, yet in SSA it is 1 in 36, contrasting sharply with 1 in 4900 in developed countries.

The distribution of maternal deaths is also unequal within countries. The difference in the MMR between rich and poor countries, and between socioeconomic classes within countries, illustrates that maternal deaths are often preventable with appropriate care. The difference is due to significant disparities in access to quality services, with poorer, less educated women receiving unacceptably low levels of access to services, due to poor health care infrastructure, a lack of availability of appropriately skilled healthcare workers, and poor understanding of danger signs by women and their families.

Further, the risk of maternal death is associated with age; girls aged 15–19 are 1.5 times more likely to die than their 20–24-year-old counterparts, and, when compared to the same group, women aged 45–49 are 9.5 times more likely to die. Parity is also important, with both nulliparous and high-parity women at increased risk of adverse maternal outcomes. This leads to important health policy considerations, particularly for contraceptive services, in terms of both adolescent health and that of women reaching the end of their reproductive years.

The timing of maternal death in relation to the pregnancy is equally important, as an understanding of when deaths occur allows for development of targeted interventions. Mortality is extremely high on the first and second days after birth (Figure 18.1). This provides strong support for prioritisation of strategies that focus on professional intrapartum care.

Maternal morbidity

The existing maternal health literature and policies focus primarily on maternal death, neglecting the increasing importance of maternal morbidity (Figure 18.2). Women who suffer from non-fatal direct obstetric complications, such as obstructed labour, puerperal sepsis, septic abortion, pre-eclampsia and eclampsia, or postnatal haemorrhage are estimated to be far higher in number than those who die, yet they are poorly documented. The global estimate of maternal morbidity is that 15% of pregnant women suffer from complications—some 20 million women annually. Skilled attendance at birth has been deemed the most important intervention that prevents unnecessary suffering of women due to maternal morbidity and eventually preventable death (Figure 18.3).

Challenges

Despite progress, societies and health systems are still failing women, most acutely in poor countries and among the poorest women in all settings. The reasons why health systems fail women

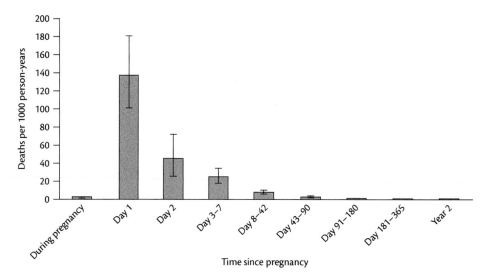

Figure 18.1 Mortality during pregnancy and by time since end of pregnancy in Matlab, Bangladesh.

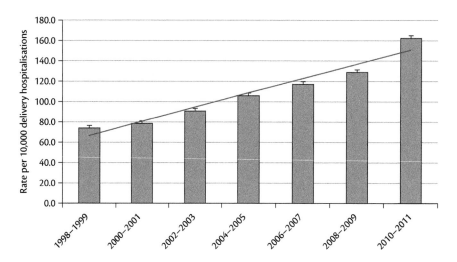

Figure 18.2 Severe maternal morbidity during delivery in the USA 1998–2011.

Source: data from Firoz, T et al. Measuring maternal health: focus on maternal morbidity. *Bulletin of the World Health Organization.* 91:794-796. doi: http://dx.doi.org/10.2471/BLT.13.117564. Geneva: World Health Organization.

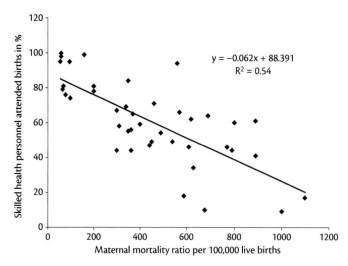

Figure 18.3 Linear regression analysis of maternal mortality ratio with skilled health personnel attended delivery using national survey data of forty-one African countries. Pearson correlation coefficient (r) = –0.7; P <0.0001.

Reproduced from Berhan, Y. Skilled Health Personnel Attended Delivery as a Proxy Indicator for Maternal and Perinatal Mortality: A Systematic Review. *Ethiopian Journal of Health Sciences.* 2014 Sep; 24(0 Suppl): 69–80. Open Access.

are often complex and are related to the biases women face in society. Women's health is profoundly affected by the ways in which women are treated and the status they are given by society as a whole. Where women continue to be discriminated against or subjected to violence, their health suffers. Gender-based discrimination leads to economic, social, and health disadvantages for women, affecting their own and their families' wellbeing in complex ways throughout the lifecourse and into the next generation. Gender equality is vital to health and to development but is determined by factors beyond the control of the health system.

Access to maternity services remains a challenge for women in low- and middle-income countries (LMICs). Economic and cultural reasons, coupled with distance and poor road networks compound the problem of access.

Even where strong public health programmes are in place across the lifecourse, they do not guarantee that women enter pregnancy in good health. Considering that women's plans change over time, encouraging women and their partners to create a reproductive health plan requires an ongoing assessment of their pregnancy desires and the provision of effective contraception or preconception care advice.

When focusing on maternal health, there is a danger that women are only considered for their reproductive capacity and their health needs are therefore only considered through the lens of maternal health. However, aside from SRH and pregnancy, women experience unique health issues and conditions, from gynaecological conditions, such as uterine fibroids and pelvic floor disorders, to menopause, and from cervical, endometrial, and ovarian cancers. Breast and cervical cancers are the most common cancers affecting women. Around half a million women die from cervical cancer and another half a million from breast cancer each year. The majority of these deaths occur in LMICs where screening, prevention, and treatment are almost non-existent, and where vaccination against human papilloma virus is yet to be implemented. Furthermore, women are more prone than men to mental health problems and more are overweight or obese. In 2012, some 4.7 million women died from non-communicable diseases before they reached the age of 70, most of them in LMICs. It is important that these non-maternal health needs are also addressed.

Future priorities

◆ Increasing numbers of women are seeking facility births and skilled birth attendants, often due to government-funded incentives. Many facilities do not have the resources to meet this increased demand and are not designated to provide higher levels of obstetric care.

◆ Facilities should, at a minimum, be able to provide basic obstetric care, that is, manage some complications, stabilise women, and be able to transfer women for appropriate care.

Conclusions

Every pregnant woman hopes for a healthy baby and an uncomplicated pregnancy. Although most pregnancies result in good maternal and foetal outcomes, for many women motherhood is associated with suffering, ill health, and even death. The global inequalities in the magnitude and causes of maternal mortality and morbidity are because girls and women do not have equal opportunities to access education, health services, and other rights recognised by law.

Opportunities to prevent and control diseases occur at multiple stages of life. Identifying which groups of women experience poorer physical and mental health and understanding which factors are most likely to influence outcomes is crucial for best practice and will enable midwives and other health professionals to better support women before, during, and after pregnancy and childbirth. Strong public health programmes that use a lifecourse perspective from infancy through childhood and adolescence to adulthood are required to improve women's health overall and support them through their reproductive and maternal health needs.

Case study: achieving maternal and child health gains in Afghanistan, a countdown to 2015 country case study

Afghanistan is one of the poorest countries in the world, affected by constant conflict and war among various groups for over three decades, leaving its health system in disarray. Despite this, Afghanistan has witnessed remarkable progress in some maternal and neonatal health indicators, providing evidence for what has and has not worked when scaling up services in Afghanistan and beyond. Between 2003 and 2015, Afghanistan witnessed improvements in the coverage and uptake of reproductive, maternal, newborn, and child health services. For example, between 2003 and 2013, antenatal care attendance increased from 16% to 53%, skilled birth attendance from 14% to 46%, and births in a health facility from 13% to 39%. Between 2005 and 2013, the number of healthcare professionals also increased, including increasing the number of midwives from 211 to 3,333 and community health workers from 2682 to 28,837. These improvements in maternal care uptake are associated with factors both within and outside the health sector, including female literacy, deployment of community midwives, and proximity to a facility. The impact of this may have been a decrease in the MMR from 1100 per 100,000 livebirths in 2000 to 396 in 2015. However, the low quality of the data on maternal mortality lends some uncertainty to these estimates.

Questions

1. Why do pregnant women not get the care they need?

2. Identify the models of maternity care that impact on maternal and neonatal health outcomes.

3. What are the social, political, environmental, and demographic factors that will transform maternal health in the next twenty years?

Key publications

World Health Organization (2015). *The Global Strategy for Women's, Children's, and Adolescent's Health (2016-2030). Every Woman Every Child*. http://www.who.int/life-course/publications/global-strategy-2016-2030/en/

An important document that advances the 2030 agenda for SDGs by guiding transformative change that enables every woman, child, and adolescent, in every setting, to realise their full potential and their human right to the highest attainable standard of health.

Miller S, Abalos E, Chamillard M, et al. (2016). Beyond too little, too late and too much, too soon: a pathway towards evidence-based, respectful maternity care worldwide. *Lancet Maternal Health Series* 388(10056): 2176–92.

This paper emphasizes that poor quality of care limits gains for improved maternal and perinatal outcomes. It highlights that a push towards births in facilities that have inadequate staff, training, infrastructure and commodities as well as insufficient evidence-based clinical practice, often results in poor quality care. This care is referred to as too little, too late (TLTL). On the other hand, the paper addresses the issue of rapid increase in facility use, accompanied by widespread over-medicalisation, termed as too much, too soon (TMTS).

Say L, Chou D, Gemmill A, et al. (2014). Global causes of maternal death: a WHO systematic analysis. *Lancet Global Health* 2: e323–33.

The paper emphasises that a key requirement for further advances in reduction of maternal deaths is to understand the causes of deaths for effective policy and health programme decisions.

Bibliography

Akseer N, Salehi A, Hossain S, et al. (2016). Achieving maternal and child health gains in Afghanistan: a countdown to 2015 country case study. *Lancet Global Health* 4(6): e395–e413.

Alkema L, Chou D, Hogan D, et al. (2015). Global, regional and national levels and trends in maternal mortality between 1990 and 2015, with scenario-based projections to 2013: a systematic analysis by the UN Maternal Mortality Estimation Inter-Agency Group. *Lancet* (387): 1–13.

Campbell O, Calvet C, Testa A, et al. (2016). The scale, scope, coverage, and capability of childbirth care. *Lancet Maternal Health Series* 3: 36–51.

Countdown to 2030 for reproductive, maternal, newborn, child, and adolescent health and nutrition. *Lancet Global Health 2016.*

Equejo J, Bryce J, Victora C, and the Countdown to 2015 writing team (2015). *A Decade of Tracking Progress for Maternal, Newborn, and Child Survival: the 2015 Report.* UNICEF and WHO: New York and Geneva.

Graham W, Woodd S, Byass P, et al (2016). Diversity and divergence: the dynamic burden of poor maternal health. *Lancet Maternal Health Series* 1: 7–35.

Kassebaum N, Bertozzi-Villa A, Coggeshall M, et al. (2014). Global, regional, and national levels and causes of maternal mortality during 1990–2013: a systematic analysis for the Global Burden of Disease Study 2013. *Lancet* 384(9947): 980–1004.

Partners in Population and Development (PPD) (2013). Promoting women's empowerment for better health outcomes for women and children. Strategy Brief for the Inter Ministerial Conference on 'South-South Cooperation in Post ICDP and MDGs', Beijing, China. http://www.who.int/pmnch/knowledge/publications/strategybriefs/sb_gender.pdf

Renfrew M, McFadden A, Bastos M, et al. (2014). Midwifery and quality care: findings from a new evidence informed framework for maternal and newborn care. *Lancet Series: Midwifery* 384: 1129–45.

Ronsmans C and Graham W (2006). Maternal mortality: who, when, where, and why. *Lancet Maternal Survival Series* 368(9542): 1189–200.

Shaw D, Guise M, and Sha N, et al. (2016). Drivers of maternity care in high-income countries: can health systems support woman centred care? *Lancet Maternal Health Series* 4: 52–65.

Say L, Chou D, Gemmill A, et al. (2014). Global causes of maternal death: a WHO systematic analysis. *Lancet Global Health* 2: e323–33.

World Health Organization (2004). *Making Pregnancy Safer—The Critical Role of the Skilled Attendant.* A joint statement by WHO, ICM and FIGO.

World Health Organization (2009). *Women and Health. Today's Evidence, Tomorrow's Agenda* http://apps.who.int/iris/bitstream/10665/70119/1/WHO_IER_MHI_STM.09.1_eng.pdf

World Health Organization (2010). *Countdown to 2015 Decade Report (2000–2010).* Geneva: WHO.

CHAPTER 19

Sexual and reproductive health

Lavanya Pillay, Jenni Smit, Mags Beksinska, and Chelsea Morroni

In this chapter we highlight current issues in and challenges to women's sexual and reproductive health (SRH) and rights (SRHR). The chapter should be read in conjunction with Chapter 12 (Adolescent sexual and reproductive health) and Chapter 20 (Family planning).

Key points

- SRHR is central to women's health and is greatly influenced by sociocultural and political factors.
- Sexually transmitted infections (STIs) represent a major health burden, with around 200 million women globally carrying one of the four major curable STIs, yet the majority do not receive any treatment. Threats to SRHR exist at individual, relationship, and societal levels.
- Investment in SRHR is critical for empowering women and for creating a world that is just, equitable, and inclusive.

Background

The imperative for universal access to SRH has been globally recognised since the 1994 International Conference on Population and Development (ICPD), where reproductive health was recognised as a human right, sexual health was included as a component of reproductive health, and a targeted call for universal SRH access by 2015 was made. Despite much progress, threats to women's SRHR, such as HIV and other sexually transmitted infections (STIs), unintended pregnancy, cervical cancer, gender-based and intimate partner violence (IPV), and female genital mutilation/cutting (FGM/C), remain. In most contexts, these threats are inter-related and are tied to gender inequality, discrimination, and vulnerability. Unequal access to education, information, and services, gender-based discrimination, female poverty, and weakened health systems contribute to poorer health outcomes for women in many areas. Improving women's SRH and advancing women's SRH care and rights is essential to improving individual-level and population-level outcomes globally, and to achieving the Sustainable Development Goals (SDGs).

SRH involves five key components:

1. Ensuring availability of contraceptive choice and infertility services.
2. Improving maternal and newborn health.
3. Reducing STIs, human immunodeficiency virus (HIV), and other SRH morbidities, including cervical cancer.
4. Eliminating unsafe abortion and providing adequate post-abortion care.
5. Promoting healthy sexuality and reducing harmful sexual practices.

Global targets

Sustainable Development Goals 2015

Goal 3 (Health)

- Ensure universal access to SRH services, including family planning, information, and education, and the integration of reproductive health into national strategies and programmes by 2030.

Goal 5 (Gender equality)

- Ensure universal access to SRH and reproductive rights as agreed in accordance with the plan of action of the ICPD.
- End all forms of discrimination against women and girls everywhere.
- Eliminate all forms of violence against women and girls.

Issues in SRH

HIV and STIs

Globally, 15–24-year-old women accounted for 20% of new HIV infections among adults in 2015, despite comprising only 11% of the population. Women's reproductive role and subordinate social standing increases their vulnerability to HIV acquisition as they have poor access to information and education, marry early, and often lack decision-making power, limiting their ability to refuse or insist on safe sex. HIV-related stigma and discrimination are further obstacles for women. Hence the calls for SRH and HIV service integration, as components of SRH are interconnected (e.g. cervical cancer and HIV; gender-based violence and HIV; unintended pregnancy; and STI transmission).

Treating and controlling the transmission of STIs is important for preventing HIV/AIDS (acquired immune deficiency syndrome) and infertility. Globally, about 200 million women of reproductive age are infected with one of four curable STIs (chlamydia, gonorrhea, syphilis, or trichomoniasis) annually, yet 83% do not receive treatment. Women are more likely to suffer complications from STIs, as they are often asymptomatic and therefore go unnoticed and untreated, and to suffer from long-term reproductive morbidities, stigma, and abuse as a result. HIV and other STIs during pregnancy can result in adverse pregnancy outcomes and transmission of the infection to the foetus or newborn.

Human papilloma virus (HPV) is the most common sexually transmitted infection. HPV causes cervical cancer, a leading cause of cancer deaths in women globally. Data from 2013 indicates 34.8 new cervical cancer cases diagnosed each year per 100,000 women in sub-Saharan Africa compared to 2.5–6.6 new cases in North America. Across sub-Saharan African countries, cervical cancer is the first or second most common cause of women's cancer, and almost 90% of cervical cancer deaths occur in low to middle-income countries (LMICs). Because pre-cancerous lesions take many years to develop, screening (recommended by the World Health Organization (WHO) every 5–10 years in women over the age of 30, or at least once in a lifetime among women aged 30–49), followed by adequate treatment, can be very effective in preventing cervical cancer-related morbidity and mortality. Screening programmes can include conventional cytological services ('Pap smear'), visual inspection of the cervix with acetic acid services, or HPV deoxyribonucleic acid (DNA) testing. The higher cervical cancer incidence and mortality rates in LMICs are due to the lack of sufficient cervical cancer screening and HPV vaccination programmes in these settings.

Gender-based violence

Gender-based violence (GBV) is a significant public health problem affecting predominantly women, across all societies and socioeconomic strata. Worldwide, 35% of women have experienced sexual violence in their lifetime. Globally, abused women are twice as likely to be depressed, to have alcohol misuse disorders, to experience unintended pregnancy, and are 1.5 times more likely to have HIV or an STI than non-abused women. FGM/C is a harmful practice continuing in many cultures. Over 125 million women and girls have experienced FGM/C in Africa, the Middle East, and Asia, exposing them to psychological and physical SRH risks.

Infertility

Infertility, most typically defined as the failure to conceive after twelve months or more of regular unprotected sexual intercourse, is estimated to affect between 15% and 25% of reproductive-aged couples worldwide. In sub-Saharan Africa, more than 30% of women aged 25–49 suffer from secondary infertility (the failure to conceive after an initial first pregnancy), and this has not declined in the past 30 years. Although male infertility has been found to be the cause of a couple's failure to conceive in up to half of all cases, the 'social burden' of infertility falls disproportionately on women, often with dire consequences. In many settings, childless women suffer violence, discrimination, stigma, and marginalisation, and this stigma often extends to the wider family. Despite its importance, infertility prevention and care remain neglected public health and clinical issues, especially for low-income countries.

Transgender issues

Transgender people have poor access to health and SRH services due to legal barriers, stigma, discrimination, and violence. According to the WHO, transgender women are 49 times more likely to be HIV-infected than other adults of reproductive age and in some places HIV rates are 80 times higher than that of the general adult population. Violence against transgender people is common (e.g. abuse by police, abuse by clients of sex workers), and transgender people may experience family rejection and violation of their rights to education, employment, and social protections. A lack of legal recognition of transgender people in most countries contributes to their exclusion and marginalisation. A comprehensive package of services is recommended to address SRHR issues in transgender people, including health-specific and structural interventions.

Interventions

Tackling gender inequity

The Microfinance for AIDS and Gender Equity (IMAGE) programme employed microfinance, gender, and HIV training to empower women and reduce IPV in Limpopo Province, South Africa. IMAGE included participatory training on gender roles, cultural beliefs, relationships, communication, domestic violence, HIV, and community mobilisation. Women who met bi-weekly to discuss business plans also educated youth and men about gender equity, IPV, and HIV. Compared to the control group, in the intervention group there was a 55% decrease in reported IPV two years following implementation.

Integrating health services

The Integra Initiative, conducted in 42 health centres in Kenya and Swaziland, explored feasibility, effectiveness, cost, and the impact of different SRH and HIV service integration models. Key findings suggest that although it may increase quality of care, integration does not necessarily result in reduced unintended pregnancies, cost, and stigma. User preference is crucial; some women favour specialised services while others prefer integrated services.

Expanding HPV vaccination

HPV vaccination is a key strategy for reducing cervical cancer. By the end of 2015, more than 65 countries had introduced the vaccine into their national immunisation programmes, including an increasing number of LMICs, but few in Africa and Asia, where the global burden of cervical cancer resides.

Challenges

The delivery of SRH services to meet SRHR is hampered by the wider health sector limitations of insufficient resources, both financial and workforce, and the socio-political context. There are also specific challenges to SRH.

Globally, women and girls have lower social status, fewer educational and economic opportunities, and less control over resources compared to men and boys. Furthermore, key populations (e.g. sex workers, youth, men who have sex with men, sero-discordant couples, gender and sexual minorities) and those who do not conform to social norms often experience stigma and discrimination, limiting their access to SRH services.

Historically SRH has been neglected and under prioritised. This is because different SRH components have been located among other health concerns, for example maternal health or child health. The wide range of services that fall under SRH also make it difficult to define the scope of integration at a practical level. Health worker shortages, inadequate infrastructure, poor training, lack of equipment, and poor management systems limit provision and scale-up of integrated services. In addition, challenges to SRH programmes persist in contexts where SRH is not openly discussed due to politics, cultural sensitivity, and stigma.

Future priorities

◆ Given that HIV/STIs and pregnancy are dynamically interconnected (unsafe sex can simultaneously lead to HIV/STI acquisition and unintended pregnancy), dual protection from unintended pregnancy and HIV/STIs is necessary. Currently, male and female condoms are the only available multipurpose prevention products. New multipurpose prevention products, particularly ones controlled by females, are needed and some are in development (e.g. intra-vaginal rings, tablets, injections, diaphragms, films, and gels).

◆ Other priorities include addressing low male participation in SRH, while enhancing female empowerment; developing services that support pregnancy planning, including safer conception for people living with HIV/AIDS and HIV sero-discordant couples, and addressing infertility.

Conclusions

Globally, threats to women's SRHR exist across multiple levels, from the individual to relationships, families, and communities, at the health systems level, and in societal structures. Multi-level and multi-sectoral commitments and political and financial investment in advancing women's SRH and rights are all required. Threats to SRH and rights are complex and cannot be considered in isolation. Without full access to SRH and rights, women's ability to lead healthy and fulfilling lives and contribute economically, socially, and politically is severely constrained.

Case study: challenging gender norms and attitudes in Africa and Asia, the Stepping Stones Programme

The Stepping Stones Programme is a life-skills training intervention designed to improve sexual health by developing stronger, more equal relationships between those of different gender. It has been implemented in Africa and Asia. Using a variety of methods, including reflection on one's attitudes and behaviour, role-play, and drama, it addresses a range of issues such as gender and peer influences impacting on actions; sex and love; conception and contraception; STIs and HIV; safer sex and condoms; GBV; motivations for behaviour (including influences of alcohol and poverty); and communication skills. While the programme did not reduce HIV incidence (its primary outcome) it did reduce the incidence of herpes simplex virus 2 (0.67 95% CI: 0.46–0.97) and improved a number of reported risk behaviours in men, including GBV, problem drinking, and transactional sex. This case study is a good example of how even if the primary outcome isn't achieved, a programme can still have very worthwhile benefits, and can be supported in further roll out.

Questions

1. What are the key components of SRH?

2. What is meant by universal access to SRH and why is it important?

3. Discuss barriers and challenges to achieving SRH and rights.

Key publications

Barot S. (2015). Sexual and reproductive health and rights are key to global development: the case for ramping up investment. *Guttmacher Policy Review* 18(1).
Documents the benefits from SRH investment.
A broad overview on the importance of prioritizing sexual and reproductive health/rights in the context of global development.
Jewkes R, Nduna M, Levin J, et al. (2008). Impact of Stepping Stones on incidence of HIV and HSV-2 and sexual behaviour in rural South Africa: cluster randomised controlled trial. *BMJ* 337: a506.
The study was key as it is one of the first HIV prevention behavioural interventions to have been subject to the most rigorous level of evaluation in Africa and to have provided some evidence of success in reducing sexually transmitted infections in women and in changing men's sexual risk-taking behaviour and reduced their use of violence.

Bibliography

Boldosser-Boesch A, Byrnes D, Carr C, et al. (2015). Briefing cards: sexual and reproductive health and rights (SRHR) and the post-2015 development agenda. Universal Access Project. Available from: http://www.unfoundation.org/what-we-do/campaigns-and-initiatives/universal-access-project/briefing-cards-srhr.pdf
Garland S, Kjaer S, Muñoz N, et al. (2016). Impact and effectiveness of the quadrivalent human papillomavirus vaccine: a systematic review of 10 years of real-world experience. *Clin Infect Dis.* 63(4): 519–27.
Integra (2013). Strengthening the evidence base for integrating HIV and sexual and reproductive health (SRH) services. Newsletter, Issue 6. Available from: www.integrainitiative.org.
International Planned Parenthood Federation (2014). Sexual and reproductive health and rights—a crucial agenda for the post-2015 framework. Available from: http://www.ippf.org/sites/default/files/report_for_web.pdf
Singh S, Darroch J, Ashford L, and Vlassoff M (2009). *Adding it up: the costs and benefits of investing in family planning and maternal and newborn health.* Guttmacher Institute and United Nations Population Fund: New York. Available from: https://www.guttmacher.org/sites/default/files/report_pdf/AddingItUp2009.pdf.
United Nations (2015). *Transforming our World: the 2030 Agenda for Sustainable Development.* United Nations. Available from: https://sustainabledevelopment.un.org/post2015/transformingourworld
United Nations (2015). *The World's Women 2015: Trends and Statistics.* United Nations, Department of Economic and Social Affairs, Statistics Division: New York. Available from: https://unstats.un.org/unsd/gender/worldswomen.html
United Nations Children's Fund (2016). *Female Genital Mutilation/Cutting: a Global Concern.* UNICEF: UNICEF. Available from: https://www.unicef.org/media/files/FGMC_2016_brochure_final_UNICEF_SPREAD.pdf
United Nations Educational, Scientific and Cultural Organisation (2015). *Emerging Evidence, Lessons and Practice in Comprehensive Sexuality Education: a Global Review.* UNESCO: UNESCO. Available from: http://www.unfpa.org/publications/emerging-evidence-lessons-and-practice-comprehensive-sexuality-education-global-review
United Nations Population Fund (2010). *How Universal is Access to Reproductive Health? A Review of the Evidence.* UNFPA. Available from: https://www.unfpa.org/sites/default/files/pub-pdf/universal_rh.pdf
United Nations Population Fund (2010). *Sexual and Reproductive Health for All. Reducing Poverty and Advancing Development and Protecting*

Human Rights. UNFPA. Available from: https://www.unfpa.org/sites/default/files/pub-pdf/uarh_report_2010.pdf

World Health Organization (2011). *Quality of Care in the Provision of Sexual and Reproductive Health Services: Evidence from a World Health Organization Research Initiative.* WHO: Geneva. Available from: http://apps.who.int/iris/bitstream/10665/44343/1/9789241501897_eng.pdf

World Health Organization (2015). The *Global Strategy for Women's, Children's, and Adolescents' Health (2016–2030). Every Woman Every Child.* Available from: http://www.who.int/pmnch/media/events/2015/gs_2016_30.pdf

World Health Organization (2017). *HIV/AIDS. Transgender People.* Available from: http://www.who.int/hiv/topics/transgender/about/en/

World Health Organization Human Reproduction Programme (2018). *Sexual and Reproductive Health. Infertility is a global public health issue.* Available from: http://www.who.int/reproductivehealth/topics/infertility/perspective/en/

CHAPTER 20

Contraception and abortion

Jennifer Hall

This chapter introduces the key concepts in the area of family planning, explains the different types of contraceptives available and their effectiveness, and considers how family planning services can be designed to better meet needs. It should be read in conjunction with Chapter 12 (Adolescent sexual and reproductive health) and Chapter 19 (Maternal sexual and reproductive health).

Key points

- Family planning is key to sexual and reproductive health rights and sustainable development. It has significant health, economic, and developmental benefits at individual, national, and global levels.

- Contraception is a cost-effective way to prevent unplanned pregnancies and reduce unsafe abortions and maternal and neonatal deaths. Despite this, 214 million women worldwide have an unmet need for family planning.

- Unsafe abortions represent a major cause of preventable mortality, especially where abortion is illegal, and there is limited post-abortion care, with abortion linked to approximately 47,000 maternal deaths a year.

- We know what makes programmes effective but the combination of interventions must be adapted to the context. The focus should be on increasing the use of long-acting reversible contraceptives (LARCs) to maximise effectiveness.

Background

'The pill' needs no introduction or explanation. It has revolutionised the lives of millions of women and is consistently recognised as one of the most significant medical and social milestones of the last 150 years. Now it is just one of the modern methods of contraception, shown in Table 20.1, alongside traditional methods such as breastfeeding and natural family planning. Each method has its own advantages, disadvantages, and side effects, making an assessment of the couple's needs essential when providing contraception. Emergency contraception, which can be taken up to three to five days after unprotected sex, is also available.

The benefits of family planning are wide-ranging. At the individual level, it allows couples to have children by choice, not by chance, meeting their sexual and reproductive health rights. Giving women control of their own bodies contributes to female empowerment. Enabling women to delay childbearing means they can complete their education, improving their long-term employment prospects, increasing their earnings, and lifting them out of poverty. It is also better for women's health, as they have fewer children with better spacing between them, and can contribute to the prevention of mother to child transmission of human immunodeficiency syndrome (HIV).

When couples can control their fertility, they tend to have fewer children. At a household level, resources are less thinly stretched, benefitting each child's health, growth, development, and education, and improving their long-term health, employment, and economic prospects. At a national level, slowing population growth will, over time, reduce the pressure on government services such as health and education. As the total fertility rate (TFR) goes down, countries' developmental indicators, such as female education and gross domestic product, tend to improve, as demonstrated in Figure 20.1. At a global level, current population growth is unsustainable; family planning is key to sustainable development.

Despite this, there are around 214 million women worldwide who have an unmet need for family planning. Consequently 43% of all pregnancies, 8.6 million a year, are 'unplanned'. Unplanned pregnancies potentially pose greater risk of adverse outcomes for both the mother and child and contribute to the 42 million abortions annually. In many countries restrictive abortion laws force women to have an unsafe abortion, causing an estimated 47,000 deaths per year and making abortion a leading cause of maternal deaths worldwide. Between 2003 and 2009 unsafe abortion caused almost 10% of maternal deaths in sub-Saharan Africa (SSA) and South America, resulting in it being called both a 'silent' and a 'preventable pandemic'. An up-to-date map of the world's abortion laws is available at: http://worldabortionlaws.com/map/

Contraception is an effective and cost-effective way of preventing unplanned pregnancies, decreasing the need for abortions and reducing maternal and neonatal mortality and morbidity. Meeting unmet need is estimated to reduce unplanned pregnancies to 22 million per year and unsafe abortions to 5.1 million, preventing the deaths of hundreds of thousands of women and millions of babies. Furthermore, every dollar spent on contraceptive services saves $2.20 in maternal and newborn healthcare costs.

Family planning has not always been high on the policy agenda: Millennium Development Goal (MDG) target 5b 'achieving universal access to reproductive health', was only added in 2007. By 2015 the global contraceptive-prevalence rate (CPR) had increased from 55% in 1990 to 64%. SSA only achieved a rate of 28%. Worldwide, unmet need for family planning among married women fell from 15% to 12% between 1990 and 2015, but in SSA it is 24%, meaning there is much more work to be done.

Table 20.1 Modern methods of family planning and their effectiveness

Frequency of use	Contraceptive method	Description	How it works	Efficacy	Effectiveness
Every act of intercourse	Male condom	Sheath that fits over man's erect penis.	Barrier preventing sperm and egg meeting. Also prevents sexually transmitted infections.	98%	85%
	Female condom	Sheath that fits inside woman's vagina.		90%	79%
	Diaphragm/cap	Latex/silicone dome fitted to cover cervix.	Barrier preventing sperm and egg meeting.	92–96%	86–94%
Daily use	Combined oral contraception (the pill)	Contains oestrogen and progestogen.	Prevents ovulation.	> 99%	92%
	Progestogen-only pills	Contains progestogen.	Thickens cervical mucous and prevents ovulation.	99%	90–97%
Weekly to 3 monthly	Combined contraceptive patch	Patch applied weekly for 3 weeks then 1 week off. Releases a progestin and an oestrogen through the skin.	Prevents ovulation.	Limited evidence, probably more effective than the pill.	
	Combined injectable contraceptives	Monthly intramuscular injection, contains oestrogen and progestogen.		> 99%	97%
	Combined contraceptive vaginal ring	Continuously releases a progestin and an oestrogen from the ring which remains *in situ* for 3 weeks then 1 week off.	Prevents ovulation.	Limited evidence, probably more effective than the pill.	
	Progestogen only injectables	Intramuscular injection every 2 or 3 months.	Thickens cervical mucous and prevents ovulation.	> 99%	97%
3–10 years	Implants	Small rods placed under the skin, contains progestogen only, lasts 3–5 years.		> 99%	
	Copper intrauterine device (IUD)	Plastic device containing copper, inserted into the uterus.	Copper damages sperm preventing fertilisation.	> 99%	
	IUD containing levonorgestrel	T-shaped plastic device inserted into the uterus, continually releases levonorgestrel.	Suppresses the growth of the lining of uterus.	> 99%	
Permanent methods	Male sterilisation (vasectomy)	Cut/block the tubes that carry sperm from the testicles.	Keeps sperm out of ejaculated semen.	> 97–99%	
	Female sterilisation (tubal ligation)	Cut/block the Fallopian tubes.	Eggs are blocked from meeting sperm.	> 99%	

Global targets

Sustainable Development Goals (SDGs) (2015)

Goal 3 (Health)

◆ By 2030, ensure universal access to sexual and reproductive healthcare services, including for family planning, information, and education, and the integration of reproductive health into national strategies and programmes.

Goal 5 (Gender equality)

◆ Ensure universal access to sexual and reproductive health and reproductive rights.

Interventions

Effective methods of contraception exist and international surveys consistently find high levels of awareness. The challenge is in providing services that meet people's needs. Experience shows us the underlying principles of effective programmes:

◆ Legitimise smaller family sizes and the use of modern contraceptives and disseminate information on all methods available.

 ◆ Mass media campaigns, for example informational radio broadcasts and soap operas, are effective and cost-effective.

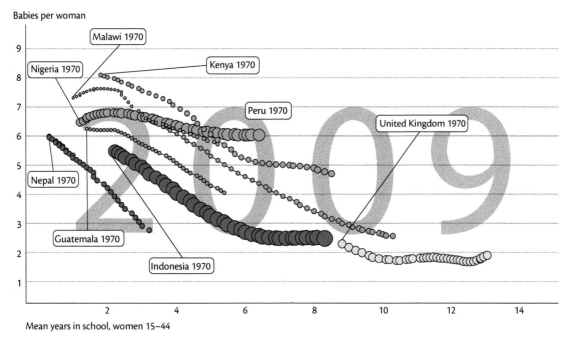

Figure 20.1 The relationship between total fertility rate and mean years in school for women aged 15–44, from 1970 to 2009.
Source: data from www.gapminder.org

◆ Address misconceptions and misinformation, particularly among men, and women's misperceptions of their partner's opinion.

  ◆ Community-based interventions, working with religious and other community leaders, and 'male-motivators'—local men trained to offer family planning counselling to their peers—can tackle this.

◆ Make a range of methods available and affordable, ideally free of charge.

  ◆ Good method mix leads to a rise in total contraceptive use and reduces the rate of discontinuation by ensuring preferences are met or offering an alternative immediately.

  ◆ Short-term supply or stock outs, of all or some methods, lead to inadvertent discontinuation and risk of unplanned pregnancies.

  ◆ Focus on maximising the use of LARCs and improving adherence to reversible methods. Approximately one third of all unintended births worldwide, and more than half of all induced abortions in some countries, are due to contraceptive failure. Shifting to LARCs will achieve greater effectiveness, yet in many settings healthcare workers are not trained in their use, limiting their uptake.

◆ Maximise the value of each health service contact.

  ◆ During pregnancy, birth, and postnatally, women are in frequent contact with services, offering ample opportunity to discuss future pregnancy plans and contraceptive needs. Postnatally, over 90% of women want to avoid a pregnancy for at least two years. The IUD can be inserted immediately post-delivery, removing the need for the woman to return to the health service.

◆ Provide high-quality services.

  ◆ This includes providing a good method mix, reliably having the products in stock, having competent staff who are present when they should be and treating patients with respect and dignity, confidentiality, and privacy.

  ◆ Ensure staff are trained to provide as many methods as possible and are kept up to date to avoid healthcare workers having misconceptions about which methods can be used and when (particularly in the postnatal period), or turning women away inappropriately.

◆ Utilise a mixture of delivery mechanism to enhance access.

  ◆ Include the public health system, private sector, community-based or outreach programmes, and non-clinicians.

  ◆ Youth-friendly services for young or unmarried men and women.

◆ Integrate with other SRH services, for example HIV testing and treatment, as per local context.

  ◆ Preventing unintended pregnancies in HIV-positive women is the most cost-effective way of preventing mother to child transmission.

Challenges

Abortion remains the major challenge to the realisation of sexual and reproductive rights globally. In some countries women's access to abortion services has become more restricted. This will increase with President Trump's expansion of the Mexico City policy or 'Global gag rule', preventing non-governmental organisations (NGOs) who receive any US-government funding from counselling about, referring to, advocating for, or providing abortion services.

Family planning has been tarnished by the implementation of coercive policies. An extreme example is China's 'One child policy', where couples faced penalities if they had more than one child. It is vital that voluntary family planning is promoted.

The progress that has been made in increasing the CPR has not been equally shared, either between or within countries. Adolescent girls in the poorest communities remain at particularly high risk of unplanned pregnancies. How to reach the poorest, most marginalised populations remains a significant challenge.

Future priorities

◆ Improving adherence to contraception will reduce contraceptive failure but is challenging; mobile health (m-health) provides some interesting research opportunities. Information technology could also be used in supply chain management.

◆ Expanding access to safe abortion requires societal attitudes to shift, a process that will take time, but that should be advocated for. Meanwhile, expanding access to contraception, including emergency contraception, and post-abortion care must be priorities.

◆ Every health service contact with women and men of reproductive age is a chance to discuss whether they are currently trying to prevent or plan a pregnancy. Appropriate contraceptive or preconception advice can then be given.

Conclusions

Family planning is highly cost-effective and is unique in the extent of its benefits at individual, household, national, and global levels. While the global TFR has fallen from around six to about three over the last fifty years, largely due to the CPR increasing from below 10% to 64%, there remain significant inequalities both within and between countries, with high levels of unmet need particularly in SSA. Without addressing these inequalities, further gains may not be achieved and progress to date could be reversed.

While most countries have appropriate policies in place, historically they have received insufficient funding, whether internally or from donors. There is some evidence that this is changing since the London 2012 Family Planning Summit and that there is recognition of the vital role family planning will play in sustainable development. Only with continued political will and funding will we realise the right of every man and woman to choose if, when, and how many children to have.

Case study: Malawi, taking action on a national level to improve family planning support

At the London Family Planning Summit in 2012, Malawi pledged to increase the country's CPR to 60% by 2020, with a focus on those aged 15–24, and stated that there would be 'no parenthood before adulthood'. The Reproductive Health Unit in Malawi was upgraded to a directorate, giving it its own resources and greater power to influence policy. A budget line for family planning was created, leading to improvements in the availability of contraceptives in health facilities. In 2015 parliament raised the minimum legal age of marriage to 18 and endorsed a new Youth Friendly Health Service Strategy. Also in 2015, 90% of health facilities submitted data to the national logistics management information system, meaning that forecasting, procurement, and supply chain issues can be better managed. In addition the government has been working to mainstream family planning and increase community participation.

This case study demonstrates a multi-party, multi-faceted intervention, with evidence of success. However, more can be done. The new law still allows girls younger than 18 to get married if they have parental consent, a loophole that needs closing. Furthermore, abortion remains illegal. Despite cross-sectoral support the government ruled out a review of the abortion law in the 2014–2019 parliament.

Questions

1. Why do you think reproductive health was originally omitted from the MDGs?

2. Describe the reasons why people aren't using family planning despite expressing a desire not to have more children.

3. What are the mechanisms by which family planning reduces maternal and child mortality?

4. For a country of your choosing describe the current contraceptive method mix and what steps you would take to diversify contraceptive use.

Key publications

United Nations (2014). *International Conference On Population And Development (ICPD) Programme of Action (PoA)*. UNFPA: New York.
  The ICPD in Cairo in 1994 was the first time that the relationships between population, development, and individual wellbeing were articulated at a global level. The PoA continues to serve as a comprehensive guide to people-centred development. It was ahead of its time in its recognition that reproductive health and rights, female empowerment, and gender equality are cornerstones of population and development programmes.

Lancet Series on Family Planning (2012). *Lancet* 380: 77–180.
  This Lancet series reviewed the evidence for the effects of population and family planning on people's wellbeing and the environment.

The Guttmacher Institute (2017). *Adding it Up: the Costs and Benefits of Investing in Sexual and Reproductive Health*. Guttmacher Institute: New York.
  Estimates the needs for and costs and benefits of sexual and reproductive health interventions at a global level.

UNFPA (2013). *Choices not Chance. UNFPA Family Planning Strategy 2012-2020*. UNFPA: New York.
  The UNFPA is the UN organisation responsible for family planning. This strategy sets out UNFPA's core commitments to the SRH of women and young people and is aligned with the ICPD PoA.

Bibliography

Bradley S, Croft T, and Rutstein S (2011). *The Impact of Contraceptive Failure on Unintended Births and Induced Abortions: Estimates and Strategies for Reduction*. DHS Analytical Studies No. 22. ICF Macro: Calverton, Maryland, USA.

Cleland J, Bernstein S, Ezeh A, et al. (2006). Family planning: the unfinished agenda. *Lancet* 368(9549):1810–27.

Gipson J, et al. (2008). The effects of unintended pregnancy on infant, child, and parental health: a review of the literature. *Stud Fam Plann* 39(1): 18–38.

Hall J, et al. (2015). Conceptual framework for pregnancy planning and prevention (P3). *J Fam Plann Reprod Health Care*.

Halpern V, et al. (2013). Strategies to improve adherence and acceptability of hormonal methods of contraception. *Cochrane Database Systematic Reviews* 10: CD004317.

Lopez L, et al. (2014). Strategies for improving postpartum contraceptive use: evidence from non-randomized studies. *Cochrane Database Systematic Reviews* 11: CD011298.

Ross J and Stover J (2013). Use of modern contraception increases when more methods become available: analysis of evidence from 1982–2009. *Glob Health Sci Pract* 1(2): 203–12.

Smith C., et al. (2015). Mobile phone-based interventions for improving contraception use. *Cochrane Database Systematic Reviews* 6: CD011159.

Tsui A, et al. (2010). Family planning and the burden of unintended pregnancies. *Epidemiologic Reviews* 32(1): 152–74.

United Nations, Department of Economic and Social Affairs, Population Division (2013). *Trends in Contraceptive Methods Used Worldwide*. Available from: http://www.un.org/en/development/desa/population/publications/pdf/popfacts/PopFacts_2013-9_new.pd.

CHAPTER 21

Direct maternal deaths

Abi Merriel, Raymond Kanthiti, and David Lissauer

This chapter introduces direct maternal deaths, what contributes to them, and where efforts should be focused to prevent mothers dying from them. It should be read alongside Chapter 22, which discusses indirect causes of maternal deaths.

Key points

◆ Ninety-nine per cent of maternal deaths occur in low-resource settings, the majority of which are direct and preventable. This tends to be highest in areas with high fertility rates and poor obstetric care.

◆ Five single causes make up approximately three-quarters of all direct maternal deaths, that is, deaths related to obstetric complications (haemorrhage, abortion-related, hypertensive disorders, sepsis, and obstructed labour).

◆ The cause of these deaths is multi-faceted, including cultural attitudes to pregnancy, quality of care, and health systems issues, and therefore a comprehensive approach is required to make substantial gains.

◆ Good quality care around the time of birth can substantially reduce direct maternal mortality.

Background

Direct maternal deaths cause nearly three quarters (258,000) of maternal deaths worldwide each year. They are attributable to obstetric complications, and much of the time these complications occur at or around the time of childbirth. Although it would be incorrect to say that all of these deaths can be prevented, almost all of them can be avoided using known and often basic interventions, for example actively managing the third stage of labour to prevent postpartum haemorrhage.

Global targets

Sustainable Development Goals (SDGs) (2015)

Goal 3 (Health)

◆ By 2030, reduce the global maternal mortality ratio (MMR) to less than 70 per 100,000 live births.

The World Health Organization (WHO) Strategies towards ending preventable maternal mortality (2015) 2030 targets

◆ All countries reduce their maternal mortality ratio (MMR) by two thirds from 2010 levels by 2030.

◆ No country to have an MMR greater than 140, meaning countries with a higher MMR than 420 need a steeper rate of decline by 2030.

◆ Progress to greater equity in MMR at a subnational level is achieved in countries with low baseline MMRs already.

◆ For countries with a MMR less than 420 in 2010 (the majority of countries worldwide): reduce the MMR by at least two thirds from the 2010 baseline by 2030.

Direct maternal deaths

There are five single causes (haemorrhage, abortion-related, hypertensive disorders, sepsis, and obstructed labour) that together make up nearly 75% of all direct maternal deaths (Figure 21.1). There is also a significant contribution from 'other direct' causes, which has become the largest single contributing group of direct deaths globally due to improvements in managing the five common causes. 'Other direct' causes include pulmonary embolism (a blood clot in the blood vessels in the lungs), amniotic fluid embolism (foetal tissue gets into the blood vessels in the lungs of the mother; this results in a severe allergic reaction), and ectopic pregnancy (when a pregnancy implants itself outside the womb, which is not compatible with ongoing pregnancy). Since 2012 the WHO considers suicide to be a direct cause of maternal death; however, this is not yet reflected in global statistics. The true burden of suicide as a direct maternal death is unknown, largely due to the lack of studies investigating the issue, especially in low- and middle-income countries (LMICs).

Why do mothers die from preventable direct causes of maternal death?

Haemorrhage

Haemorrahge can occur during or after pregnancy, but is most common around the time of delivery. Known as postpartum haemorrhage (PPH), it occurs in approximately 2% of women. Whilst some women are at increased risk, it is largely unpredictable. If a woman is given a drug to contract her womb after delivery, the incidence is reduced by about 60%. If she goes on to bleed heavily, the presence of a skilled provider to initiate further management and access adequate resources, such as blood transfusion, can save women in all but a very few cases. Women who have had many pregnancies are at higher risk of haemorrhage, as are women who are anaemic.

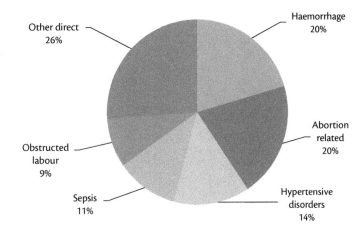

Figure 21.1 Causes of direct maternal death.
Source: data from Say, L. et al, 2014. Global causes of maternal death: a WHO systematic analysis. *The Lancet Global Health*. 2(6), 323–e333. Copyright © 2014 World Health Organization. Published by Elsevier Ltd.

Abortion-related deaths

There are estimated to be 22 million abortions annually; between 2010 and 2014 this led to over 47,000 deaths. In countries where abortion is not legal or is highly restricted, women, especially poorer women, are forced to seek abortions from unregulated providers, which means having an unsafe abortion. Deaths are usually due to haemorrhage or sepsis. However, because there are specific policy issues to tackle with unsafe abortion, these abortion-related deaths are separated from the haemorrhage/sepsis statistics and included in this specific category. In addition to the maternal deaths, it is estimated that five million women are admitted to hospital with complications of abortion and a further three million women do not access care. Access to safe, legally available abortion care, alongside a package of sexual health education and access to family planning, could end almost all abortion-related deaths.

Hypertensive disorders

About 10% of pregnant women suffer from hypertensive disorders. Access to high quality antenatal care enables identification of high blood pressure, referral, and treatment before complications occur. If women do not have these conditions diagnosed due to lack of attendance at antenatal care, or poor quality of care at a facility (e.g. lack of monitoring of blood pressure), the consequences can be catastrophic for her and her baby. Pre-eclampsia and eclampsia can cause women severe morbidity (e.g. stroke or organ failure) or death. Pre-eclampsia also affects the growth of the foetus and, if untreated, it can be fatal for the baby too. Appropriate management includes monitoring, anti-hypertensive drugs, the use of magnesium sulphate to prevent and treat seizures, and, when appropriate, delivery of the baby and intensive care.

Sepsis

Up to 10% of women suffer from some form of morbidity from infection in low-income countries, although the true prevalence of sepsis is difficult to determine. The infections women experience can include pregnancy specific infections (e.g. chorioamnionitis, an infection inside the womb) or non-pregnancy specific infections (e.g. urinary tract infections), which may be more common and are often more serious due to the physiological changes of pregnancy.

There are many risk factors for sepsis, including cleanliness of place of delivery, poor maternal nutritional state, human immunodeficiency virus (HIV) infection, and anaemia. The most important risk factor is having had a Caesarean section. A comprehensive package of interventions is required, from community-based interventions for nutrition and anaemia, through to referral, access to appropriate resources, and high-quality clinical care. Tools to identify sepsis and aid early initiation of appropriate antibiotics can support this. A particular challenge is that many infections occur postnatally, when women are in the community, which makes them a particularly difficult group to access and treat appropriately.

Obstructed labour

This remains a significant contributor to maternal deaths, mainly due to uterine rupture and as a precipitating factor for sepsis. Undernutrition in childhood is a risk factor for obstructed labour as it can lead to a small pelvis in affected women. This is compounded when a girl marries young and/or pregnancy occurs before the girl is fully grown. The partogram is a simple decision support tool to help identify prolonged labour and prompt action. It provides a pictorial overview of progress and facilitates the transfer of care when labour is delayed and is thus strongly recommended by the WHO. A Caesarean section is needed in obstructed labour. This necessitates appropriately skilled staff to perform the procedure and the required health infrastructure and resources to be available.

The three delays model

The three delays model (Figure 21.2) is a widely accepted approach to considering maternity care and why women die. Delay one, of a woman and her family deciding to seek health care, needs to be addressed through health education, policy, and cultural shifts. Delay two, of reaching a medical facility, needs to be addressed through policies targeting infrastructure, for example roads and transport links, as well as community level programmes to educate women and their families about birth preparedness. The third delay is focused on receiving appropriate care on arrival at a facility.

The third delay is receiving increasing attention, as addressing it is vitally important in ensuring that women receive high-quality

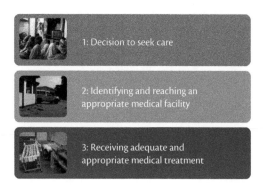

Figure 21.2 The Three Delays Model.

Source: data from Thaddeus, S. et al. Too far to walk: maternal mortality in context. *Social Science & Medicine*. 38(8), .1091–1110. Coyright © 1994 Elsevier Science Ltd; and photographs reproduced courtesy of Abi Merriel.

care. The cornerstone for high-quality care is having a skilled attendant at birth. Reducing much maternal mortality depends upon the immediate actions of a skilled individual in response to deteriorating maternal condition. Furthermore, these individuals need to be equipped with the tools to make these decisions, for example simple decision support tools such as partograms.

In addition to being accredited and competent, a provider must also have access to the necessary equipment and systems, including transport and referral facilities for emergency obstetric care. This is encompassed in the WHO definition of skilled birth attendance. It is also becoming increasingly important that care is provided in a respectful way, such as labour wards being equipped with curtains.

What approaches have been taken to address direct maternal deaths?

Many interventions have been developed and refined as the advocacy around safe motherhood has been strengthened over the last thirty years. Women's groups have proven to be a useful community intervention to empower women, encourage health-seeking behaviours, and encourage birth preparedness. In doing this, Prost et al. (2013) showed that they have reduced maternal mortality by 37%. Skills training for healthcare workers has been undertaken globally to improve the recognition and response to management of obstetric emergencies by health providers. Health policy has been altered to encourage women to deliver in facilities. For example, in Nepal there is a maternity incentive scheme to provide women with transport costs for delivering in an institution.

Building on a 'Beyond the Numbers' approach, Maternal Death Surveillance and Response was launched by the WHO in 2012. This aims to reduce preventable maternal mortality through a continuous cycle of action and surveillance to identify, quantify, notify, and review maternal deaths on a local and national level. This information is then aggregated and interpreted to make recommendations for ways to prevent maternal deaths.

Challenges

There are challenges in the measurement of maternal mortality, synonymous with the measurement of indicators in any resource-poor setting. For example, the large reliance on facility-based data collection despite many of the events of interest occurring in the

community. Even when deaths occur in the facility, there is the challenge of ascribing the correct cause to each woman. When community methods are employed it can be difficult to collect accurate data as data collection is often retrospective and therefore based upon people's recall of the situation.

To increase the number of births attended by skilled providers there has been a concerted effort to encourage women to deliver in facilities. However, this has resulted in the number of women attending facilities burgeoning, with little extra-investment in staff, resources, or infrastructure. This has placed huge pressure on the health system and staff within it, and is increasing demand without improving supply, which has a negative effect on quality.

Traditional birth attendants (TBAs) have been a source of controversy. TBAs have historically provided much of the delivery care in communities, despite having no formal training. When the movement for skilled birth attendance came, there was a move away from TBAs and in some countries they were, temporarily at least, banned. However, they continued to provide delivery care. There is some evidence that TBAs who are trained can be a useful adjunct to facility-based delivery in cases where there are too few staff or the facilities are difficult to access.

Future priorities

♦ Reducing maternal deaths further poses a significant challenge. The deaths which are easiest to prevent are likely to have been averted during the Millennium Development Goals (MDGs) era. Now efforts must be concentrated on the harder to reach women, and also on the parts of the reproductive lifecourse that are harder to access, for example preconception and postnatal care.

♦ The approach needs to be comprehensive. In addition to focusing on improving quality of care for women in facilities, there must be a focus at a policy level on the broader determinants of health, including gender, poverty, and culture.

♦ Women must be empowered to take control of their reproductive health through improved access to education and appropriate community mobilisation strategies.

♦ Researchers need to concentrate on the 'messy' health system issues to enable women to seek and receive the care they deserve.

Conclusions

It is possible to significantly reduce direct maternal deaths, but to do this most effectively a comprehensive approach crossing community, health, and political boundaries is required. Education of women and health workers, health system strengthening to provide skilled birth attendance and forward thinking, cross-sectoral policy is needed to address direct maternal mortality at its core.

Case study: a typical story of unacceptable health care being associated with maternal death

Chifundu attends a rural health centre in Malawi. The midwife is extremely busy, but eventually she diagnoses prolonged labour. An ambulance is called and after several hours she arrives at the hospital, late in the evening. A midwife decides she needs a Caesarean section.

A clinical officer (non-physician clinician) is called in; when he arrives over an hour later, he agrees and theatre is prepared. There is no electricity and it takes time to find fuel for the generator. A healthy baby is delivered; however, the clinical officer struggles to stop Chifundu's bleeding. He has no one to call for help. They try to find a pint of blood, but there is none in the blood bank. They continue to try to save Chifundu but she dies on the operating table. This death could have been prevented with more rapid assessment, a referral and transfer system, and better management of supplies such as blood.

Questions

1. What are the most important causes of direct maternal death?

2. What factors, other than medical issues, contribute to these deaths?

3. What potential strategies could you design to reduce maternal deaths?

Key publications

Say L, Chou D, Gemmill A, et al. (2014). Global causes of maternal death: a WHO systematic analysis. *Lancet Global Health* 2(6): e323–33.
Provides estimates of the causes of maternal deaths worldwide.

World Health Organization (2015). *Trends in Maternal Mortality: 1990 to 2015.* World Health Organization: Geneva.
Presents trends on maternal mortality over the MDG era.

Temmerman M, Khosla R, Laslki L, et al. (2015). Women's health priorities and interventions. *BMJ* h4147–6.
Provides a general overview of maternal health issues.

Thaddeus S and Maine D (1994). Too far to walk: maternal mortality in context. *Social Science & Medicine* 38(8): 1091–110.
A seminal paper reviewing the factors contributing to maternal mortality in the developing world, and outlining the 'Three Delays Model'.

Bibliography

Ana J (2011). Are traditional birth attendants good for improving maternal and perinatal health? Yes. *BMJ* 342: d3310.

Bailey P, Paxton A, Lobis S, and Fry D (2006). The availability of life-saving obstetric services in developing countries: an in-depth look at the signal functions for emergency obstetric care. *International Journal of Gynecology & Obstetrics* 93(3): 285–91.

Draycott T, Sibanda T, Owen L, et al. (2006). Does training in obstetric emergencies improve neonatal outcome? *BJOG* 113(2): 177–82.

Graham W and Campbell O (1992). Maternal health and the measurement trap. *Social Science & Medicine* 35(8): 967–77.

Liang J, Dai L, Zhu J, et al. (2011). Preventable maternal mortality: geographic/rural-urban differences and associated factors from the population-based Maternal Mortality Surveillance System in China. *BMC Public Health* 11(1): 243.

Prost A, Colbourn T, Seward N, et al. (2013). Women's groups practising participatory learning and action to improve maternal and newborn health in low-resource settings: a systematic review and meta-analysis. *Lancet* 381(9879): 1736–46.

Say L and Chou D (2011). Better understanding of maternal deaths—the new WHO cause classification system. *BJOG: An International Journal of Obstetrics & Gynaecology* 118: 15–17.

World Health Organization (2004). *Beyond the Numbers: Reviewing Maternal Deaths and Complications to Make Pregnancy Safer.* World Health Organization: Geneva.

World Health Organization (2004). *Making Pregnancy Safer: the Critical Role of the Skilled Attendant. A Joint Statement by WHO, ICM and FIGO.* World Health Organization: Geneva.

World Health Organization (2011). *WHO Recommendations for Prevention and Ttreatment of Pre-eclampsia and Eclampsia.* World Health Organization: Geneva.

World Health Organization (2012). *The WHO Application of ICD-10 to Deaths During Pregnancy, Childbirth and the Puerperium: ICD-MM.* World Health Organization: Geneva.

World Health Organization (2012). *Safe Abortion: Technical and Policy Guidance for Health Systems.* World Health Organization: Geneva.

CHAPTER 22

Indirect maternal deaths

Heather Lytle, Beatrice Chikaphonya-Phiri, and Abi Merriel

This chapter introduces indirect maternal deaths and briefly discusses late and incidental deaths of pregnant women. It should be read in conjunction with Chapter 21 (Direct maternal deaths) and Chapter 23 (Maternal morbidity).

Key points

◆ Indirect maternal deaths account for an increasing proportion of maternal deaths, particularly in countries with a low overall maternal mortality ratio (MMR).

◆ Indirect deaths have causes rooted in chronic and communicable diseases. This impact is strongest in high-income countries, where over 90% of the indirect deaths are due to pre-existing medical conditions.

◆ Preventing these deaths can be difficult, particularly given that historically the focus has been on direct causes of maternal death. A robust health system is required to identify and treat at-risk women. Further targeted research and interventions are needed to combat these deaths.

Background

Indirect maternal deaths are of increasing significance and account for over a quarter of maternal deaths worldwide. The majority of interventions to prevent maternal deaths to date have focused on addressing direct causes, primarily targeting interventions around the time of delivery. This has reduced maternal mortality, but consequently the relative contribution of indirect causes has increased. In addition, the health status and risk profile of pregnant women is changing. More pregnancies are complicated by women's pre-existing health status and therefore the number of indirect maternal deaths is rising. The human immunodeficiency virus (HIV) epidemic has also been a major cause of indirect maternal mortality.

The role of obstetric transition

Countries with minimal obstetric care and high fertility rates have a high maternal mortality ratio due to both direct and indirect deaths, with most indirect deaths being due to communicable diseases. With improved medical infrastructure and increased uptake of reproductive health services and obstetric care, fertility rates and maternal mortality fall, in particular direct deaths and indirect deaths due to communicable disease. As the country develops economically, the ability to treat chronic conditions in childhood improves. Additionally, as women can access education and family planning they may postpone childbearing. Thus, women are more likely to have pre-existing medical conditions when they become pregnant and indirect non-communicable maternal deaths rise. Consequently, strategies aimed at preventing indirect, non-communicable causes of maternal death will play a larger role in reducing maternal deaths globally from now on.

Global targets

Sustainable Development Goals (SDGs) (2015)

Goal 3 (Health)

◆ Reduce the global maternal mortality ratio to less than 70 per 100,000 live births by 2030.

Why is pregnancy a risk period?

The physiology of a mother is unique during pregnancy (Figure 22.1). Normal physiological changes occur due to hormonal stimuli from the placenta or foetus and are typically well tolerated by healthy women. Some medical conditions, such as autoimmune diseases, like multiple sclerosis or rheumatoid arthritis, can improve during pregnancy. However, physiological changes during pregnancy can worsen some pre-existing health conditions and impact a woman's ability to tolerate new illnesses that develop during pregnancy. For example the volume of blood is increased during pregnancy, meaning that the heart must pump more blood. This increases the risk of mortality from congenital heart malformations, rheumatic heart disease, or cardiovascular diseases. Other chronic diseases such as epilepsy, sickle cell anaemia, asthma, and diabetes can be exacerbated by pregnancy, increasing risks for pregnant women.

Distribution of indirect maternal deaths

In total, indirect deaths account for 27.5% of all maternal deaths. The global trends seen in Figure 22.2 are driven by low- and middle-income countries (LMICs) where the majority of the world's maternal deaths occur, but indirect deaths have a significant impact in both LMICs and high-income countries (HICs).

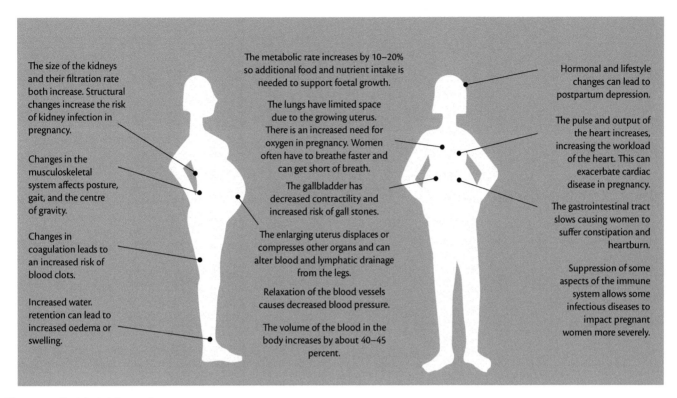

Figure 22.1 Physiological changes that accompany pregnancy.
Reproduced courtesy of the authors.

What causes indirect maternal deaths?

The lack of data about specific causes of indirect maternal mortality means we have limited knowledge on the global impact of many individual diseases leading to indirect deaths. Indirect causes are likely to vary by geographical region, and within and between countries.

Globally, pre-existing medical conditions are responsible for 53.8% of indirect deaths, a further 20% are HIV related, and the remaining 26.2% are due to other causes, such as infectious diseases acquired during pregnancy. In other words, over 70% of indirect maternal deaths worldwide are due to chronic medical conditions, including HIV, that pre-date the pregnancy. This impact is strongest in HICs, where over 90% of the indirect deaths are due to pre-existing medical conditions. In contrast, in sub-Saharan Africa, nearly a third of indirect deaths were due to conditions that arose during pregnancy.

Communicable causes

Pregnant women are at increased risk of mortality from a variety of infectious diseases due to pregnancy-induced changes in the immune response to infection. What are normally non-life threatening illnesses can result in the death of a pregnant woman. The impact of communicable diseases on maternal mortality is largest in LMICs where infectious diseases are more prevalent. The three infectious diseases: influenza, HIV/AIDS (acquired immune deficiency syndrome, and malaria, demonstrate how significantly an area's maternal mortality ratio (MMR) can be impacted by endemic disease, outbreaks, and seasonality.

Influenza

Influenza is a virus causing cough, fever, and systemic symptoms. Mortality in healthy adults is typically low; however, pregnant women are more likely to suffer severe pulmonary complications and death. For example, pregnant women represent 1% of the US population but were responsible for 5% of deaths from the 2009 influenza A(H1N1) epidemic. These deaths also contributed to an overall increase in infection-related maternal deaths during this time, illustrating the effect that disease outbreaks can have on maternal mortality trends. Many countries now recommend influenza vaccination for pregnant women.

HIV/AIDS

HIV is a leading cause of communicable maternal deaths, accounting for 1.6% of total global maternal deaths in 2015. AIDS-related maternal deaths in sub-Saharan Africa have risen from about 1500 in 1990, to 4000 in 2015, with a peak of 12,000 in 2005. While maternal mortality ratios were decreasing in other LMICs between 1990 and 2013, the MMRs of many countries in sub-Saharan Africa increased because of HIV/AIDS. About 85% of the global AIDS-related maternal deaths occur in sub-Saharan Africa. In five countries, HIV accounts for over 10% of all maternal deaths: South Africa, Swaziland, Botswana, Lesotho, and Mozambique.

Malaria

Malaria is caused by an infection of the red blood cells with *Plasmodium* parasites. Annually, more than 25 million pregnant women are at risk of infection. Malaria may be asymptomatic or mild but pregnant women are three times more likely to have severe disease than non-pregnant women. Malaria's disproportionate impact on pregnant

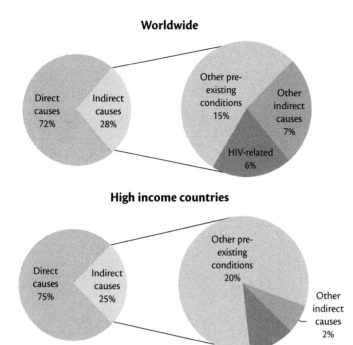

Worldwide

High income countries

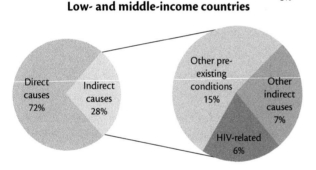

Low- and middle-income countries

Figure 22.2 The distribution of indirect maternal deaths worldwide.
Source: data from Say, L. et al. Global causes of maternal death: a WHO systematic analysis. *The Lancet Global Health*. 2(6), 323–333. Copyright © 2014 World Health Organization. Published by Elsevier Ltd.

women makes it a significant contributor to indirect maternal mortality. Transmission rates vary seasonally or annually, and these variations impact maternal mortality rates. In Rwanda, for example, the most common cause of an indirect maternal death was malaria (7.5%), but with rates fluctuating year by year from 0.5% to 11.2%, in keeping with the general population's malaria morbidity trends.

Non-communicable causes

In regions with high indirect maternal mortality due to chronic conditions, the MMR may indicate the underlying risk profile and health status of reproductive-aged women more than the quality of obstetric care. Cardiovascular disease and sickle cell disease, which are discussed below, exemplify how the underlying health status of pregnant women can impact maternal deaths. Preconception counselling to optimise women's health and comprehensive medical care of pregnant women with chronic conditions is increasingly important as the risk profile of the population of reproductive-aged women changes.

Cardiovascular disease

Cardiovascular diseases are the leading cause of maternal mortality in HICs. For example in the US they are responsible for 14.6% of

maternal deaths. Over 1% of pregnancies in the USA are now complicated by heart disease. The increasing prevalence of risk factors for cardiovascular disease in the pregnant population, including obesity, hypertension, diabetes, and advanced age, plays a significant role, as does the increased survival and fertility of women with congenital heart disease.

Sickle cell disease

Sickle cell disease is a genetic disease affecting red blood cells, which can be fatal without treatment. However, with good supportive medical care, affected girls can survive into adulthood and go on to become pregnant. In Jamaica, improvements in medical care have resulted in more affected, high-risk pregnancies associated with greater maternal mortality. Asnani et al. (2011) found that women have a maternal mortality rate 7–11 times higher than the general population, with sickle cell disease directly causing 41% of their deaths.

Late maternal deaths

Late maternal deaths, which occur between 43 and 365 days after the end of a pregnancy, are often excluded from the traditional definition of maternal mortality. However, they can be due to causes exacerbated by pregnancy, such as malignancy, heart disease, diabetes, and stroke. This could lead to underestimation of the importance of indirect obstetric deaths.

Coincidental deaths

Deaths considered accidental or incidental to the pregnancy, such as those resulting from accidents, homicide, and cancers, are coincidental deaths. Although not considered maternal deaths by classic definitions, and thus not reported in most MMRs, coincidental deaths are important causes of death in some settings. A study in the US by Chang et al. (2005) looking at deaths of women while pregnant or within a year postpartum found that over a quarter of the deaths (27.1%) were related to trauma, with the motor vehicle accidents, homicide, and other unintentional injuries being the leading traumatic events.

Challenges

The increased attention on maternal mortality has resulted in improved data collection relating to maternal deaths. However, much is still unknown. Unfortunately, gaining accurate knowledge about the nature and magnitude of these deaths, particularly indirect deaths, continues to be problematic. In settings without accurate diagnostics, underlying medical conditions may go unrecognised, meaning the correct attribution of cause of death is not possible. In other cases, the pregnancy status may not be mentioned because it was unknown or believed to be unrelated to the death. Even in HICs, underestimation of maternal deaths is common, in part due to failure to properly identify the cause of maternal deaths in the national reporting mechanisms. Use of these imperfectly applied causes of death to determine maternal mortality resulted in underestimation of maternal deaths by 22–93% in one study in the USA and Europe.

An important consideration in HIV/AIDS-related deaths is the difficulty in determining the proportion of deaths that should be classified as maternal versus incidental. Some women may have been dying irrespective of their pregnancy (incidental), whereas for others, pregnancy resulted in their death due to HIV/AIDS (maternal). Furthermore, direct obstetric deaths in HIV positive individuals may be misclassified as indirect if HIV was listed as the cause of death. For example, if an HIV positive woman dies of sepsis, it is the bacterial infection (direct) that killed her, not the HIV (indirect).

Future priorities

◆ Current strategies have largely focused on prevention of direct obstetric deaths. To continue progress toward the SDGs, additional, innovative strategies need to be devised to target indirect maternal deaths.

◆ This requires an improved understanding of the individual causes of indirect maternal deaths.

◆ Strengthening of primary care and health systems is required, as indirect deaths reflect the increase in underlying medical conditions amongst women of reproductive age.

◆ Focus will need to be placed on preconception care so that high-risk women can be identified and assisted to either avoid pregnancy or optimise their health prior to pregnancy.

◆ Universal health coverage is needed to ensure the progress toward improving maternal health leaves no one behind.

Conclusions

Indirect obstetric deaths account for over a quarter of maternal deaths and are becoming increasingly important. Compared to direct causes of maternal deaths relatively little is known about the specifics of indirect maternal mortality. Timely research and increased attention from policy and programme-makers will be necessary to effectively target and prevent indirect maternal deaths.

Case study: a maternal death from a potentially preventable heart attack

Maria, a 42-year-old obese undocumented migrant from Mexico became unexpectedly pregnant while working in the USA. With no health insurance she had not been to see a doctor since arriving ten years previously. Her hypertension, heart disease, and diabetes had gone undiagnosed and untreated. She had little time off work and did not speak English. She had not yet found a clinic to obtain antenatal care. Her immigration status was a pressing concern and so, in the seventh month of her pregnancy, when she began experiencing chest pain, leg swelling, and shortness of breath, she was hesitant to go to the emergency room. Her sister told her that heartburn and swelling are common in pregnancy, so she took some antacids and tried to ignore her problems. Later that evening the pain worsened, she became sweaty and collapsed. Her family called an ambulance and resuscitation was attempted, but she was pronounced dead. Autopsy revealed that her undiagnosed chronic health problems were exacerbated by her pregnancy, leading to heart failure and ultimately death. This was a preventable death, triggered by poor engagement with health care and underlying migration policies, and lack of management of risk factors for indirect maternal death.

Questions

1. How would strategies for reducing indirect maternal deaths differ from those that have focused on reducing direct causes of maternal mortality?

2. What trends are expected in the causes of maternal mortality as a country goes through the 'obstetric transition'?

3. What challenges face researchers who seek to gather additional data on the frequency and causes of indirect maternal deaths?

Key publications

Say L, Chou D, Gemmill A, et al. (2014). Global causes of maternal death: a WHO systematic analysis. *Lancet Global Health* (World Health Organization) 2(6): e323–33.
This recent WHO systematic review of the causes of maternal deaths in 2003–2009 highlighted that indirect maternal deaths are now responsible for over a quarter of global maternal deaths.

Souza J, Tunçalpö, Vogel J, et al. (2014). Obstetric transition: the pathway towards ending preventable maternal deaths. *BJOG, An International Journal of Obstetrics & Gynaecology* 18(121): 1–4.
This commentary introduces readers to the conceptual framework of the 'obstetric transition'.

Bibliography

Asnani M, McCaw-Binns A, and Reid M (2011). Excess risk of maternal death from sickle cell disease in Jamaica: 1998–2007. D Covas (ed.). *PLoS ONE* 6(10): e26281–9.

Chang J, Berg C, Saltzman L, et al. (2005). Homicide: a leading cause of injury deaths among pregnant and postpartum women in the United States, 1991–1999. *Am J Public Health* 95(3): 471–7.

Creanga A, Berg C, Syverson C, et al. (2015). Pregnancy-related mortality in the United States, 2006–2010. *Obstetrics and Gynecology* 125(1): 5–12.

Deneux-Tharaux C, Berg C, Bouvier-Colle M, et al. (2005). Underreporting of pregnancy-related mortality in the United States and Europe. *Obstetrics & Gynaecology* 106(4): 684–92.

Desai M, ter Kuile F, Nosten F, et al. (2007). Epidemiology and burden of malaria in pregnancy. *Lancet Infect Dis* 7(2): 93–104.

Graham W, Woodd S, Byass P, et al. (2016). Diversity and divergence: the dynamic burden of poor maternal health. *Lancet* 388(10056): 2164–75.

Kaaja R (2005). Manifestations of chronic disease during pregnancy. *JAMA* 294(21): 2751.

Kassebaum N, Bertozzi-Villa A, Coggeshall M, et al. (2014). Global, regional, and national levels and causes of maternal mortality during 1990–2013: a systematic analysis for the Global Burden of Disease Study 2013. *Lancet* 384(9947): 980–1004.

Sayinzoga F, Bijlmakers L, van Dillen J, et al. (2016). Maternal death audit in Rwanda 2009–2013: a nationwide facility-based retrospective cohort study. *BMJ Open* 6(1): e009734–9.

Simpson L (2012). Maternal cardiac disease. *Obstetrics and Gynecology* 119(2, Part 1): 345–59.

Siston A, Rasmussen S, Honein M, et al. (2010). Pandemic 2009 influenza A(H1N1) virus illness among pregnant women in the United States. *JAMA* 303(15): 1517–25.

World Health Organization (2012). *The WHO Application of ICD-10 to Deaths During Pregnancy, Childbirth and the Puerperium: ICD-MM.* World Health Organizsation: Geneva.

World Health Organization (2010). *Trends in Maternal Mortality: 1990–2010.* World Health Organization: Geneva.

Zaba B, Calvert C, Marston M, et al. (2013). Effect of HIV infection on pregnancy-related mortality in sub-Saharan Africa: secondary analyses of pooled community-based data from the network for analysing longitudinal population-based HIV/AIDS data on Africa (ALPHA). *Lancet,* 381(9879), 1763–71.

CHAPTER 23

Maternal morbidity

Mary McCauley and Nynke van den Broek

This chapter introduces the concept of maternal morbidity, describes how it is defined and measured, and summarises what is known about the burden of maternal morbidity globally. It should be read in conjunction with Chapters 21 and 22 (Direct and indirect causes of maternal mortality) and Chapter 25 (Maternal mental health).

Key points

- Most pregnancies have positive outcomes for both mother and baby. However, globally up to twenty million women each year experience ill health associated with pregnancy, ranging from mild anaemia to life-threatening conditions, such as obstructed labour.

- There are criteria in place to identify women who have severe acute maternal morbidity and conditions that are life threatening, such as eclampsia. In contrast, identification and support for those with morbidities that are not immediately life threatening, such as fistula, is still largely overlooked.

- There is a global need to further define, understand, and measure non-life-threatening maternal morbidity using a comprehensive, holistic approach in order to inform screening and targeted, effective care packages.

Background

The number of women who die during or after pregnancy and childbirth is often referred to as the 'tip of the iceberg' as it does not represent the overall burden of poor maternal health. The true extent and burden of maternal morbidity is currently unknown, but it is estimated that annually, up to 10% of pregnant women (twenty million) worldwide suffer morbidity related to pregnancy and/or childbirth. There is an assumption that there is a continuum from health to maternal morbidity to life-threatening or severe morbidity and, if undiagnosed or untreated, maternal death (Figure 23.1). However, at present there is a lack of clarity regarding the proportion of women who have either minor maternal morbidity, potentially life-threatening conditions, or severe acute maternal morbidity (SAMM), and of the ratios between these, which will clearly vary depending on the condition in question. Overall it has been suggested that for every woman who dies during or after pregnancy, 20–30 more women will suffer complications, disability, and ill health.

The definition of maternal morbidity, 'any condition that is attributed to, or aggravated by, pregnancy or childbirth which has a negative impact on the woman's wellbeing and/or functioning', is imprecise and does not lend itself to objective study without clearer refinement. It is also extremely broad; a World Health Organization (WHO) working group on maternal morbidity has listed more than 180 diagnoses, divided into 14 organ dysfunction categories, ranging from obstetric to cardiorespiratory and rheumatology conditions.

Non-life-threatening maternal morbidity is a neglected area of research, especially in low- and middle-income countries (LMICs), that deserves attention on a global scale. At present, non-life-threatening maternal morbidity, such as leakage of urine or abnormal vaginal bleeding, which may be recognised at primary level by a healthcare provider or perceived as ill health by the woman herself, is poorly

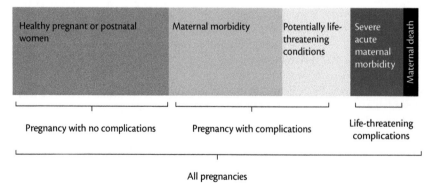

Figure 23.1 Spectrum demonstrating continuum from maternal health to maternal death.

Note: proportions are not known.

Adapted with permission from Say. L, et al. on behalf of the WHO Working Group on Maternal Mortality and Morbidity Classifications. Maternal near miss - towards a standard tool for monitoring quality of maternal health care. *Best Practice & Research Clinical Obstetrics & Gynaecology.* 23(3), 287–296. doi: 10.1016/jbpobgyn.2009.01.007. Copyright © 2009 World Health Organization.

documented. There are no specific global health indicators to measure non-life-threatening maternal morbidity in a way that is comprehensive, standardised, or comparable between country settings.

In contrast, SAMM, or maternal near miss (MNM), is well defined as: 'the case of a woman who nearly died but survived a complication that occurred during pregnancy, childbirth or within 42 days of termination of pregnancy'. It is generally assessed at secondary or tertiary healthcare levels using internationally accepted criteria (Table 23.1). Recent research on maternal morbidity has focused on SAMM and has been used to investigate deficiencies in maternal care as a complementary measure into the investigations of the causes of maternal deaths.

While physical complications during pregnancy and childbirth are recognised as a leading cause of death, disability, and ill health among women of reproductive age, the importance of psychological and social health during and after pregnancy is increasingly being highlighted. This includes issues such as depression, suicidal ideation, domestic violence, and substance misuse. Recognising and addressing all the components of maternal morbidity before they become severe, and improving general maternal health should be international priorities to improve the survival of mothers and their babies and to improve their overall health and wellbeing during and after pregnancy.

The scope of global maternal health targets has been expanded recently, moving from a focus on preventing death to emphasising the importance of health and wellbeing, as evidenced by the Global Strategy for Women's, Children's, and Adolescents' Health (2016–2030). The current international aim is to ensure that every woman in every setting has an equal chance to survive, thrive, and contribute to the transformative change envisioned by the Sustainable Development Goals (SDGs). This is only possible if all women have access to good quality healthcare during and after pregnancy, including screening for all preventable ill health and being treated with evidence-based medicine once the ill health is detected, preventing progression to more serious conditions.

Table 23.1 Severe acute maternal morbidity (SAMM) criteria

Organ system dysfunction	Clinical criteria
Cardiovascular	Shock
	Cardiac arrest (no heart beat and loss of consciousness)
Respiratory	Very fast or very slow breathing
	Turning blue
Kidney	Low urine output that does not respond to fluids or drugs
Blood	Failure to form blood clots
Liver	Jaundice in the presence of pre-eclampsia
Neurological	Any loss of consciousness lasting >12 h
	Coma
	Stroke
	Uncontrollable fits
	Total paralysis
Uterine	Uterine haemorrhage or infection leading to hysterectomy

Global targets

Sustainable Development Goals (2015)

Goal 3 (Health)

♦ Ensure healthy lives and promote wellbeing for all.

Global Strategy for Women's, Children's, and Adolescents' Health (2016–2030)

♦ All women have the right to the highest attainable standard of health and wellbeing, including physical, mental and social aspects.

What is the burden of maternal morbidity?

The Global Burden of Disease Study reported in 2016 that non-fatal dimensions of disease and injury are more important than ever before. However, limited information was available for maternal health specifically. It has been estimated that reproductive ill health accounts for 22% of the global disease burden among women of reproductive age. This is likely to be an underestimate as much of the research assessing maternal morbidity has been carried out in high-level care settings and/or in high-income countries (HICs) and usually refers only to the time around delivery and not to the whole antenatal and postnatal period. There are a few published community-based studies conducted in LMICs in which self-reported maternal morbidity ranges from 12–78%, suggesting a large proportion of women suffer significant ill health during pregnancy and the postnatal period. The limitations of self-reporting are well recognised, but it could be argued that these are signs and symptoms which women themselves consider as significantly contributing to 'non-health' or are associated with an adverse pregnancy outcome.

What causes maternal morbidity?

The causes of maternal morbidity can be mapped to the WHO categorisation of causes of maternal death in the *International Classification of Diseases—Maternal Mortality* (ICD-MM) (Table 23.2). The full extent of how common these conditions are and how these conditions affect the health and wellbeing of women during and after pregnancy is currently unknown.

Normal physiological changes

Some maternal morbidity is due to the normal physiological changes of pregnancy, including nausea and vomiting, heartburn, constipation, breast tenderness, or backache. Nausea and vomiting are both very common, affecting 50% of women (known as 'morning sickness'), although the severe form, hyperemesis gravida only occurs in 0.1–1.0% of pregnancies.

Communicable causes

Urinary tract infection, chorio-amnionitis, endometritis, and mastitis are common infections related to pregnancy. Asymptomatic bacteriuria and urinary tract infection in pregnancy is the most common infective condition, with estimated median rates of 3–35%. Other infective conditions include the following: human immunodeficiency virus (HIV), malaria, tuberculosis, syphilis, dengue fever and Ebola virus, the prevalences of which vary enormously geographically, but are highest in sub-Saharan African countries.

Non-communicable causes

Medical conditions complicating pregnancy include: anaemia, asthma, diabetes, venous thrombosis disease, cardiac disease, liver disease, epilepsy, malnutrition, and obesity. Anaemia in pregnancy is very common, with a global prevalence of 41.8% (affecting an estimated 56.4 million pregnant women per year). Pre-existing hypertension complicates 10–15% of all pregnancies, and asthma affects an estimated 10% of pregnant women globally. The risk of venous thrombosis disease is estimated to be increased five-fold during pregnancy, and up to twenty-fold in the six weeks after pregnancy. Type 1 diabetes mellitus affects an estimated 0.5% and type 2 diabetes mellitus affects 2% of pregnant women. Gestational diabetes is more common, complicating an estimated one in seven births. Epilepsy affects 0.5% of women of childbearing age and is the most common chronic neurological disorder to complicate pregnancy. Pre-existing conditions such as diabetes and epilepsy can increase the risk of maternal and foetal complications, including presenting a risk of teratogenicity from medications. Preconception care is vital to stabilise the condition, review medications, and reduce the risk for mother and child.

Obstetric complications

Obstetric complications can include: hypertensive disorders, haemorrhage, polyhydramnios, intrauterine growth restriction, premature rupture of membranes, threatened preterm labour, preterm birth, malpresentations, multiple pregnancy, obstructed labour, retained placenta, complications of Caesarean section, vaginal tears, wound infections, urinary incontinence, fistulae, postpartum depression, and psychosis.

The current challenge is that the prevalence estimates of many of the conditions that affect the health, wellbeing, and/or functioning of women during and after pregnancy, are derived from high-income countries. Available estimates of global prevalence of obstetric complications include: pre-eclampsia 4.6%, sepsis 2.7–5.2%, prolonged and/or obstructed labour 8.7%, Caesarean section 18.6%, postpartum haemorrhage 10.8%, severe haemorrhage 2.8%, postpartum depression 15%, and incontinence 29–33%. However, these estimates do not represent the prevalence in LMICs. For example a study in Ethiopia by Fantu et al. (2010) found an incidence of obstructed labour of 12.2%. The most common maternal complications in cases of obstruction were uterine rupture, sepsis, haemorrhage, and fistula, and only 45% of the babies were born alive. Obstructed labour is the most common cause of fistula, which affects two million women worldwide (see case study).

Many of the conditions that contribute to maternal morbidity are not routinely screened for during antenatal or postnatal care and are neither recognised nor treated and therefore have the potential to result in more severe ill health and disability.

Table 23.2 Groups of underlying causes of non-life threatening maternal morbidity during and after pregnancy

Type of maternal ill health	Categorisation of maternal death	Possible related morbidities
Direct	Pregnancies with abortive outcome	Complications of abortion, miscarriage, ectopic pregnancy.
Direct	Hypertensive disorders during and after pregnancy	Complications from pregnancy induced hypertension, pre-eclampsia, eclampsia.
Direct	Obstetric haemorrhage	Antenatal and/or postnatal bleeding.
Direct	Pregnancy-related infection	Infection in the womb during or after pregnancy, breast infection.
Direct	Other obstetric complications	Obstructed labour, pre-term labour, complications of breech presentation.
Direct	Unanticipated complications of management	Complications of medical and surgical care, side effects of medication, Caesarean section wound infection.
Indirect	Non-obstetric complications	◆ Cardiac disease ◆ Endocrine conditions ◆ Gastrointestinal tract conditions ◆ Central nervous system conditions ◆ Respiratory conditions ◆ Genitourinary conditions ◆ Autoimmune disorders ◆ Skeletal diseases ◆ Psychiatric disorders ◆ Neoplasms ◆ Infections (HIV, malaria, syphilis, tuberculosis).
Indirect	Psycho-social complications	◆ Depression, anxiety, thoughts of self-harm ◆ Domestic violence ◆ Substance misuse
Unspecified	Unknown /undetermined	Ill health where underlying cause is unknown

Challenges

There are many challenges in measuring maternal morbidity, particularly in LMICs. These include poor health system infrastructures, limited documentation in medical records, and lack of routine data collection. These difficulties are most pronounced for physical and psychosocial morbidities that are not life-threatening and that are in rural areas, as these cases may never present to health services, yet still impact on women's quality of life. A major difficulty in the documentation and understanding of non-life-threatening maternal morbidity has been the lack of a standard methodology for the measurement of this type of maternal morbidity, including both subjective and objective components. Furthermore, while the origins of maternal morbidity lie in pregnancy, the consequences might take several months to manifest themselves, posing a further challenge for data collection. There are new studies underway which will provide better data in future.

Future priorities

◆ Good data on women's wellbeing and morbidity, during and after pregnancy is vital. It should be used to inform targeted, effective antenatal and postnatal care packages, and to support and monitor the implementation of policies such as routine screening for anaemia, diabetes, hypertension, infection, unplanned pregnancy, depression, domestic violence, and substance misuse, both ante- and postnatally.

◆ Agreement must be reached on a narrower definition of maternal morbidity. This could mirror that of maternal mortality, for example limiting the timeframe to forty-two days after the end of the pregnancy, at least in first instance, though recognising that morbidity can continue for months or years after birth. There is a need for qualitative research to enable a better understanding of what women, their families, and their healthcare providers consider maternal morbidity to be, to inform this definition and understand the cultural context of how women report and describe ill health.

◆ Additionally, there is a need for an internationally accepted and user-friendly data collection tool to measure maternal morbidity in a comprehensive and holistic manner. Once such estimates of maternal morbidity are conducted, modelling can be used to develop a composite maternal morbidity score. This would be useful as a baseline measurement at antenatal booking and to monitor changes in a woman's health over time. Subsequent research would be required to assess this score as a clinical outcome measure and a strategic and programmatic key performance indicator in different health systems and in different populations, both in a clinical and research capacity.

Conclusions

It has been estimated that three out of every four women will suffer ill health because of pregnancy. This has a detrimental effect on a women's wellbeing and functioning and is not currently well recognised, documented, or treated. Indeed, there are no specific targets for maternal morbidity in the SDGs.

There have been significant advances in monitoring and improving women's quality of care related to SAMM or 'near miss' events; however, standardised measurements of less severe maternal morbidity are lacking. Better measures to document and monitor maternal morbidity will help inform policy and programme decisions and resource allocations to improve maternal health, especially in LMICs. Better information on women's wellbeing and morbidity during and after pregnancy is important to be able to plan targeted, effective antenatal and postnatal care and education, ensuring that all women to not only survive, but also thrive during and after pregnancy.

Case study: obstructed, unassisted labour leading to obstetric fistula resulting in physical, psychological, and social morbidity

Tigist is an 18-year-old farmer's wife who has travelled a long way to a district general hospital clinic in Ethiopia complaining of leakage of urine, a constant foul smell, and persistent fever. Tigist is exhausted from her difficult journey. She had to borrow money from relatives for the journey to hospital. Tigist tells the doctor that she delivered a stillborn baby boy and lost a lot of blood two months ago after labouring at home for three days. The leakage of urine started soon after the delivery of her dead baby. She has tried to insert herbs and cloth into her vagina to stop the leakage but with no effect. Tigist breaks down and starts to cry, telling the doctor that her husband no longer wants her to be his wife due to the constant foul smell. She has lost hope and does not know if she will ever be well again. Fortunately, the doctor knows a surgeon based in the capital city who is skilled to perform fistula surgery and arrangements are made for Tigist to go to the hospital for specialist care.

Questions

1. What is meant by maternal ill health?

2. How well do current maternal health indicators measure and reflect the health needs of women during and after pregnancy in LMICs?

3. How can existing antenatal and postnatal care packages in LMICs be adapted to meet women's health needs in a holistic approach?

Key publications

Say L, Souza J, Pattinson R, and the WHO working group on Maternal Mortality and Morbidity classifications. (2009). Maternal near miss—towards a standard tool for monitoring quality of maternal health care. *Best Pract Res Clin Obstet Gynaecol* 23: 287–96.
First paper to describe severe acute maternal morbidity.

Firoz T, Chou D, von Dadelszen P, et al., and Maternal Morbidity Working Group (2013). Measuring maternal health: focus on maternal morbidity. *Bull World Health Organ* 91(10): 794–6.
First paper to define maternal morbidity.

Zafar S, Jean-Baptiste R, Rahman A, et al. (2015). Non-life threatening maternal morbidity: cross sectional surveys from Malawi and Pakistan. *PLoS ONE* 10(9): e0138026.
First study to attempt to measure maternal morbidity in a subjective way in low resource settings.

Bibliography

Bang R, Bang A, Reddy M, Deshmukh M, Baitule S, and Filippi V (2004). Maternal morbidity during labour and the puerperium in rural homes and the need for medical attention: a prospective observational study in Gadchiroli, India. *BJOG*111(3): 231–8.

Bhatia J (1995) Levels and determinants of maternal morbidity: results from a community-based study in southern India. *International Journal of Gynecology and Obstetrics* 50(2): S153.

Datta K, Sharma R, Razack P, Ghosh T, and Arora R (1980) Morbidity pattern among rural women in Alwar-Rajasthan—a cohort study. *Health and Population—Perspectives & Issues* 3(4): 282–92.

Fantu S, Segni F, and Alemseged F (2010). Incidence, causes and outcome of obstructed labor in Jimma University Specialized Hospital. *Ethiop J Health Sci* 20(3): 145–51.

Fortney J and Smith J (eds) (1997). *The Base of the Iceberg: Prevalence and Perceptions of Maternal Morbidity in Four Developing Countries: the Maternal Morbidity Network*. Family Health International, Maternal and Neonatal Health Center: Research Triangle Park, NC. Available at: http://pdf.usaid.gov/pdf_docs/Pnacg698.pdf

Nelson-Piercy C (2015). *Handbook of Obstetric Medicine*. Fifth edition. CRC Press: Boca Raton.

Osman-Hassan E (1995). *Study of the Prevalence and Perception of Maternal Morbidity in Menoufeya Governmate, Egypt*. The Egyptian Fertility Care Society: Cairo.

Vos T, Barber R, Bell B, et al. (2015). Global, regional, and national incidence, prevalence, and years lived with disability for 301 acute and chronic diseases and injuries in 188 countries, 1990–2013: a systematic analysis for the Global Burden of Disease Study 2013. *Lancet* 386: 743–800.

World Health Organization (2005) *The World Health Report 2005: Make Every Mother and Child Count*. World Health Organization: Geneva.

World Health Organization (2011). *Evaluating the Quality of Care for Severe Pregnancy Complications: the WHO Near-miss Approach for Maternal Health*. Available at: http://apps.who.int/iris/bitstream/10665/44692/1/9789241502221_eng.pdf

World Health Organization (2016). *Health Statistics and Information Systems*. Available at: http://www.who.int/healthinfo/statistics/indmaternalmortality/en/

CHAPTER 24

Maternal nutrition

Delan Devakumar and Patricia Rondó

This chapter will address the public health importance of improving maternal nutrition for both mother and child in both the short and long term. It should be read in conjunction with Chapter 7 (Developmental Origins of Health and Disease (DOHaD)) and Chapter 37 (Child nutrition).

Key points

◆ Reducing under and over nutrition in pregnancy is important for improving the health of the woman and foetus.

◆ Rapid foetal growth takes place in early pregnancy. Changing this growth trajectory can have an impact not just on the foetus immediately, but also when they become a child, adult, and a parent. This is mediated through epigenetic and hormonal changes.

◆ Improving the overall maternal diet (quantity, diversity, and availability) is paramount, but the ways to do this are still to be elucidated.

Background

Optimising maternal nutrition is important for both mother and offspring for three reasons: it can improve (1) the health of the mother; (2) the health of the foetus; and (3) the long-term health of the child or adult decades later (Figure 24.1). From conception until ideally six months of age, the foetus/infant is dependent on their mother for nutrition. Impaired antenatal nutrition can affect foetal development and growth, increasing the risk of premature birth and birth defects and, in the medium-term, growth and cognitive development.

The link between maternal nutrition and foetal nutrition is mediated by the woman's metabolism and hormonal levels that alter how nutrients are used and stored in the body. Pregnancy places greater demands on the woman in terms of energy requirements and micronutrients. For most well-nourished women, extra food is not needed but in areas where malnutrition is common, changes to the diet may be required. In low-resource settings, women's diets are likely to be deficient in both quantity and quality. Even if women get enough to eat, as in developed countries, they may become malnourished if the food does not provide adequate quantities of micronutrients to meet daily nutritional requirements. For women already suffering from malnutrition or with limited stores of nutrients, pregnancy can lead to deficiency-related disease.

Maternal nutrition is one of the most important environmental cues that result in epigenetic changes in the offspring. It may alter foetal nutrients in the short term but this is unlikely to lead to lasting changes in stores. Long-term effects are due to epigenetic or hormonal changes in the offspring or the result of altered growth trajectories. As described in Chapter 7, the DOHaD hypothesis proposes critical or sensitive periods in early development in which environmental influences can have lasting effects on growth and physiology. Inadequate nutrition can result in stunting and short stature as an adult and is linked to poor educational performance. In women it is a risk factor for complications in labour and Caesarean section.

Improving maternal nutrition should start before conception. The diet needs to meet the requirements of the individual, to respond to the woman's increased demand at different stages of pregnancy and infection or other increases in demands (Table 24.1) and depends on her nutritional status prior to pregnancy (and growth as a child). If the diet does not meet these needs, because of suboptimal energy intake (inadequate or excessive calories) or poor quality, it can result in malnutrition with its subsequent consequences (Table 24.2). For many, especially those in conflict-affected regions of the world, improving food security (i.e. access to food) and dietary diversity is most important, but this is easier said than done (Figure 24.2). In high-income countries improving the quality, not quantity, of food is important.

Global targets

Sustainable Development Goals (SDGs) (2015)

Goal 2 (Hunger and food security)

◆ By 2030, end all forms of malnutrition, including achieving, by 2025, the internationally agreed targets on stunting and wasting in children under five years of age, and address the nutritional needs of adolescent girls, pregnant and lactating women, and older persons.

The World Health Organization (WHO) global nutrition targets 2025 (2014)

Directly related to maternal nutrition:

◆ Achieve a 50% reduction of anaemia in women of reproductive age.

◆ Achieve a 30% reduction in low birthweight.

Indirectly related to maternal nutrition:

◆ Achieve a 40% reduction in the number of children under five who are stunted.

◆ Ensure that there is no increase in childhood overweight.

◆ Reduce and maintain childhood wasting to less than 5%.

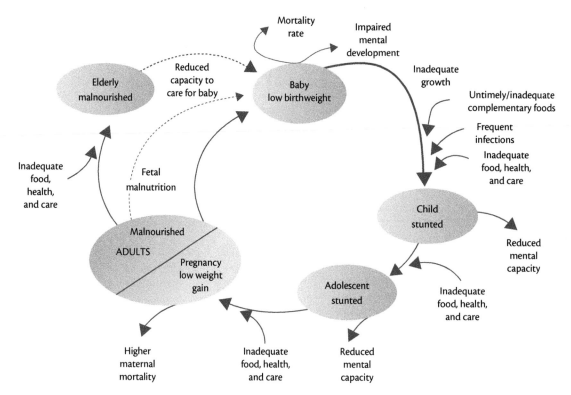

Figure 24.1 Nutrition throughout the lifecycle.
Reproduced with permission from ACC/SCN (2000) Fourth Report on the World Nutrition Situation. Geneva: ACC/SCN in collaboration with IFPRI, https://www.unscn.org/web/archives_resources/files/rwns4.pdf.

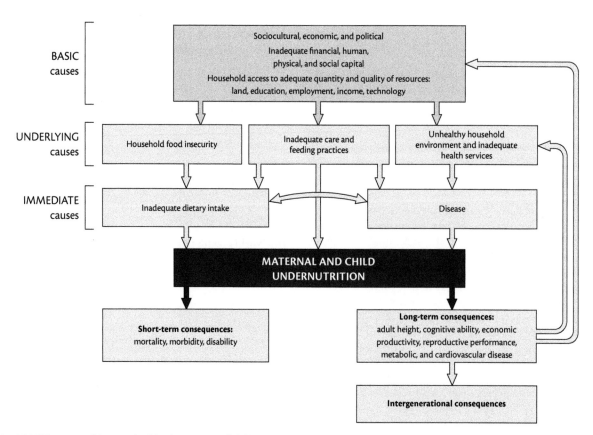

Figure 24.2 UNICEF conceptual framework of the determinants of child nutrition.
Source: data from UNICEF. Improving child nutrition; The achievable imperative for global progress. UNICEF, April 2013. Copyright © 2013 UNICEF.

Table 24.1 Pregnancy requirements

Energy (kcal)	2200–2900
Protein (g)	71
Lysine (mg/kg)	51
Omega-3 fatty acids (g)	1.4
Folate (µg)	600
Iron (mg)	27
Iodine (µg)	200

Table 24.2 Consequences of maternal malnutrition

Mother	Foetus and child
Complications in labour, leading to morbidity and mortality	Miscarriage, stillbirth, and neonatal death
Anaemia	Intrauterine growth restriction
Infection	Infection
Lethargy and weakness	Congenital abnormalities
	Brain damage

Macronutrients

Macronutrients are required for the formation of cells for foetal growth. Nine of the twenty amino acids that are the building blocks for proteins are 'essential', that is, need to be obtained from the diet. Fats are required for energy (15–30% of daily energy intake) and omega-6 and omega-3 fatty acids are essential components in the diet. Extra energy is required during pregnancy for foetal growth and the growth of organs such as the placenta and uterus. Recommendations vary but, for example, the Food and Agriculture Organization/WHO/United Nations University suggest an 85 kcal/day increase in energy intake in the first trimester, followed by 285 kcal/day and 475 kcal/day increases in the second and third trimesters respectively. The exact recommendation for an individual may vary and depends on her starting body mass index (BMI).

In undernourished populations, nutrition education, and balanced energy and protein dietary supplementation are recommended for pregnant women. Many different protein and energy interventions have been tried. The best evidence exists for balanced protein/energy supplementation, where protein provides ~25% of total energy content. Ota et al. (2015) found that this was found to reduce the risk of stillbirth (RR 0.60; 95% CI: 0.39–0.94) and increase birthweight (+40.96 g; 95% CI: 4.66–77.26) with a reduction in small for gestational age (RR 0.79; 95% CI: 0.69–0.90). Receiving nutritional education in pregnancy may lead to increased protein intake, a lower risk of preterm births and, in undernourished women, increase birthweight.

Micronutrients

Micronutrient deficiency is believed to affect approximately two billion people worldwide and pregnant women are at particular risk because of their high metabolic demands. Assessment of micronutrient status is by biomarkers but these can be altered by a number of factors, such as inflammation and infection, and cut-off points are not always clear. Prescription of micronutrients

for women who have a micronutrient deficiency-related disease is clearly of benefit. At a population level, improving nutrition is normally by supplementation or fortification. The WHO currently recommends folic acid and iron supplementation, and calcium and vitamin A in context with deficiency. The main micronutrients are described in Table 24.3. There has been long-standing debate on the benefit of multiple micronutrients supplementation. It has been shown to increase birthweight by a small amount (~50 g) and is hypothesized to lead to future health benefits but the evidence does not support this.

Overweight and obesity

In 2014, more than 1.3 billion adults were overweight and 600 million obese. Rather than being an inert store of energy, fat is a metabolically active tissue, for example increasing the risk of insulin resistance. Overweight or obesity in pregnancy is a risk factor for the mother and child. In the woman, it can increase the risk of glucose intolerance and pre-eclampsia, increasing her risk of diabetes and hypertension respectively in later life. Around the time of labour, there is an increased risk of Caesarean section and postpartum haemorrhage. For the foetus/infant, there is an increased risk of chorioamnionitis, preterm birth, and miscarriage, neural tube malformations, congenital heart defects and gastrointestinal malformations. The increased exposure to sugar leads to an increase in birthweight that can result in birth trauma, for example shoulder dystocia. Longer term, there is increased risk of obesity in the child.

Interventions for obesity include:

◆ Reducing calorie intake (depending on the starting BMI) and ensuring it is of adequate quality.

◆ Exercise: a combination of diet and exercise has been shown in many trials to reduce the risk of excessive gestational weight gain, but generally no difference in other maternal or neonatal outcomes have been observed.

Food safety

The diet of pregnant women needs to be free from bacteria and toxins. In pregnancy there are instances where heavy metals such as mercury, arsenic, lead, and cadmium can have detrimental effects on foetal growth and development. It is important for pregnant women to avoid certain foods, for example fish that contain mercury (such as shark or marlin), soft cheese that may have listeria, and raw eggs that can contain salmonella. Fruit and vegetables need to be washed to remove parasites such as toxoplasmosis.

Paternal nutrition

While this chapter focuses on the nutrition of the mother, it is important to consider improvements in health that can be gained by optimising paternal nutrition. The mother's egg cells are formed before she is born but the sperm cells of the father are created daily. Via epigenetic modifications, sperm cells can react to immediate changes in the environment. Exposure to nutrients and toxins in the sperm and seminal fluid can alter offspring physiology.

Challenges

One of the main challenges is in enabling women in resource-poor settings to get an optimal diet. The reasons for a poor diet can range

Table 24.3 Micronutrients

Micronutrient	What it does	Deficiency-related illness	Intervention (supplementation)
Folate (B$_9$)	Acts a cofactor for many essential cellular reactions, including DNA and nucleic acid synthesis, and is a potent DNA methylser.	Neural tube defects.	Preconception and in early gestation reduces neural tube defects and the associated mortality. Fortification of staples, e.g. flour, cereals
Iron	Needed for oxygen transport and cellular respiration. Found in haemoglobin, myoglobin, enzymes, and cytochromes.	38% of pregnant women have iron deficiency leading to anaemia and it is estimated by Bhutta et al. (2013) to cause 20% of maternal deaths. Deficiency in early pregnancy increases the risk of preterm birth and low birthweight.	Pena-Rosas et al. (2012) found a mean increase in birthweight of 57.7 g (95% CI: 7.7–107.8 g). Treatment for other causes of anaemia, such as hookworm infection, may be required.
Vitamin A	Multiple roles including cell differentiation, immune function, organ and bone formation, and is important for vision, reproduction, and growth.	Deficiency found in 15% of pregnant women, causes night blindness and increases the risk of infection.	Recommendations differ according to the region of world. High-income countries usually do not recommend vitamin A due to the risk of foetal teratogenicity, but it is thought to be advantageous overall in low-income countries. Supplementation can reduce maternal anaemia, night blindness and maternal infection, but does not improve neonatal outcomes.
Iodine	Needed for growth, development, and metabolism, in particular nerve cell growth and synapse formation.	Foetal hypothyroidism can result in intellectual impairment. It is the most common preventable cause of impaired brain development and mental function.	Iodine can be found in seafood but most foods have low quantities. Iodine fortification of food, such as salt, is common worldwide.
Calcium	Acts in nerve and muscle cells, and maintains cell membranes; required for bone mineralisation.	Essential for foetal development and bone formation.	Buppasiri et al. (2015) found an increase in mean birthweight (+56 g) and there is some evidence for a reduction in the proportion of preterm births.
Vitamin D	Needed for bone integrity and calcium homeostasis. Increasingly other functions, such as its effect on immune status are being discovered.	Associated with abnormal foetal bone development, pre-eclampsia and possibly preterm birth.	May reduce the proportion born with low birthweight, increase birth length and head circumference. When combined with calcium could reduce the risk of pre-eclampsia.

from a lack of agricultural production to policies that favour one food over another. While it is clear that improving maternal nutrition is a good thing, the best way to do this is less clear. It is generally believed that improving food security and enabling the population to have a diverse diet at low cost is best. However, this is complicated to achieve and some say supplementation, especially for micronutrients, is the best approach as it can deliver the correct dose. Others argue that mass supplementation cannot be effective. Instead, it is better to respond to clinical manifestations of deficiency. To overcome some of the issues in supplementation, fortification of food has been suggested. This can be done centrally by the manufacturer, or sachets with sprinkles can be provided to families. There is a lack of evidence to indicate if this approach is effective and it is not clear whether adherence to sprinkles is better than supplements. However, it is difficult to maintain both supplementation and fortification programmes on a large scale for an indefinite period. Nutrition education has to be linked with the nutritional programmes, alongside improvements in women's physical and mental health, and with empowerment.

Future priorities

◆ Carrying out more detailed studies into the effects of nutrients on mother and child will allow better understanding of nutritional needs. Coupled with this, there is a need to look at more than just individual nutrients and be more focused on an understanding of assessing and fulfilling overall nutritional needs.

◆ Identifying ways to improve food security to enable a diverse, available, and sustainable diet for all.

◆ It is becoming increasingly important to understand the effects of over-nutrition and the best ways to reduce this.

Conclusions

Improving nutrition before and during pregnancy can break the intergenerational cycle of malnutrition. For the mother it can reduce deficiency-related disease and reduce long-term health risks. For the foetus/newborn improved nutrition can optimise growth in the short term and has long-term health benefits.

Case study: Dutch famine, World War II 1944–45, effects still seen two generations on

The German blockade of food into the Netherlands and the subsequent harsh winter conditions led to a dramatically reduced food supply (rations dropped to 400 calories per person per day). The food supply then improved rapidly after liberation in May 1945. The long-term effects on the children conceived during this time depended on when in gestation it occurred. Those affected in early gestation were found to have a higher risk of coronary heart disease, while those affected in mid to late gestation had reduced glucose tolerance. Peri-conceptional exposure was associated with hypomethylation of the insulin-like growth factor II gene in adults, important in growth-related processes; for example regulating placental growth and nutrient transport. The detrimental effects of the Dutch famine extended into the next generation, with the offspring of women born in the famine found to have lower birthweight.

Questions

1. What are the advantages and disadvantages of focusing on nutrition in pregnancy compared to other time points in the lifecourse?

2. What interventions in pregnancy have been shown to be of benefit in improving maternal and newborn outcomes?

3. What are the pros and cons of:

   a) supplementation with nutrients?

   b) fortification with micronutrients?

Key publications

Abu-Saad K and Fraser D (2010). Maternal nutrition and birth outcomes. *Epidemiologic Reviews* 32: 5–25.

Black R, Victora C, Walker S, et al. (2013). Maternal and child undernutrition and overweight in low-income and middle-income countries. *Lancet* 382: 427–51.
Reviews of maternal nutrition, covering epidemiology and causes of ill health.

Hanson M, Bardsley A, De-Regil L, et al. (2015). The International Federation of Gynecology and Obstetrics (FIGO) recommendations on adolescent, preconception, and maternal nutrition: 'Think Nutrition First'. *International Journal of Gynaecology and Obstetrics* 131(Suppl 4): S213–53.
Comprehensive summary of maternal nutrition and potential interventions.

Mason J, Shrimpton R, Saldanha L, et al. (2014). The first 500 days of life: policies to support maternal nutrition. *Global Health Action* 7: 23623.
Policy implications of changes to maternal nutrition.

Bibliography

Bailey R, West K, Black R, et al. (2015). The epidemiology of global micronutrient deficiencies. *Ann Nutr Metab* 66(Suppl 2): 22–33.

Bhutta Z, Das J, Rizvi A, al. (2013). Evidence-based interventions for improvement of maternal and child nutrition: what can be done and at what cost? *Lancet* 382: 452–77.

Blencowe H, Cousens S, Modell B, and Lawn J (2010). Folic acid to reduce neonatal mortality from neural tube disorders. *Int J Epidemiol* 39(Suppl 1): i110–21.

Buppasiri P, Lumbiganon P, Thinkhamrop J, et al. (2015). Calcium supplementation (other than for preventing or treating hypertension) for improving pregnancy and infant outcomes. *Cochrane Database Systematic Reviews* 2: CD007079.

Curley J, Mashoodh R, and Champagne F (2011). Epigenetics and the origins of paternal effects. *Horm Behav* 59: 306–14.

De-Regil L, Fernandez-Gaxiola A, Dowswell T, and Pena-Rosas J (2010). Effects and safety of periconceptional folate supplementation for preventing birth defects. *Cochrane Database Systematic Reviews* CD007950.

De-Regil L, Palacios C, Lombardo L, and Pena-Rosas J (2016). Vitamin D supplementation for women during pregnancy. *Cochrane Database Systematic Reviews* 1: CD008873.

Fleming T, Watkins A, Velazquez M, Mathers J, Prentice A, Stephenson J, et al. (2018). Origins of lifetime health around the time of conception: causes and consequences. *Lancet* 391: 1842–52.

McCauley M, Van Den Broek N, Dou L, and Othman M (2015). Vitamin A supplementation during pregnancy for maternal and newborn outcomes. *Cochrane Database Systematic Reviews* 10: CD008666.

Muktabhant B, Lawrie T, Lumbiganon P, and Laopaiboon M (2015). Diet or exercise, or both, for preventing excessive weight gain in pregnancy. *Cochrane Database Systematic Reviews* 6: CD007145.

Ota E, Hori H, Mori R, Tobe-Gai R, and Farrar D (2015). Antenatal dietary education and supplementation to increase energy and protein intake. *Cochrane Database Systematic Reviews* 6: CD000032.

Pena-Rosas J, De-Regil L, Dowswell T, and Viteri F (2012). Daily oral iron supplementation during pregnancy. *Cochrane Database Systematic Reviews* 12: CD004736.

Stevens G, Finucane M, De-Regil L, et al. (2013). Global, regional, and national trends in haemoglobin concentration and prevalence of total and severe anaemia in children and pregnant and non-pregnant women for 1995–2011: a systematic analysis of population-representative data. *Lancet Global Health* 1: e16–25.

United Nations Children's Fund (2013). *Improving Child Nutrition: the Achievable Imperative for Global Progress.* UNICEF: New York, US.

Waller D, Shaw G, Rasmussen S, et al. (2007). Prepregnancy obesity as a risk factor for structural birth defects. *Arch Pediatrics & Adol Med* 161: 745–50.

World Health Organization (2016). *WHO Recommendations on Antenatal Care for a Positive Pregnancy Experience.* WHO: Geneva.

World Health Organization (2018). *WHO global database on vitamin A deficiency.* WHO: Geneva.

CHAPTER 25

Maternal mental health

Robert Stewart and Selena Gleadow Ware

This chapter will highlight the importance of maternal mental health, provide an outline of the major clinical conditions and their impact on both the mother and child, and describe bio-psychosocial approaches to intervention. It should be read in conjunction with Chapter 14 (Adolescent mental health), and Chapter 23 (Maternal morbidity).

Key points

♦ Mental health conditions affect one in five women during the perinatal period, and suicide is now the leading cause of maternal death in high-income countries.

♦ Maternal mental illness is associated with adverse maternal and infant outcomes, particularly if no intervention is provided. It has been estimated that the long-term costs of just the perinatal mental health burden across births over one year in the UK is £8.1 billion.

♦ Psychosocial and pharmacological interventions are cost-effective and acceptable. They should be provided, even in low-resource settings.

Background

Efforts to improve global women's, children's, and adolescents' health will not succeed if we do not pay attention to the mental health of mothers. One in five women will experience a mental health problem during pregnancy and/or the postnatal period. This includes depression, anxiety, post-traumatic stress disorder, postpartum psychosis, and exacerbation of pre-existing disorders such as bipolar disorder. The prevalence of perinatal mental health problems is higher in low- and middle-income countries (LMIC) than high-income countries (HICs); this may be because women in LMICs have greater exposure to risk factors such as poverty, violence, malnutrition, and obstetric complications. Stigma and discrimination add to the suffering and impairment.

The consequences of untreated perinatal mental health problems can be catastrophic for both mother and baby. Suicide is a leading cause of maternal death in high-income countries (HICs). In the UK, one in seven women who died between six weeks and one year after pregnancy died from suicide (2011–2013 data). Maternal suicide is also likely to be an important health issue in LMICs, although there is limited current evidence because insufficient attention has been paid to mental disorder in studies of maternal morbidity and mortality. Maternal mental illness can affect foetal and infant growth and development and, in rare cases, severe perinatal mental disorder can lead to infanticide.

Despite the burden of mental illness, up to 90% of people with a mental health problem in LMICs do not have access to appropriate treatment. There are effective evidence-based interventions for perinatal mental disorders, but considerable ongoing efforts will be required to bring these to scale. The World Health Organization (WHO) recommends that maternal mental health is 'integrated into general health care, including women's health, maternal and child health care, reproductive health care, and other relevant services'. Although only one Sustainable Development Goal (SDG) explicitly mentions mental health, SDGs focused on poverty, education, gender equality, child mortality, and maternal health are relevant to maternal mental health.

Global targets
Sustainable Development Goals (2015)
Goal 3 (Health)

♦ 'By 2030, reduce by one third premature mortality from noncommunicable diseases through prevention and treatment, and promote mental health and well-being.'

Psychiatric disorders affecting women during the perinatal period

Table 25.1 summarises the epidemiology and clinical features of perinatal psychiatric disorders. Perinatal depression affects 10–20% of women worldwide and often starts antenatally. Severe depression can lead to infant rejection, abandonment, and neglect. Pregnancy is a natural time of heightened anxiety; for some women this develops into an anxiety or obsessive compulsive disorder. Women with a history of childhood trauma are at increased risk of post-traumatic stress disorder (PTSD). Fear of childbirth- tokophobia-can lead to avoidance of antenatal care. In postpartum psychosis, delusional beliefs may focus on the unborn child or infant (e.g. that the baby is possessed by the devil). During the antenatal and postnatal period, medical complications can mimic mental illness and should be excluded first to prevent fatality.

Aetiology of perinatal mental disorder

Biological, psychological, and social factors interact to determine the risk of onset and persistence of perinatal mental disorders. Genetic factors play a particular role in postpartum psychosis; personal or family history of either postpartum psychosis or bipolar affective disorder increases risk. Other biological factors include rapid changes in reproductive hormones following childbirth, and maternal nutritional deficits, though the results of studies

Table 25.1 Epidemiology and clinical features of maternal mental disorders

	Prevalence	Typical onset	Clinical features
Baby blues	50%	3–5 days postnatal.	Self-limiting emotional distress.
Antenatal depression	11–15%	Continuation of pre-existing episode or onset during pregnancy.	Feelings of guilt; 'thinking too much'; negative thoughts; hopelessness; suicidal ideation.
Postnatal depression	10–20%	6–8 weeks postnatal.	As antenatal depression. Mother-infant relationship may become impaired.
Anxiety disorders	13%	Antenatal or postnatal onset.	Catastrophisation; rumination; feelings of tension, palpitations, and agitation. Marked avoidance.
Obsessive compulsive disorder	2–4% of primiparous women	Antenatal or postnatal onset.	Distressing obsessions (thoughts and images), e.g. fears of illness, contamination. Compulsions such as excessive checking, handwashing; avoidance of potential threats.
Post-traumatic stress disorder	4–6%	Postnatal or pre-existing.	Intrusive images and thoughts of traumatic event.
Tokophobia	Up to 8%	Primary tokophobia may lead to avoidance of pregnancy; secondary tokophobia— following traumatic delivery.	Intense fear and anxiety provoked by thoughts and/or reminders of childbirth.
Postpartum psychosis	1 in 500	Peak onset: first three months postnatally.	Fluctuating symptoms, irritability, elation or depression, hallucinations and delusional beliefs, which can focus on infant.
Delirium and organic causes of mental health symptoms	Determined by prevalence of e.g. infection (inc HIV) haemorrhage, anaemia, pulmonary embolism.	Antenatal or postnatal.	Clouding of consciousness, sudden change in mental state, associated with other signs of physical illness.
Pre-existing major mental disorder	Bipolar affective disorder (1–2% lifetime risk), Schizophrenia (0.5–1% lifetime risk).	May relapse at any time perinatally, but particularly high risk of bipolar affective disorder relapse postnatally.	Relapse can start suddenly and evolve rapidly.

investigating these have been mixed. There is robust evidence that psychosocial stressors are important risk factors for perinatal depression and anxiety. These stressors include a lack of social support, socioeconomic disadvantage, unplanned pregnancy, experience of intimate partner violence, and reproductive and child health problems.

Perinatal mental disorder and child outcomes

Postnatal depression is associated with delay in child cognitive, behavioural, and socio-emotional development. Depressed mothers may be less emotionally sensitive and attuned, leading to apathy and withdrawal among their infants. There is also evidence that antenatal depression and anxiety is associated with heightened risk of mental disorder in the offspring. Antenatal depression is associated with preterm birth and intrauterine growth restriction, with associations more likely to be found in socioeconomically deprived populations. Regarding postnatal growth, a meta-analysis of studies from LMICs by Surkan et al. (2011) showed that children of mothers with depression were more likely to be underweight (OR 1.5; 95% CI 1.2–1.8) or short for their age (OR 1.4; 95% CI 1.2–1.7). Other outcomes associated with perinatal depression/anxiety include prolonged labour, delayed initiation of breastfeeding, and increased infant diarrhoeal illness. Antenatal depression and anxiety may exert an effect on the foetus through physiological pathways (e.g. altered cortisol release) and epigenetic effects, or through

associated lifestyle behaviours (e.g. smoking). Symptoms of depression may lead to functional impairment affecting health care-seeking behaviours, breastfeeding, weaning, and hygiene. The association between infant health and perinatal depression may be bi-directional; caring for a sick child is a significant stressor for postnatal depression.

Interventions

Multi-level intervention is required to improve maternal and infant mental health and mitigate the impact of illness on the mother, infant, and extended family. Table 25.2 outlines examples of interventions.

Awareness raising can make it easier for women and families to seek help, as stigma remains a significant barrier to care. Community-based interventions can influence some of the risk factors for illness, such as intimate partner violence. Effective screening tools for common mental disorders, for example the Edinburgh Postnatal Depression Scale, have been validated in a number of different countries.

Once a maternal mental health condition is suspected, it is important that a woman and her family receive accessible and non-judgemental assessment and care. There is evidence for both psychosocial and pharmacological interventions during the perinatal period. For example, provision of counselling during the antenatal period improves symptoms of depression/anxiety and

Table 25.2 Population interventions for maternal mental health

Type of intervention		Target	Example(s)
Global		Public awareness campaigns.	Anti-stigma campaigns, online resources that enable women and families to recognise illness.
Community		Reduce risk factors for perinatal mental disorder; community-based treatment interventions.	Community-based counselling to improve relationships; peer support for vulnerable women; positive parenting programmes with mental health support component; participatory women's groups.
Primary care	Screening	Improve early detection and assessment of perinatal mental disorder.	Screening programme undertaken by primary care workers, midwives, or health visitors to identify anxiety and depression.
	Management	Optimise early intervention and treatment of mental disorders.	Primary care healthcare workers trained in cognitive behavioural therapy-based intervention.
Secondary care		Specialist mental health services—district or national level.	Mother and baby units for women with postpartum psychosis.

reduces risk of postnatal depression. Participatory women's groups have been demonstrated to improve symptoms of anxiety and depression, alongside improvements in other indicators of maternal and child health. Psychoeducation groups using cognitive behavioural, problem solving, or interpersonal therapy approaches have been found to support recovery. Primary healthcare workers can provide effective treatment for perinatal depression (see case study).

Women experiencing severe mental illness, such as postpartum psychosis, require treatment under specialist supervision and should be able to access psychiatric mother-and-baby units designed to support the mother-infant relationship. Women who have a pre-existing major mental disorder, particularly bipolar affective disorder, should be able to access preconception advice and prophylactic treatment if needed.

Challenges

The greatest challenge to improving maternal mental health is the low priority given to it by governments and other policymakers. Mental health receives less than 1% of health budgets in many countries. This reflects long-standing and entrenched stigmatising beliefs around mental illness. There is also a perception that interventions may not be cost-effective; however, perinatal mental disorder has been estimated to carry a long-term cost to society of £8.1 billion for each one-year cohort of births in the UK, thus easily justifying investment in treatment.

Future priorities

- Investigating the processes that underlie the in-utero and postnatal effects of maternal mental disorder on offspring, including epigenetic effects.
- Interventions shown to improve maternal mood have not had the expected effect on child outcomes so there is a need to refine these to include a greater focus on functioning and mother-infant interaction.

- Globally, a key challenge is to investigate how maternal mental health interventions can be scaled up to reach the 90% of women who do not have access to the treatment they need, thus reducing the suffering and intergenerational impact of these important conditions.

Conclusions

Maternal mental health problems are common, cause significant morbidity and mortality, and have long-term impacts on child development. Evidence-based interventions are available, but not effectively implemented, especially in LMICs. There is an urgent need to integrate mental health into maternal and child health research and service provision.

Case study: managing maternal mental health in a low-resource setting through cognitive behavioural therapy

The Thinking Healthy Programme is a manualised psychological intervention for perinatal depression that can be delivered by non-specialist community health workers in low-resource settings. It is based on the principles of cognitive behavioural therapy, problem solving, and promotion of family support. Rahman et al. (2008) carried out a large randomised controlled trial of the programme in rural Pakistan. The intervention was delivered by female health workers as part of their usual duties. Women receiving treatment were twice as likely to recover than those in the control group. They were also more likely to use contraception and to play with their infants. The infants were more likely to have complete immunisation and had fewer episodes of diarrhoea. The programme has since been adopted by the WHO as a recommended intervention for perinatal depression in LMICs. The case demonstrated how people in rural Pakistan not only engaged with the intended intervention for depression, but also became more widely engaged in health care as result, potentially related to improved mood, and potentially due to greater awareness of healthcare services.

Questions

1. What are the main perinatal mental disorders and what affects their prevalence within a community?

2. What are the potential negative outcomes of perinatal mental disorder for the mothers, their children, and wider society?

3. What interventions for perinatal depression are effective and what resources are required in a country to ensure that women receive appropriate perinatal mental health care?

Key publications

Perinatal mental health Lancet (2014) 384

> Howard L, Molyneaux E, Dennis C, Rochat T, Stein A, and Milgrom J (2014). Non-psychotic mental disorders in the perinatal period. *Lancet* 384(9956): 1775–88.

> Jones I, Chandra P, Dazzan P, and Howard L (2014). Bipolar disorder, affective psychosis, and schizophrenia in pregnancy and the post-partum period. *Lancet* 384(9956): 1789–99.

> Stein A, Pearson R, Goodman S, et al. (2014). Effects of perinatal mental disorders on the foetus and child. *Lancet* 384(9956): 1800–19.
> This series summarises the evidence in relation to the burden of perinatal mental disorders and argues that there can be no health without perinatal mental health.

National Institute for Health and Care Excellence (2014). *Clinical Guideline (CG192) Antenatal and Postnatal Mental Health: Clinical Management and Service Guidance*. NICE: London, UK.
Evidence-based advice on the recognition, assessment, care, and treatment of perinatal mental disorders.

Surkan P, Kennedy C, Hurley K, and Black M (2011). Maternal depression and early childhood growth in developing countries: systematic review and meta-analysis. *Bull World Health Organ* 89(8): 608–15.
This paper synthesises the evidence for the association between maternal depression and child growth in LMICs.

Chowdhary N, Sikander S, Atif N, et al. (2014). Psychosocial interventions for perinatal depression by non-specialist health workers in LMIC: a systematic review. Best *Practice & Research Clinical Obstetrics & Gynaecology* 28(1): 113–33.
This paper reviews the evidence for community-based psychosocial interventions deliverable in LMICs.

Bibliography

Cantwell R, Knight M, Oates M, and Shakespeare J on behalf of the MBRRACE-UK mental health chapter writing group. (2015). Lessons on maternal mental health. In Knight M, Tuffnell D, Kenyon S, Shakespeare J, Gray R, and Kurinczuk J (eds) on behalf of MBRRACE-UK. *Saving Lives, Improving Mothers' Care—Surveillance of Maternal Deaths in the UK 2011–13 and Lessons Learned to Inform Maternity Care from the UK and Ireland Confidential Enquiries into Maternal Deaths and Morbidity 2009–13*. National Perinatal Epidemiology Unit, University of Oxford: Oxford, UK. pp. 22–41.

Centre for Mental Health and London School of Economics (2014). *The Costs of Perinatal Mental Health Problems*. Centre for Mental Health: London.

Fisher J, Cabral de Mello M, Patel V, et al. (2012). Prevalence and determinants of common perinatal mental disorders in women in low- and lower-middle-income countries: a systematic review. *Bull World Health Organ* 90(2): 139G–149G.

Glover V (2014). Maternal depression, anxiety and stress during pregnancy and child outcome; what needs to be done. *Best Practice & Research. Clinical Obstetrics & Gynaecology* 28(1): 25–35.

Grote N, Bridge J, Gavin A, Melville J, Iyengar S, and Katon W (2010). A meta-analysis of depression during pregnancy and the risk of preterm birth, low birth weight, and intrauterine growth restriction. *Archives of General Psychiatry* 67(10): 1012–24.

Honikman S, van Heyningen T, Field S, Baron E, and Tomlinson M (2012). Stepped care for maternal mental health: a case study of the perinatal mental health project in South Africa. *PLoS Med* 9(5): e1001222.

Murray L, Halligan S, and Cooper P (2010). Effects of postnatal depression on mother-infant interactions and child development. In Wachs T and Bremner G (eds). *Handbook of Infant Development*. Wiley-Blackwell: Oxford, UK. pp. 192–220.

Rahman A, Malik A, Sikander S, Roberts C, and Creed F (2008). Cognitive behaviour therapy-based intervention by community health workers for mothers with depression and their infants in rural Pakistan: a cluster-randomised controlled trial. *Lancet* 372(9642): 902–9.

Rahman A, Fisher J, Bower P, et al. (2013). Interventions for common perinatal mental disorders in women in low- and middle-income countries: a systematic review and meta-analysis. *Bull World Health Organ* 91: 593–601.

Rojas G, Fritsch R, Solis J, et al. (2007). Treatment of postnatal depression in low-income mothers in primary care clinics in Santiago, Chile: a randomised controlled trial. *Lancet* 370: 1629–37.

Seng J, Sperlich M, Low L, Ronis D, Muzik M, and Liberzon I (2013). Childhood abuse history, posttraumatic stress disorder, postpartum mental health, and bonding: a prospective cohort study. *Journal of Midwifery & Women's Health* 58: 57–68.

Tripathy P, Nair N, Barnett S, et al. (2010). Effect of a participatory intervention with women's groups on birth outcomes and maternal depression in Jharkhand and Orissa, India: a cluster-randomised controlled trial. *Lancet* 375(9721): 1182–92.

World Health Organization. *Maternal Mental Health*. Available at: http://www.who.int/mental_health/maternal-child/maternal_mental_health/en/.

World Health Organization (2008). *MHGAP: Mental Health Gap Action Programme: Scaling Up Care for Mental, Neurological and Substance Use Disorders*. WHO: Geneva.

CHAPTER 26

Strategies to improve maternal and reproductive health

Address Malata, Jennifer Hall, and Martha Kamanga

This chapter provides an overview of key priorities and strategies to improve maternal and reproductive health and reduce maternal mortality. There are many interventions to enhance the access to and quality of maternal and reproductive health services. However, challenges exist that must be addressed across the continuum of care and within society to create a supportive environment for better maternal health outcomes.

Key points

- Many single interventions are available, but none alone can reduce the rate of maternal mortality in a population—packages of interventions delivered across the continuum of care at high levels of coverage and quality are required.

- Strategies for empowering women in the context of their reproductive and maternal health care must ensure that they not only have the power of decision making but also the availability of affordable options that allows them to exercise their choices.

- Women's access to quality preconception and antenatal care, skilled attendance at childbirth with referral to emergency obstetric services and postnatal care can prevent most maternal deaths and adverse perinatal outcomes, and should be at the heart of the drive to provide universal healthcare coverage.

Background

While there have been significant improvements in maternal health around the world, progress was not fast enough to achieve the Millennium Development Goal (MDG) target on maternal mortality. The Sustainable Development Goal (SDG) target for maternal mortality is highly ambitious, and will require a faster rate of reduction than was achieved between 1990–2015 and is complemented by the breadth of the SDGs, tackling many of the determinants of maternal and child health.

Strategies to improve maternal and reproductive health, such as the Global Strategy for Women's, Children's, and Adolescents' Health (2016–2030), act as a roadmap to ensure that every woman and her newborn survive. The concept of knowing what works is complicated by a huge diversity of country contexts, the broad determinants of maternal health, and the need to improve the health and status of women in general. The strategic objectives of the World Health Organization's (WHO's) strategy for Ending Preventable Maternal

Mortality (EPMM), which should underpin all efforts to improve reproductive, maternal and neonatal health, are:

- Address inequities in access to and quality of sexual, reproductive, maternal, and newborn health care.

- Ensure universal health coverage for comprehensive sexual, reproductive, maternal, and newborn health care.

- Address all causes of maternal mortality, reproductive and maternal morbidities, and related disabilities.

- Strengthen health systems to respond to the needs and priorities of women and girls.

- Ensure accountability to improve quality of care and equity.

The strategy also has guiding principles, such as the empowerment of women, girls, and communities, country ownership, and human rights, and crosscutting actions, such as adequate resources, financing, and measurement systems, to support the achievement of these objectives.

Intervention packages across the continuum of care

To improve maternal health, it is vital that both the whole continuum of care and all levels of health care, from community to tertiary settings are considered, as shown in Figure 26.1. These interventions target adolescent health; reproductive health; care in pregnancy, labour, and childbirth; postnatal maternal and newborn care; and child health care. Further, the theory of change (Figure 26.2) by Darmstadt et al. (2013), identifies a pathway towards impact on maternal and neonatal survival. This theory of change enhances interactions between families and front-line workers which is critical for increasing the effective coverage of life-saving interventions. The theory includes initiatives that work across the continuum, from discovery and development of tools and technologies, to the implementation of delivery strategies that lead to high, equitable, and cost-effective coverage of key interventions. Addressing both supply and demand is also crucial, as is a supportive policy environment.

Preconception

The importance of preconception interventions for improving maternal, perinatal, and neonatal and child health outcomes is being increasingly recognised. In couples who are planning a pregnancy, preconception nutritional status and other lifestyle factors should

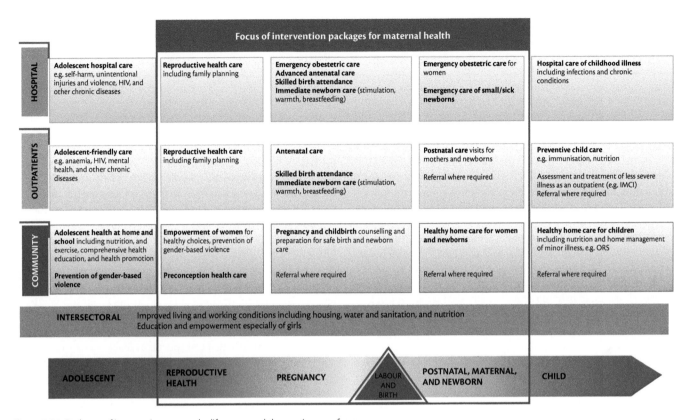

Figure 26.1 Packages of interventions across the lifecourse and the continuum of care.

be optimised. This includes appropriate supplementation, such as folic acid to prevent neural tube defects, stopping or cutting down smoking, alcohol, and substance abuse, optimising the management of any pre-existing conditions, including safe conception for those with human immunodeficiency virus (HIV), and achieving a healthy weight. Undernourished mothers are more likely to give birth to preterm or small for gestational age (SGA) babies, and obese mothers are at increased risk of gestational diabetes and other complications. The uterine environment and sperm condition around conception are increasingly being associated with a

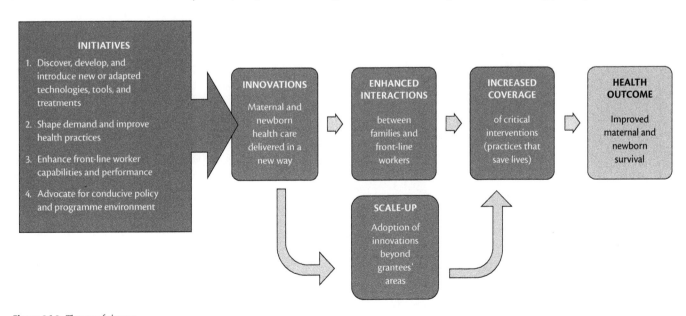

Figure 26.2 Theory of change.

child's long-term health and development, making preconception care an important part of tackling the non-communicable disease agenda. Investigations and treatment for couples experiencing infertility should also be available.

For couples who do not wish to become pregnant, they should be counselled on their family planning options, and testing and treatment for sexually transmitted infections (STIs) should be available. Contraception can delay the age of the first pregnancy, reducing adolescent pregnancies which are high risk for both mother and baby, optimise the spacing of pregnancies (12–60 months), and limit births once desired family size is achieved. Addressing the unmet need for family planning has the potential to prevent 7600 maternal deaths per year and halve the numbers of neonatal deaths and stillbirths, as well as improving the health of other children and allowing adolescents to complete their education. For couples with an unplanned pregnancy, safe abortion services should be available to the full extent possible within the law. Post-abortion care must be provided, regardless of the legality of abortion, to help to reduce the significant contribution of unsafe abortion to maternal mortality.

Pregnancy

Eighty per cent of women receive antenatal care at least once during pregnancy, but only 55% receive the previously recommended minimum of four visits or more (eight visits are now recommended), and the quality of care is often suboptimal. The salient antenatal interventions include the screening and management of infection, particularly malaria, HIV, tuberculosis, syphilis, and other sexually transmitted infections. Malaria can be targeted with intermittent preventive treatment and insecticide-treated

bednets; antiretroviral drugs decrease mother-to-child transmission of HIV; antenatal syphilis screening combined with penicillin treatment can reduce neonatal mortality, preterm births, and stillbirths.

While these, and other interventions during antenatal care, are primarily aimed at improving outcomes for the neonate, as countries progress through the obstetric transition pre-existing chronic diseases, notably diabetes, hypertension, and mental health, require increased attention and management during pregnancy to reduce the risk of indirect maternal deaths and maternal morbidity. For example pregnancy-induced disorders such as hypertensive diseases (hypertension, pre-eclampsia, eclampsia) and gestational diabetes should be assessed for and treated. Administration of magnesium sulphate significantly reduces the risk of eclampsia.

Labour and birth

The day of birth is the most dangerous for mothers and babies, resulting in nearly half of maternal and newborn deaths and stillbirths. Care around the time of birth has the greatest potential for impact, averting 41% of deaths. The most important intervention for safe motherhood is to make sure that a skilled birth attendant is present at every birth, that transport is available to referral services, and that quality emergency obstetric care is available. Birth preparedness, clean birth kits, and education regarding clean birth practices, such as handwashing and the use of sterile cord cutting, can reduce maternal and neonatal tetanus and other infections.

Postnatal care

Postnatal care has long been a gap in the continuum of care (Figure 26.3) but it is important that both women and newborns are

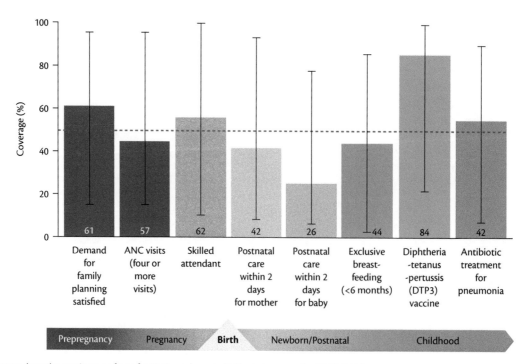

Figure 26.3 Coverage along the continuum of care for 75 Countdown to 2015 priority countries (2007–2012).
Source: Lawn, JE. et al. Born Too Soon: Accelerating actions for prevention and care of 15 million newborns born too soon. *Reproductive Health*. 10(Suppl 1): S6. Copyright © 2013 Lawn et al; licensee BioMed Central Ltd. 2013; and source: data from Requejo, JH. et al. Accountability for maternal, newborn and child survival: The 2013 Update. Geneva: World Health Organization and UNICEF. Copyright © 2013 World Health Organization and UNICEF.

properly assessed and monitored, as many complications occur in the first 24 hours. This is also a crucial time to support the establishment of breastfeeding and address any difficulties with attachment and positioning.

Mother and baby should be examined in the first 24 hours, whether the birth occurred at a facility or at home, and the mother should be advised of the danger signs to be aware of during the postnatal period. For the mother, these include increasing vaginal bleeding, fever, calf pain, shortness of breath, wound infection, or smelly vaginal discharge. The World Health Organization (WHO) recommends that they should also be visited at home by a trained health worker within the first week after birth. At this visit information can be provided on a range of issues, from child care and immunisation schedules to postpartum family planning, hygiene, and feeding, as well as being a chance to address any questions the woman and family may have. In addition, the mother's mental health status should be assessed, and while the 'baby blues' may occur in the first week or two, postnatal depression is more severe, more persistent, and can lead to suicide or infanticide.

Delivery of interventions across the health system

Effective delivery of these interventions requires implementation from community to hospital settings, with strong links between them.

Community care

Improving access to health care is feasible if women are empowered to take decisions about their own health in a supportive environment and can receive care in their own communities, when appropriate. Community-based, demand-side interventions, such as financial incentives/direct subsidies, patient transfer systems, and community involvement such as women's groups (Figure 26.4),

can improve access to and uptake of health care by addressing the first and second delays of the three delay model (delay in danger sign recognition and delay in care seeking) (Chapter 21). To create a supportive environment in which these demand-side strategies can be effective there is an urgent need to address gender-based, decision-making norms, engage in dialogue, and design contextually appropriate communication strategies in collaboration with communities and local leaders. Health promotion messages around hygiene, feeding practices, and danger signs in pregnancy, childbirth, and children can be disseminated at this level.

Facility care

Most sexual and reproductive health services, antenatal, and postnatal care can be delivered through primary care and outreach services.

Skilled attendance for normal delivery should be available at every birth facility. This must be backed up with referral systems and access to emergency obstetric care to reduce the third delay (delay in receiving high-quality, facility-based care) in the three delay model. At primary care level, services should provide Basic Emergency Obstetric Care (BEmOC), which includes the ability to:

1. Administer antibiotics, uterotonic drugs (oxytocin), and anti-convulsants (magnesium sulphate).

2. Manually remove the placenta.

3. Remove retained products after miscarriage or abortion (manual vacuum extraction, dilation, and curettage).

4. Perform assisted vaginal delivery (vacuum extraction, forceps delivery).

5. Perform basic neonatal resuscitation (bag and mask).

Primary care facilities should have referral and transportation systems in place to transfer women to higher level facilities for

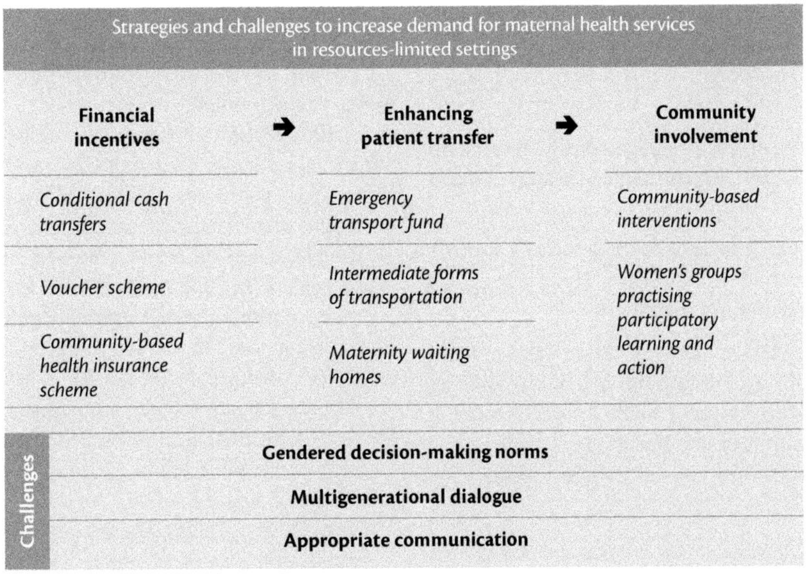

Figure 26.4 Strategies and challenges for maternal health services in resource-limited settings.

Source: Elmusharaf, K. et al. Strategies to increase demand for maternal health services in resource-limited settings: challenges to be addressed. *BMC Public Health* 15(870). https://doi.org/10.1186/s12889-015-2222-3. Copyright © 2015 Elmusharaf et al; licensee BioMed Central Ltd. 2015.

Comprehensive Emergency Obstetric Care (CEmOC), including surgery, such as Caesarean sections, blood transfusions, and the care and resuscitation of sick and low birthweight babies.

Challenges

The focus has often been either on the woman or on her baby; however, a collaborative approach is needed in supporting and managing women and babies together around the time of birth and after birth. Interventions for both mother and baby delivered at the same time, in the same place, and by the same health worker will have the greatest impact on health outcomes. This needs to translate into the integrated design of services, the responsibilities of health workers, and funding. It is also important that neonatal and maternal health estimates converge and are interpreted together.

The shortage of health workers worldwide is a barrier to achieving targeted health goals. The WHO recommends task shifting to increase access to trained and skilled birth attendants. Task shifting is the 'rational redistribution of tasks among health workforce teams'. Specific tasks are moved, where appropriate, from highly qualified health workers to health workers with shorter training and fewer qualifications in order to make more efficient use of available human resources for health. One example of task shifting is the use of clinical officers to conduct Caesarean sections in the absence of obstetricians.

There are challenges in the provision of quality maternal health care at the facility level. There is both 'too little too late', where care is inadequate, inaccessible, and under-resourced, and 'too much too soon', where care is unnecessary, inappropriate, and potentially harmful. As more women give birth in health facilities the issue of 'too much too soon' is increasing, for example in Latin America and the Caribbean over 40% of births are by Caesarean section, which has short and long-term risks and costs.

Future priorities

♦ According to the WHO, factors such as rapid urbanisation, political unrest in conflict areas, changes in fertility rates, or growing numbers of institutional births change the scenario of maternal risk and call for reappraisal of a country's maternal health strategy and programme priorities.

♦ Countries need to identify current programme priorities based on the most frequent causes and determinants of maternal death in their context.

♦ The obstetric transition model can be used to identify a country's current obstetric stage, which in turn indicates which strategies a country can use to make further improvements.

♦ The paradox that it is low-risk women who experience most of the complications, due to the greater number of low-risk women, highlights the urgent need for improvements in the assessment of risk and the early detection of complications. This is linked to understanding the utilisation and content of appropriate antenatal care.

Conclusions

Each year pregnancy and childbirth affects the lives of millions of women and their families. The causes of maternal mortality and morbidity are complex and context specific. Despite making global progress in maternal mortality reduction, countries need to adhere to best practices that are context specific. A global approach that supports implementation of evidence-based care packages for routine care from preconception to the postpartum period, tailored to the setting, is required to impact on maternal and neonatal health outcomes. High-quality care should be safe, effective, woman-centred, timely, efficient, and equitable. Scaling up existing and new health interventions and improving the health systems in most low-income and lower-middle-income countries could reduce maternal deaths to levels seen in the best-performing middle-income countries.

Case study: Mexico's obstetric transition over 30 years

Between 1980 and 2009, Mexico experienced stage 3 of the obstetric transition, a decline in maternal mortality from 124 to 52/100,000 live births, one of the lowest in Latin America.

In the late 1990s to early 2000s two observations were made. First, progress to MDG 5 was slow and inequitable and there were significant problems with the data, and second, more than half of health expenditure was paid out of pocket and this often pushed families further into poverty.

Improving maternal, neonatal, and child health became a priority and in 2001 the *Arranque Parejo en la Vida* (Fair Start in Life) initiative was launched. Specific budget allocations were made to strengthen health services, improve commodity supplies, including blood, and increase the availability of skilled birth attendants. Antenatal care and institutional delivery provision was expanded and the prompt diagnosis and treatment of obstetric emergencies was highlighted. A new system to improve the detection and recording of maternal deaths was established, including clinical audits and verbal autopsy. The national family planning policy was revised and new contraceptive methods, including emergency contraception were made available, despite opposition from the Catholic Church. A wellness model of maternity care covering the whole continuum, from preconception to postnatal, focusing on prevention and wellness to improve birth outcomes and reduce costs, was promoted.

In 2003 legislative reform increased public funding to provide universal health insurance through *Seguro Popular* (Popular Health Insurance), guaranteeing access to over 250 essential interventions as well as cervical and breast cancer treatment.

The National Center of Gender Equity and Reproductive Health was created in 2003, with a mandate to suggest, monitor and evaluate national sexual and reproductive health policies, promoting a gender-sensitive approach to address equality and the position of women in society. In 2003 the first National Survey on Violence against Women found that one in five women had experienced intimate partner violence in the last year, leading to the passing of the general law guaranteeing access for all women to a life free of violence in 2006.

From 2006 to 2007, there was high political commitment to eliminating barriers to reach health services through Healthy Pregnancy Programmes. In 2008, Mexico incorporated national strategies to reduce maternal mortality based on the three delays model: improving detection of complications, timely referral, and receipt of appropriate care, while Universal Coverage of Emergency Obstetric care was achieved in 2009.

As a result of all this, the rate of decline during the period 2000–2009 was significantly faster than 1980–2000 and was also more equitable, due to the strategies that were implemented to promote maternal health during this time. The case study shows how even when the maternal mortality rate is already going down, more can potentially be done to bring it down faster and more equitably.

Questions

1. What are the advantages of having a global versus a national strategy or policy statement on the right of every woman to have access to skilled care at childbirth?

2. What is the ideal antenatal care strategy to maximise maternal mortality reduction?

3. What are the barriers that lead to women dying of preventable disease during pregnancy, labour, and the postpartum period?

Key publications

Chaves S, Cecatti J, Carroli G, et al. (2015). Obstetric transition in the World Health Organization Multicountry Survey on Maternal and Newborn Health: exploring pathways for maternal mortality reduction. *Rev Panam Salud Public*, 37(4/5): 203–10.
This analysis developed the theory of obstetric transition using multicountry data. The Obstetric Transition Model could provide justification for customising strategies for reducing maternal mortality according to a country's stage in the obstetric transition.

Darmstadt G, Marchant T, Claeson M, et al. (2013). A strategy for reducing maternal and newborn deaths by 2015 and beyond. *BMC Pregnancy and Childbirth* 13: 216.
This strategy takes into account current trends in coverage and cause-specific mortality, builds on lessons learned about what works in large-scale implementation programmes, and charts a course to reach those who do not yet access services.

Elmusharaf K, Byrneet E, and O'Donovan D (2015). Strategies to increase demand for maternal health services in resource-limited settings: challenges to be addressed. *BMC Public Health* 15: 870.

This strategy proposes that universal health access will not be achieved unless women are cared for in their own communities and are empowered to take decisions about their own health in a supportive environment.

World Health Organization (2015). *Strategies Toward Ending Preventable Maternal Mortality (EPMM)*. WHO: Geneva.
In this strategy, the WHO stipulates that ending preventable maternal mortality remains an unfinished agenda and one of the world's most critical challenges. Maternal health, wellbeing, and survival must remain a central goal and investment priority in the post-2015 framework for sustainable development.

Bibliography

Campbell O and Graham W (2006). Strategies for reducing maternal mortality: getting on with what works. *Lancet Maternal Survival Series* 368: 1284–99.

Global Campaign for the Health MDGs (2013). Accelerating progress in saving the lives of women and children. http://www.norad.no/en/thematic-areas/global-health/maternal-child-and-womens-health/accelerating-process-2013-report

Hubert C (2013). *Maternal mortality trends in Mexico: state differences*. Population Research Center: University of Texas, Austin, US.

Hunt P and De Mesquita J (2016). *Reducing Maternal Mortality: the Contribution of the Right to the Highest Attainable Standard of Health*. Human Rights Centre: University of Essex, UK. https://www.unfpa.org/sites/default/files/pub-pdf/reducing_mm.pdf

Lozano R, Wang H, Foreman K, et al. (2011). Progress towards Millennium Development Goals 4 and 5 on maternal and child mortality: an updated systematic analysis. *Lancet* 378(9797): 1139–65.

Miller S, Abalos E, Chamillard M, Ciapponi A, Colaci D, Comandé D, et al. (2016). Beyond too little, too late and too much, too soon: a pathway towards evidence-based, respectful maternity care worldwide. *Lancet Maternal Health Series* 388:2176–92.

UNICEF, WHO The World Bank, UNFPA (2012). *Levels and Trends in Child Mortality*. UNICEF: New York, US.

Victora C, Requejo J, Boerma T, et al. on behalf of Countdown to 2030 (2016). Countdown to 2030 for reproductive, maternal, newborn, child, and adolescent health and nutrition. *Lancet Global Health* 4(11), e775–e776.

Villalobos J.(2010). *Strategies to Improve Maternal and Child Health*. Presentation given by the Minister of Health of Mexico at the PMNCH Partner's Forum in New Delhi, India 14 November 2010. http://www.who.int/pmnch/events/partners_forum/3_plenary_cordova.pdf

Newborn health

CHAPTER 27

Introduction to newborn health

Samantha Sadoo, Hannah Blencowe, Shefali Oza, and Joy Lawn

This chapter highlights the trends and policy changes in newborn health over the last few decades, and the ongoing burden of disease.

Key points

- Around 2.6 million babies die in the neonatal period, now accounting for 46% of child deaths under five.

- Sustainable Development Goal (SDG) targets have been set to end preventable neonatal deaths (≤12 neonatal deaths per 1000 livebirths in every country by 2030).

- Over a third of deaths occur on the day of birth; targeting care around the time of birth provides a quadruple return on investment, reducing maternal deaths, stillbirths, and newborn deaths and disability.

- Data regarding neonatal mortality and morbidity need to be strengthened to improve tracking of progress towards SDG targets and to prioritise programmatic action. Currently less than 5% of all neonatal deaths have a death certificate.

Background

Since 1990 and the start of the Millennium Development Goals (MDGs), child and maternal mortality rates have halved worldwide; however, the progress for neonatal mortality has been much slower and neonatal deaths now account for 46% of all child deaths under the age of five. The estimated 2.6 million stillbirths every year were entirely invisible in the MDGs, and rates of reduction have been even slower. Neonatal mortality rates (NMR) vary greatly from <5 deaths per 1000 livebirths in most high-income countries (HICs), to over 40 per 1000 livebirths in some low-income countries (Figure 27.1). Up to three quarters of these deaths could be prevented with public health and low-technology measures.

Where?

The countries with the most neonatal deaths tend to be those with the most births and also with the slowest progress in reducing mortality. 97% of all neonatal deaths occur in low- and middle-income countries, with more than 75% of newborn deaths occurring in South Asia and sub-Saharan Africa (Figure 27.1). More than half of neonatal deaths occur in the five highest burden countries: India, Nigeria, Pakistan, China, and Democratic Republic of Congo. There is often a significant equity gap in countries with a high NMR; addressing this gap will reduce neonatal deaths. South Asia has the highest small for gestational age rates, and sub-Saharan Africa has the highest preterm birth rates. Long-term impairment and disability following neonatal conditions (especially preterm birth) occurs mostly in middle-income countries where there has been a scale up of neonatal intensive care but with varying standards of quality; rates are double that of HICs. However, some countries have achieved rapid reductions in mortality rates, such as Malawi and Saudi Arabia.

When?

Nearly three-quarters of all neonatal deaths are estimated to occur in the first week of life, with a third of all deaths occurring on the day of birth. Labour and childbirth also account for 46% of all maternal deaths and 40% of stillbirths, and this is the time period when babies face the highest risk of disability. Therefore investment in care around the time of birth can achieve the greatest impact, yielding a quadruple return. Alongside crucial timepoints, interventions should be targeted across the lifecourse in order to optimise newborn and stillbirth outcomes.

Why?

Three conditions account for >80% of all neonatal deaths; direct complications of prematurity, intrapartum-related events (previously referred to as birth asphyxia), and infection (Figure 27.2). A further 5% of deaths are due to congenital disorders. Suboptimal intrauterine foetal growth and low birthweight is an important underlying risk factor in many of these deaths. These important causes for neonatal mortality and morbidity will be discussed in detail in the subsequent chapters; see Table 27.1 for an overview. Looking beyond survival, an estimated 1.5 million newborns develop long-term disabilities every year; these can arise from preterm birth, intrapartum-related neurological injury, severe bacterial infection, and severe jaundice.

Who?

Targeting preterm and small babies is crucial, as they account for over 80% of neonatal deaths. Babies who are small, either due to being small for gestational age or prematurity, have an increased risk of death, stunting, and adult-onset, non-communicable diseases. Boys have a higher biological risk; however, girls have a higher risk associated with social practices (including foeticide, infanticide and reduced access to health care).

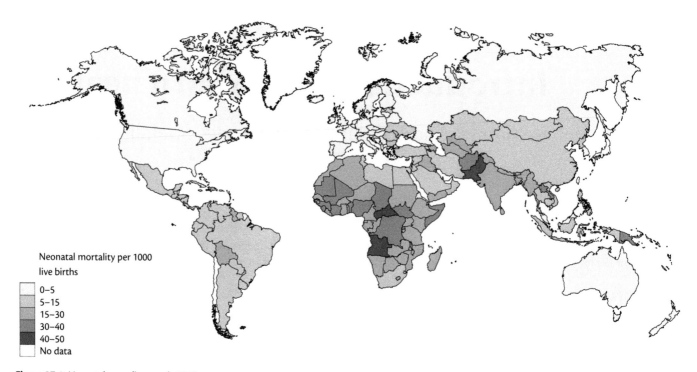

Figure 27.1 Neonatal mortality rates in 2015.

Source: data from UN Inter-agency Group for Child Mortality Estimation (UN IGME). Levels and Trends in Child Mortality, Report 2015: Estimates Developed by the UN Inter-agency Group for Child Mortality Estimation. Copyright © 2015 UN IGME

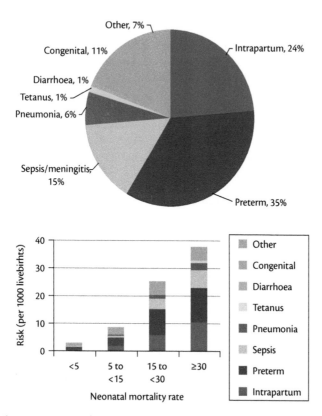

Figure 27.2 Causes of neonatal death worldwide in the year 2015.

Adapted with permission from Lawn, JE. et al. on behalf of Lancet Every Newborn Study Group. Every Newborn: progress, priorities, and potential beyond survival. *The Lancet*. 384(9938), 189–205. doi: 10.1016/S0140-6736(14)60496-7. Copyright © 2014 Elsevier Ltd. All rights reserved.

Policy change and history

During the 1990s, over four million neonatal deaths worldwide each year were neglected on the global health agenda. It was assumed that an improvement in women and children would trickle down to benefit newborn health, and there was a perception that newborn care was technical and expensive, and not feasible for low-resource settings. However, in 1999, Abhay Bang published findings that a community-based package for mothers and newborns in rural India could reduce neonatal mortality by 62%. In 2000, the Bill and Melinda Gates Foundation established the Save the Children's 'Saving Newborn Lives' initiative, aiming to develop evidence, policy, and programmes to improve global newborn survival. In 2003, the *Lancet* published the landmark Child Survival Series, highlighting the burden of newborn deaths, and the gaps in our knowledge regarding the causes of newborn deaths, interventions especially at the community level, and how to deliver newborn care in low-resource settings. Subsequently in 2005, the *Lancet Neonatal Survival Series* discussed the causes, timing, and location of neonatal deaths, and high-impact, cost-effective interventions, about a third of which could be provided through community care. It emphasised that Millennium Development Goal (MDG) 4 for child survival could not be achieved unless greater focus was placed on newborn survival, and therefore called for the integration of newborn health across the continuum of care. Several important policy changes and programmatic shifts occurred during a relatively brief period, for example global guidance from the World Health Organization (WHO) and United Nations Children's Fund (UNICEF) in 2009 on the content and timing of postnatal home visits for newborn care, and recommendations for the implementation of women's groups. Progress had also been made regarding estimates for burden of disease, and evidence for interventions for the three leading causes of newborn deaths; preterm

Table 27.1 Clinical presentations of newborn illness, with long-term mobidity and associated classication of death

Clinical presentation	Long-term morbidity/impairment	Cause of death
Respiratory distress syndrome (RDS), neonatal infections, hyper bilirubinaemia, feeding difficulties; necrotising enterocolitis (NEC), patent ductus arteriosis (PDA)	Cerebral palsy, cognitive impairment, epilepsy, retinopathy of prematurity, chronic lung disease, specific learning needs, mental health disorders	Direct complications of preterm birth
Feeding difficulties, seizures, multi-organ failure	Cerebral palsy, cognitive impairment, epilepsy	Intrapartum related events (birth asphyxia)
Feeding difficulties, seizures, multi-organ failure	Cerebral palsy, cognitive impairment, epilepsy, hearing impairment	Neonatal infections (sepsis, meningitis)

birth, intrapartum-related events, and infection. In 2013, the United Nations Every Woman Every Child movement highlighted that neonatal deaths accounted for an increasing proportion of deaths of children under five, and that country commitments, plans, and budgets had been variable and poorly monitored, and needed more systematic attention and political mobilisation. Where progress in countries had occurred, it had been enabled by strong leadership and partnerships, effective use of data, linking of community and facility-based care, and locally generated and adapted evidence to inform policy and programme design and implementation.

The Every Newborn Action Plan (ENAP) was launched and endorsed by all member countries in a World Health Assembly resolution. The target for neonatal mortality reduction was included in the SDGs, and the target for stillbirth reduction included in the UN strategy for women, children and adolescent health.

Global targets

Sustainable Development Goals (2015)

Goal 3 (Health)

♦ By 2030, end preventable deaths of newborns . . . with all countries aiming to reduce neonatal mortality to at least as low as 12 per 1000 live births.

UN Global Strategy for Women's, Children's, and Adolescents' Health (2016–2030), and ENAP

♦ By 2030, reduce neonatal mortality to at least as low as 12 per 1000 live births.

♦ By 2030, reduce stillbirth rate to at least as low as 12 per 1000 births.

Implications for programme priorities

After decades of research, the burden and causes of neonatal mortality have been identified, and there are cost-effective interventions that are available to address the majority of these deaths. The great challenge is to deliver and scale up these services, and ensure quality of care. Based on the above epidemiology, interventions must be targeted at the main causes of newborn deaths, and a lifecourse approach should be taken to address the entire continuum of care, with a focus on high-impact interventions such as care around the time of birth, and the care of small and sick newborns.

Challenges

The estimates presented in this chapter are based on available data, combined, where necessary, with statistical models. Neonatal

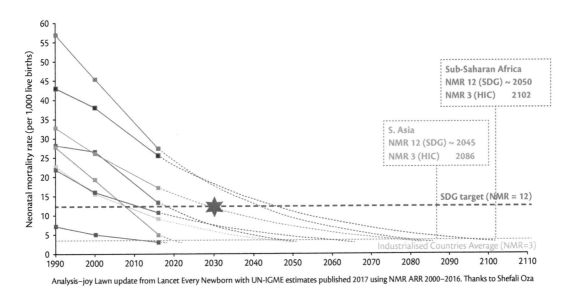

Analysis–joy Lawn update from Lancet Every Newborn with UN-IGME estimates published 2017 using NMR ARR 2000-2016. Thanks to Shefali Oza

Figure 27.3 Global progress towards SDG Goal 3 for neonatal mortality (Blue line = NMR 12; green line = global equity with NMR of 3 as per industrialised countries).

ARR = average annual rate of reduction. NMR = neonatal mortality rate (per 1000 live births)

Source: Lawn JE, et al. Every newborn: progress, priorities, and potential beyond survival. *Lancet* 2014; 384: 189–205. Updated with data from UN Interagency Group for Child Mortality Estimation: Estimates for NMR ARR 2000-2016 (7).

deaths are frequently unrecorded in many countries, especially from high-risk groups such as ethnic minorities and populations affected by conflict. Half of the world's newborns are not registered at birth, and >95% of neonatal deaths and nearly all stillbirths have no death certificate. Data on the rates, distribution, and causes of neonatal deaths need to be strengthened to improve the tracking of coverage and progress towards SDG targets, and to design context-specific community and health system strategies.

Partnerships across the reproductive, maternal, newborn, and child health (RMNCH) continuum of care have been weak, and there has been a tendency towards single-issue advocacy and funding, taking a more vertical commodity-driven approach in which newborn survival has not been a priority. Links with maternal health, family planning, child health, and nutrition are imperative, and have been demonstrated by countries that have been successful in reducing neonatal mortality rates.

Leadership and advocacy for newborn health has been poor. In high-income and middle-income countries, the voices of parents and professional groups (especially neonatologists) have supported the agenda for newborn health. However, in low-income countries, women often do not have powerful voices, and neonatologists are a cadre that does not exist in healthcare systems in much of the world; clinical cadres are often not clear on who is responsible for newborn care.

Looking beyond survival, disability following neonatal conditions is high and occurs mostly in middle-income countries where there has been scale-up of neonatal services without due attention to ensuring quality of care. It is imperative that as the coverage of advanced neonatal care increases, measures to ensure its quality are also implemented and monitored. There is a need for more standardised and simplified assessments of disability, particularly in countries in which neonatal intensive care is expanding.

Future priorities

♦ There is a research gap regarding the prevention and care for preterm birth and poor foetal growth this is important not only to reduce the large burden of deaths in this cohort, but also to reduce the long-term consequences (disability, growth failure, adolescent and adult-onset non-communicable diseases).

♦ Clear indicators and data collection platforms for newborn health need to be developed. Improved vital registration and facility-based information management systems will help to ensure that every birth and death is registered. Audit and feedback mechanisms should be established in institutions to monitor progress and hold health professionals accountable to their practice.

♦ Until recently much of the focus on neonatal health has been on reducing neonatal mortality; however, the three largest causes of death are also important causes of both short-term morbidity and long-term impairment. Greater attention should be placed on monitoring and treating these important outcomes.

Conclusions

The data highlight that the burden of stillbirths, neonatal mortality, and disability is significant and that progress has been lacking. Whilst there has been positive transition with regards to newborn health on the global agenda, from being neglected in the MDGs to being a key element in the RMNCH continuum of care, this needs to translate into action. It requires more investment, political commitment, and attention in policies and programmes, alongside the mobilisation of communities and civil society.

Case study: using perinatal audit to improve birth outcomes and accountability

Perinatal audits can be used at the community, facility, and the national level to inform policy and measure successes. At a community level, trained workers can visit households after a death, and feed back into a data collection system, using verbal and/or social autopsy. At a facility level, each site can collect data on births and deaths, including the causes, with a subset examined in more detail. More in-depth support can be provided through facilities, from a multi-disciplinary team, and with mechanisms to follow up on action points and recommendations from investigation. On a national level, trends can be identified to inform priorities, planning, and resource allocation. This typically involves the health minister, but might go as far as the head of state, and is likely to link multiple professional organisations and stakeholders. National information, in particular, ought to be disseminated at all levels in reports or meetings, with follow-up on recommendations put in place. Having such systems in place at the community, facility, and national level ensures that there is clear identification of the scale of any problem, measurement of the impact of any interventions, and accountability if things go awry.

Questions

1. Why are there such differences in neonatal mortality rates within and between countries?

2. What are the leading causes of newborn death during the neonatal period?

3. What are the most effective packages of care for improving neonatal health?

Key publications

Lawn J, et al. (2014). Lancet Every Newborn Study Group. Every Newborn series. *Lancet* 384.
   The five papers in this important series present the ongoing slow progress in newborn survival and stillbirths, providing new focus beyond survival and setting targets to ensure that every newborn has a healthy start in life.

Healthy Newborn Network: Numbers (http://www.healthynewbornnetwork.org/numbers/)
   This website provides updated global, country, and regional level estimates relating to newborn health.

Bibliography

Darmstadt G, Bhutta Z, and Cousens S (2005). Evidence-based, cost-effective interventions: how many newborn babies can we save? *Lancet* 365(9463): 977–88.

Darmstadt G, Kinney M, Chopra M, et al. (2014). Who has been caring for the baby? *Lancet* 384(9938): 174–88.

de Bernis L, Kinney M, Stones W, et al. (2016). Stillbirths: ending preventable deaths by 2030. *Lancet* 387(10019): 703–16.

Knippenberg R, Lawn J, and Darmstadt G (2005). Systematic scaling up of neonatal care in countries. *Lancet* 365(9464): 1087–98.

Lawn J, Cousens S, and Zupan J (2005). Four million neonatal deaths: When? Where? Why? *Lancet* 365(9462): 891–900.

Lawn J, Cousens S, and Darmstadt G (2006). One year after the Lancet, Neonatal Survival Series—was the call for action heard? *Lancet* 367: 1541–7.

Martines J, Paul V, and Bhutta Z (2005). Neonatal survival: a call for action. *Lancet* 365: 1189–97.

UN Inter-agency Group for Child Mortality Estimation (IGME) (2013). *Levels and Trends in Child Mortality: Report 2013.* UNICEF: New York, US.

CHAPTER 28

Stillbirths

Hannah Blencowe, Samantha Sadoo, and Joy Lawn

This chapter highlights the burden of stillbirths worldwide, the impact of stillbirths on families, the importance of monitoring these deaths, and the available interventions that could prevent most of these deaths.

Key points

- An estimated 2.6 million stillbirths occur annually, 98% in low- and middle-income countries (LMICs).

- Half of all stillbirths occur during labour and birth, and most of these deaths can be prevented through high-quality antenatal and intrapartum care.

- Most result from preventable conditions (contrary to widespread fatalism), such as maternal syphilis and malaria, non-communicable diseases, and obstetric complications.

- Stillbirths have received significantly less policy attention than other maternal and child health outcomes, and work is needed to integrate them into global and national maternal and child health agendas.

- Data on stillbirths need to be improved, applying standard definitions, to track progress towards 2030 targets.

Background

Burden

Stillbirths have been neglected on the global health agenda, being entirely invisible in the Millennium Development Goals (MDGs), and progress has been substantially slower than for maternal mortality, children under five, or neonatal mortality. In 2015 there were an estimated 2.6 million third trimester stillbirths globally; the number has remained unchanged since 2011. Ninety-eight per cent of these were in LMICs, with three quarters in sub-Saharan Africa and South Asia. National stillbirth rates (SBR) range from <5 per 1000 total births in high-income countries to nearly 50 per 1000 in some low-income countries (Figure 28.1). Sub-Saharan Africa has the highest SBR and the slowest rates of progress worldwide. Even in countries where the overall SBR is low, the equity divide is great with regards to ethnicity, age, poverty, and geographical location; 60% occur in rural areas and more than half in conflict and emergency zones, affecting the families most underserved by heath systems. Despite this, there was no target for stillbirths in the Sustainable Development Goals (SDGs).

Causes

Many disorders associated with stillbirths are potentially modifiable and often coexist. These include maternal factors, notably infection such as malaria and syphilis, non-communicable diseases such as diabetes and hypertension, and placental disorders, including pre-eclampsia and eclampsia. Both maternal age >35 years and adolescent pregnancies are at higher risk of stillbirth; short inter-pregnancy intervals are also thought to increase the risk. Also important and modifiable are maternal nutrition-both obesity and undernutrition-, lifestyle factors such as smoking and alcohol use, indoor air pollution, and gender-based violence. Foetal factors such as prolonged pregnancy >42 weeks and rhesus disease can increase the risk of stillbirth. Despite widespread fatalism around stillbirth, less than 10% of stillbirths are due to congenital abnormalities, and some of these are preventable, for example neural tube defects. Half of all stillbirths are estimated to occur during labour, most due to complications of childbirth and are associated with a lack of timely, good-quality intrapartum care. Underlying socioeconomic factors and lack of maternal empowerment and education are also associated with increased risk. Box 28.1 shows the five most important causes of stillbirth. Figure 28.2 shows the number of stillbirths globally, attributed to seven potentially modifiable causes.

Effects

Stillbirths are associated with significant direct, indirect, psychological, and social costs to women, families, society, and governments, which are often underappreciated. These include the costs of medical care and investigation at the time of a stillbirth and in subsequent pregnancies, and funeral and burial costs. There may be an effect on women's physical health, for example if there is a higher risk of obstetric fistula or death. The intangible costs are great; due to the taboo of stillbirths, women frequently feel stigmatised and socially isolated. In some cases they may be subject to abuse and violence, and there may be family and relationship disruption or breakdown. Women are at higher risk of mental health disorders particularly depression, and due to subsequent reduced level of functioning, there may be an effect on employment and productivity.

Global targets

Every Newborn Action Plan (2014) and Global Strategy for Women's, Children's, and Adolescents' Health (2016–2030)

- Less than 12 stillbirths per 1000 total births in every country by 2030.

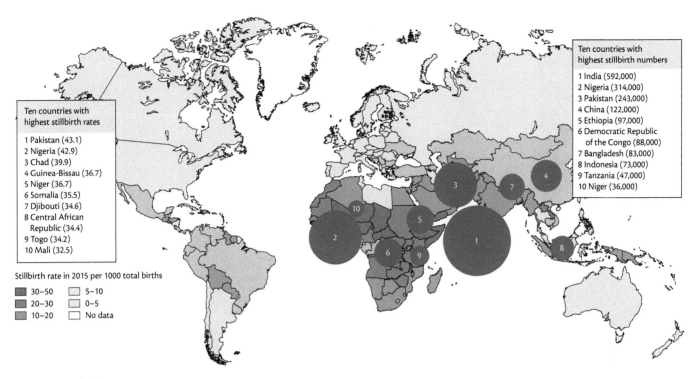

Ten countries with highest stillbirth rates

1 Pakistan (43.1)
2 Nigeria (42.9)
3 Chad (39.9)
4 Guinea-Bissau (36.7)
5 Niger (36.7)
6 Somalia (35.5)
7 Djibouti (34.6)
8 Central African Republic (34.4)
9 Togo (34.2)
10 Mali (32.5)

Ten countries with highest stillbirth numbers

1 India (592,000)
2 Nigeria (314,000)
3 Pakistan (243,000)
4 China (122,000)
5 Ethiopia (97,000)
6 Democratic Republic of the Congo (88,000)
7 Bangladesh (83,000)
8 Indonesia (73,000)
9 Tanzania (47,000)
10 Niger (36,000)

Stillbirth rate in 2015 per 1000 total births

- 30–50
- 20–30
- 10–20
- 5–10
- 0–5
- No data

Figure 28.1 Stillbirth rates in 2015.

Adapted with permission from Lawn, JE. et al. on behalf of The Lancet Ending Preventable Stillbirths Series Study Group with *The Lancet* Stillbirth Epidemiology Investigator Group. Stillbirths: rates, risk factors, and acceleration towards 2030. *The Lancet* 387(10018), 587–603. Copyright © 2016 Elsevier Ltd. All rights reserved.

Interventions

Ambitious change will be required to reach <12 stillbirths per 1000 total births by 2030, with fifty-six countries needing to more than double their progress from 2000–2015. The Global Strategy for Women's, Children's, and Adolescents' Health (2016–2030) identified stillbirths as a neglected area requiring priority action, and included both neonatal mortality rate and stillbirth rate as core indicators; these are to be achieved by 2030.

Ending preventable stillbirths cannot be achieved without an integrated approach, providing interventions across the continuum of care from before conception and throughout the pregnancy to birth. Specific interventions to reduce stillbirths target the major causes of stillbirth (Table 28.1).

Prepregnancy

Interventions before conception involve optimising the nutritional and physical health of the woman, and where possible reducing harmful exposures such as tobacco, alcohol, substance use, and household air pollution. Neural tube defects can be prevented with folic acid supplementation, or fortification requiring a public health approach. Access to family planning (counselling, contraception, safe abortion) can delay, space, and limit pregnancies, all reducing the risk of stillbirth. Community mobilisation and gender empowerment, targeting social discrimination, violence, and unequal access to education and health care, play a role in women's general health and wellbeing and thus can contribute to a reduction of stillbirths; this requires concerted social and political efforts.

Pregnancy

High-impact interventions in pregnancy to reduce stillbirths include the prevention of malaria with insecticide-treated bednets or intermittent preventive treatment, and syphilis detection and treatment with penicillin. The World Health Organization (WHO) recommends eight antenatal care visits; however, optimising the timing and quality of these visits and attention to the disadvantaged, including those with mental health conditions, is vital. Care provided for common non-communicable diseases needs to be improved in low-resource settings, including the 6% of pregnancies complicated by severe hypertensive disorders of pregnancy, and the increasing number of pregnancies affected by pre-existing and gestational diabetes associated with the global epidemic of obesity. Stillbirths due to foetal growth restriction can be reduced by reliable detection and monitoring with serial ultrasound scans, and the availability of timely induction of labour or Caesarean section; however, this is currently not feasible in many settings. Likewise, the management of pregnancies lasting longer than forty-one weeks can reduce stillbirths secondary to an increased risk of placental failure; however, without accurate dating of pregnancies

---

Box 28.1 Major underlying causes for stillbirth.

Complications of childbirth
Maternal infections in pregnancy, e.g. syphilis, malaria
Non-communicable disorders, e.g. hypertension and diabetes
Other placental disorders, e.g. pre-eclampsia
Congenital abnormalities

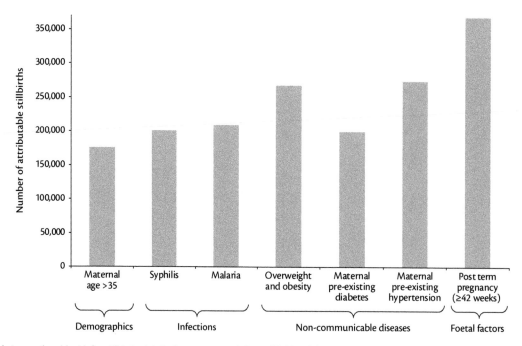

Figure 28.2 Population attributable risk for stillbirth, globally, for seven potentially modifiable risk factors.
Adapted with permission from Lawn, JE. et al. on behalf of The Lancet Ending Preventable Stillbirths Series Study Group with *The Lancet* Stillbirth Epidemiology Investigator Group. Stillbirths: rates, risk factors, and acceleration towards 2030. The Lancet 387(10018), 587–603. Copyright © 2016 Elsevier Ltd. All rights reserved.

Table 28.1 Effective interventions to prevent stillbirths

Period	Intervention	Notes
Preconception	Folic acid supplementation or fortification to reduce neural tube defects	Limited evidence to support the impact as most women commence too late. A public health approach using fortification is recommended.
	Family planning	To delay the first pregnancy, prevent unintended pregnancies in older women, and optimise inter-pregnancy interval.
	Smoking cessation	Addressing other harmful lifestyle factors including alcohol and substance use.
	Optimising the clinical management of maternal pre-existing diseases	Including diabetes, hypertensive disorders, infectious diseases.
Pregnancy	Malaria prevention	Including insecticide treated bednets, and in endemic areas, intermittent preventative treatment.
	Syphilis detection and treatment	One or three doses of penicillin.
	Detection and optimising the clinical management of maternal disorders during pregnancy	Focus to high burden conditions with high morbidity and mortality in mothers and babies, including diabetes and hypertensive disorders of pregnancy.
	Foetal growth restriction detection and management	Routinely undertaken in many high-income countries; currently limited feasibility of screening and management in most low-income settings.
Birth	High-quality respectful intrapartum-care	Including monitoring and timely access to safe emergency obstetric care, including Caesarean section if required.
	Induction of labour for pregnancies lasting >41 weeks	Applicable only in settings with availability of early ultrasound for accurate dating of pregnancies, and safe emergency obstetric care. Without these, there is potential for harm to women and their babies through increased risk of Caesarean section and preterm birth in cases of mistaken gestational age.

through early ultrasound and safe emergency obstetric care, this can be unsafe and worsen outcomes.

Labour and birth

The three delays model developed for maternal deaths is relevant for stillbirths: delays in danger sign recognition, delays in care seeking due to social or economic barriers, distance and lack of transport, and delays in receiving high-quality, facility-based care. High coverage of skilled birth attendance is strongly associated with lower intrapartum stillbirth rates. Availability of timely high quality emergency obstetric care including assisted vaginal delivery or Caesarean section for foetal indication if required can further reduce stillbirth rates.

Psychosocial

Addressing the negative psychosocial consequences of stillbirth can be mitigated through improving the voice of women and openly addressing stillbirths, as well as culturally appropriate respectful care during labour, childbirth, and after death. Providing access to bereavement and support groups, engaging women's rights and mental health groups, and actions to reduce stigma are crucial. Also beneficial are staff who have been trained in providing support and communication following a stillbirth, employers who provide effective leave arrangements, and governments who provide support such as funeral costs and paid leave from work commitments. However, these resources are rarely available outside high-income settings.

Challenges

There has been a false assumption that stillbirths would automatically decline in parallel with maternal and neonatal mortality; this has not been seen in recent trends. It is necessary to have national targets and funding specifically for stillbirth, whilst ensuring its integration within maternal and newborn health plans and research.

Data for stillbirths is currently weak in many high burden settings. There needs to be greater investment in national health information systems and data collection, particularly for registering stillbirths routinely, and tracking the coverage and quality of programmes; present estimates are largely based on household surveys. Additionally, data is needed to assess the stigma associated with stillbirths and to measure the provision of bereavement care and support. Accountability should be improved, for example through perinatal mortality audit, investigating the causes and preventability of stillbirths. Measurable indicators for burden and monitoring, and a universally adopted definition and classification system of stillbirth, are urgently required. Indicators for high quality antenatal and intrapartum care should include antepartum and intrapartum stillbirths respectively.

In the event of any death in pregnancy or childbirth, contextual, respectful, and supportive care is an important yet still neglected component of care. Strengthening the voices of women and the community can help to address issues of stigma associated with stillbirth.

Future priorities

◆ Close the equity divide by supporting governments in their development of strategies to improve access to high quality antenatal and intrapartum care for all women.

◆ We need to improve our understanding of the placental pathways leading to stillbirth and investigate causal pathways of unexplained stillbirth, in order to be able to predict them. We also need to improve methods to avoid stillbirth through the application of tests and development of novel investigations to decide on the optimum timing of delivery.

◆ Enhancing strategies to reduce the prevalence of obesity and smoking in women of reproductive age can help reduce the risk of stillbirth. Further investigation into the effectiveness of primary healthcare prepregnancy visits to improve maternal morbidity and reduce stillbirth will also be beneficial.

◆ Regarding care following a stillbirth, further research is needed into optimising bereavement care, and into improving guidelines for subsequent pregnancy care.

◆ Standardising definitions and classifications of causes of stillbirths will help to strengthen the data needed to develop recommendations, policies, and services to prevent them.

Conclusions

Stillbirths have been neglected on the global agenda, and the burden worldwide remains unacceptably high. Whilst global attention to stillbirths is now increasing, for many countries the accomplishment of the SBR target by 2030 will need concerted efforts. There needs to be a shift in thinking that stillbirths are not inevitable and that many can be prevented through high-quality obstetric care, and integrating stillbirths into the maternal and newborn health agenda. The burden, causes, and costs of stillbirths need to be recognised and monitored with clearer indicators, and research is needed to improve crucial knowledge gaps. This cannot be done without the support, funding, and leadership from governments in collaboration with other stakeholders.

Case study: difficulties in accessing high-quality, facility-based care in rural Nigeria leading to a stillbirth

Abebi is a twenty-one-year-old girl who lives on a farm in rural Nigeria, and became pregnant with her first baby shortly after getting married. At nine months into the pregnancy, she developed stomach cramps whilst at home alone. She managed to walk to the main road, and take a minibus to the nearest facility 5 km away. When she arrived, there was no one available to help, and an hour later she delivered her baby on the floor in the corridor without anyone in attendance. The baby had the cord wrapped around the neck and was pale and not breathing or moving. A midwife eventually came and took her dead baby away. Abebi took a bus home; her husband later blamed her for what had happened. There was a delay in care seeking, and a delay in receiving high-quality, facility-based care, resulting in a potentially preventable stillbirth.

Questions

1. What are the factors that can affect health and survival of the foetus during pregnancy?

2. Why are there such differences in stillbirth rates across countries?

3. What are the challenges faced for researchers estimating the burden and impact of stillbirths worldwide?

Key publications

The Lancet series on Ending Preventable Stillbirths (2016). *Lancet Ending Preventable Stillbirth Studies* 387: 515–716. See: https://www.thelancet.com/series/ending-preventable-stillbirths

The five papers in this series report on the present state of stillbirths, highlight missed opportunities, and identify actions for accelerated progress to end preventable stillbirths.

Bibliography

Allanson E, Tunçalp Ö, Gardosi J, et al. (2016). The WHO application of ICD-10 to deaths during the perinatal period (ICD-PM): results from pilot database testing in South Africa and United Kingdom. *BJOG* 123(12): 2019–28.

Bhutta Z, Das J, Bahl R, et al. (2014). What will it take to avert preventable newborn deaths and stillbirths and at what cost? *Lancet* 384: 347–70.

Blencowe H, Cousens S, Jassir F, et al. (2016). National, regional, and worldwide estimates of stillbirth rates in 2015, with trends from 2000: a systematic analysis. *Lancet Global Health* 4(2): e98–108.

de Bernis L, Kinney M, Stones W, et al. (2016). Stillbirths: ending preventable deaths by 2030. *Lancet Ending Preventable Stillbirth Studies* 387(10019): 703–16.

Flenady V, Wojcieszek A, Middleton P, for the Lancet Ending Preventable Stillbirths study group, and the Lancet Stillbirths In High-Income Countries Investigator Group (2016). Stillbirths: recall to action in high-income countries (2016). *Lancet Ending Preventable Stillbirth Studies* 387: 691–702.

Goldenberg R, McClure E, and Bann C (2009). The relationship of intrapartum and antepartum stillbirth rates to measures of obstetric care in developed and developing countries. *Acta Obstet Gynecol Scand* 86(11): 1303–9.

Goldenberg R, McClure E, Bhutta Z, et al. (2011). Lancet's Stillbirths Series steering committee. Stillbirths: the vision for 2020. *Lancet Ending Preventable Stillbirth Studies* 377(9779): 1798–805.

Harrison M, Ali S, Pasha O, et al. (2015). A prospective population-based study of maternal, fetal, and neonatal outcomes in the setting of prolonged labor, obstructed labor and failure to progress in low- and middle-income countries. *Reprod Health* 12: S9.

Heazell AE, Siassakos D, Blencowe H, et al. (2016). Stillbirths: economic and psychosocial consequences. *Lancet* 387: 604–16.

Kerber K, Mathai M, Lewis G, et al. (2015). Counting every stillbirth and neonatal death to improve quality of care for every pregnant woman and her baby. *BMC Pregnancy & Childbirth* 15: S9.

Lawn J, Blencowe H, Waiswa P, and for the Lancet Ending Preventable Stillbirths Series study group with the Lancet Stillbirth Epidemiology investigator group. Stillbirths: rates, risk factors, and acceleration towards 2030 (2016). *Lancet Ending Preventable Stillbirth Studies* 387: 587–603.

McClure E and Goldenberg R (2009). Stillbirth in developing countries: a review of causes, risk factors and prevention strategies. *J Matern Fetal Neonatal Med* 22(3): 183–90.

Michalow J, Chola L, McGee S, et al. (2015). Triple return on investment: the cost and impact of 13 interventions that could prevent stillbirths and save the lives of mothers and babies in South Africa. *BMC Pregnancy & Childbirth* 15: 39.

Qureshi Z, Millum J, Blencowe H, et al. (2015). A silenced cry: should stillbirth be given greater priority on the global health agenda? *BMJ* 23: 351.

United Nations (2015). *Every Woman Every Child. The Global Strategy for Women's, Children's and Adolescents' Health*. UN: New York, US.

CHAPTER 29

Preterm births

Sarah Moxon, Samantha Sadoo, and Tom Lissauer

This chapter will describe the global health issues relating to prematurity; its epidemiology, clinical features, and some of the health system requirements for immediate and longer-term care to reduce its associated mortality and morbidity.

Key points

◆ Direct complications from preterm birth are now the leading cause of death in children under the age of five.

◆ Prevention of prematurity is complex, with some target interventions available across preconception, antenatal, and obstetric care, but with limited impact.

◆ Improving the care of preterm infants has resulted in major reductions in mortality and disability in high-income countries (HICs), and has a major potential impact in low- and middle-income countries (LMICs), but requires more investment in skilled personnel and robust technology.

◆ When scaling up inpatient care for small and sick newborns, attention must be paid to improving measurement, follow up to prevent/ manage impairment, and providing family support.

Background

Burden

Each year there are approximately fifteen million babies born preterm (before 37 completed weeks). Direct complications of preterm birth are now the leading cause of neonatal mortality, and also child mortality under five, worldwide. They account for over a third of newborn deaths; this comprises 1.1 million deaths a year, and there are approximately a further one million where preterm birth is a risk factor (e.g. for infection). South Asia and sub-Saharan Africa account for 60% of the world's preterm babies, and over three quarters of the world's newborn deaths due to preterm birth complications. Prematurity can lead to a range of long-term sequelae in survivors, including impairment of vision, hearing, and neurodevelopment.

Causes/risk factors

Preterm birth is not a single condition, but a case definition based on one point in time with a wide variety of biological, clinical, behavioural, and social risk factors. Mortality and morbidity are closely related to gestational age, especially in infants less than 32 weeks' gestation. However, 84% of premature babies are moderate to late preterm (i.e. between 32 and 37 weeks of gestation); see Figure 29.1.

The rate of preterm birth is increased by a mix of demographic (mothers age of <20 years or >35 years, short inter-pregnancy interval of <6 months), parity, environmental (lifestyle factors and infections), and genetic factors. Some preterm births are provider-initiated, with early induction of labour or Caesarean section (for medical or non-medical criteria). Other common causes are multiple pregnancy (i.e. twins, triplets or more), pre-existing maternal non-communicable disease such as hypertension, diabetes, and disorders of pregnancy, including pre-eclampsia. However, most preterm births occur spontaneously, with unknown cause in up to half of cases. Estimates of prematurity rates vary widely between countries, from 5% in several European countries to 18% in some African countries, which markedly influences their neonatal mortality rates. Without major reductions in deaths from preterm birth complications, it will be difficult for countries to meet the global targets for child health by 2030.

Global targets

Born Too Soon (2012)

◆ Reduce the preterm-birth attributable mortality by 50% for the period 2010–2025 in all countries with a neonatal mortality rate (NMR) >5 per 1000 live births in 2010 by focusing on equitable, quality care, and minimising long-term impairment.

Every Newborn Action Plan (ENAP) (2015)

◆ Halve hospital deaths of all newborns by 2020.

Interventions

Preterm birthrelated mortality and morbidity can be reduced through clinical interventions targeted across the continuum of care, from optimising preconception and pregnancy care, to postnatal care of a premature baby. With universal coverage (>95%) of these newborn interventions for small and sick newborns, it has been estimated that countries could achieve an 84% reduction in the 1.1 million deaths due to complications of preterm birth. A small proportion of preterm newborns will require more advanced care, such as respiratory support with CPAP (continuous positive airway pressure) and mechanical ventilation. Figure 29.2 summarises health system requirements for small and sick newborns by different levels of care.

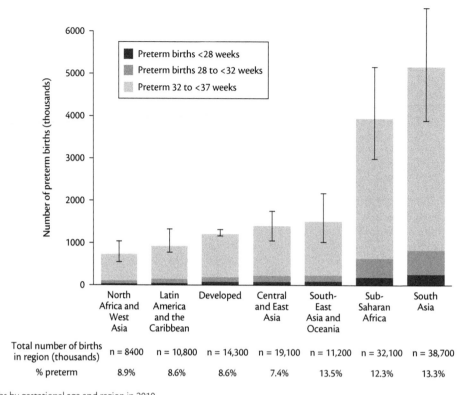

Figure 29.1 Preterm births by gestational age and region in 2010.

Preconception and pregnancy

The greater a woman's standard of health and nutrition before and during pregnancy the greater the chance of a healthy term birth. Monitoring and treatment of pregnancy complications such as pre-eclampsia, infections, smoking, or illicit substance abuse are important for reducing the risk of preterm birth. Family planning in order to reduce the number of pregnancies, adolescent pregnancies, and increase birth spacing can reduce rates of preterm birth. For mothers at higher risk (short cervix on ultrasound and previous spontaneous preterm birth), cervical cerclage or vaginal progesterone are used in HICs, but are not widely available in LMICs, and their potential impact in LMICs has not been determined.

Labour and birth

In preterm labour, administration of antenatal corticosteroids to the mother is standard care in HIC to reduce the risk of breathing difficulties for babies <34 weeks' gestation. In LMICs, the World Health Organization (WHO) recommends steroids for pregnant women at risk of preterm birth at 24–34 weeks' gestation, where this can be accurately assessed, with no clinical evidence of maternal infection, to accelerate lung maturation and reduce the risk of respiratory failure. The use of magnesium sulfate is recommended for women at risk of imminent preterm birth before 32 weeks' gestation, to reduce the risk of cerebral palsy in the infant. Intrapartum antibiotics for preterm premature rupture of the membranes (PPROM) are also recommended to cover an increased risk of infection to the baby. Access to adequate facility care for delivery is essential, with the level of care appropriate to the gestation of the baby (i.e. the more premature the baby, the greater the likelihood of need for more advanced care).

Care of the preterm newborn

Basic newborn care (resuscitation, temperature control, and feeding support)

The more premature the infant, the more likely resuscitation will be required. International guidelines (International Liaison Committee on Resuscitation (LCOR)) have been adapted for low-income countries in the 'Helping Babies Breathe' programme by the American Academy of Pediatrics and partners, which concentrates on effective breathing using a bag and mask.

Preterm babies are vulnerable to hypothermia (especially <32 weeks); they should be delivered into a warm and draught-free environment and placed under a radiant warmer. Every 1°C below normal body temperature on admission to the neonatal unit increases mortality by 28%. They may subsequently require nursing in an incubator if their condition is unstable or they are extremely preterm. Once stable, they can be nursed clothed in cots on heated mattresses or preferably by kangaroo mother care (KMC).

Preterm babies have high nutritional requirements and breast milk should be introduced as soon as possible. Most premature babies under 34 weeks' gestation cannot coordinate sucking and swallowing and need to be fed via gastric tubes followed by a feeding syringe, cup, or spoon. Assistance for the mother is required to successfully express breast milk. Preterm infants may require intravenous fluids whilst milk feeds are established. If this is likely to be prolonged, parenteral nutrition may be needed but this requires intensive care facilities. Fluid requirements will vary depending on gestational and chronological age, clinical condition, and success with feeding. Necrotising entero-colitis, a serious bowel condition in preterm infants, is reduced

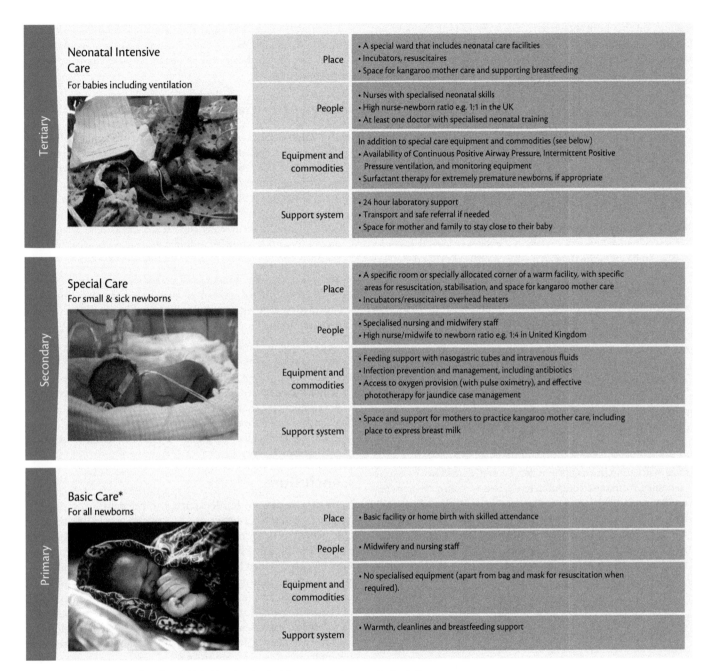

Figure 29.2 Inpatient care of small and sick babies, showing health system requirements by level of care.
Adapted from Lee, AC. Et al. Intrapartum-related neonatal encephalopathy incidence and impairment at regional and global levels for 2010 with trends from 1990. *Pediatric Research.* 74(Suppl 1), 50–72. doi:10.1038/pr.2013.206. Copyright © 2013 Nature Publishing Group. Open Access.

by exclusive breastmilk feeding. Vitamin K should be given at birth to reduce the risk of bleeding, which is higher in preterm compared to term babies. Supplementation is advised for some low birthweight infants with phosphorus, calcium, vitamin D, and iron when older.

Kangaroo mother care

KMC should be initiated in a health facility as soon as the baby is clinically stable. KMC involves continuous direct skin-to-skin contact with the mother (or sometimes other caregiver) to provide warmth, encourage breastfeeding, reduce infection, and promote maternal-infant bonding. Lawn et al. (2010) have shown that KMC leads to a 51% reduction in neonatal mortality for stable babies weighing <2000 g in comparison to conventional care. A Cochrane review by Conde-Agudelo et al. (2011) also reported a 40% reduction in deaths at discharge and approximately 60% reduction in neonatal infections. It may also improve long-term developmental outcomes. Other benefits include a shorter hospital stay and reduced nursing workload. Despite the evidence of its cost-effectiveness, KMC is still under-utilised in most settings.

Alongside KMC, there needs to be greater attention towards 'baby-friendly' care, using a minimal handling approach, maximising comfort, and further increasing the involvement of families in the care of newborns on neonatal units, including feeding. This has been shown to reduce stress of both the newborn and their families, and facilitate greater family confidence to care for the vulnerable infant after discharge from the facility.

Infection prevention and management

Premature babies are particularly vulnerable to infection, either acquired from the mother, at delivery, or after birth. They should be given a course of intravenous antibiotics from birth, according to local guidelines. As preterm babies are handled by many health professionals and often have invasive procedures, for example intravenous lines and blood tests, strict hygiene and infection control procedures are critical. Infections prolong hospital stay and increase the risk of mortality, short and longer-term morbidities.

Respiratory support and more comprehensive care

Surfactant, which lines the airways of the lungs to keep them open, is only produced in the third trimester of pregnancy. Its deficiency results in respiratory distress syndrome, a significant cause of morbidity and mortality in preterm infants. Respiratory support can be provided with additional oxygen therapy or CPAP, where air and oxygen are delivered via nasal cannulae or face mask and pressure is applied to the airway to prevent collapse of the lungs after each breath. Oxygen should be monitored to maintain oxygen saturation at 91–95%. Unregulated use of oxygen must be avoided as it can lead to retinopathy of prematurity, a leading cause of blindness in LMICs. Additional respiratory support can be provided by surfactant therapy but this costly intervention necessitates instilling surfactant directly into the trachea via an endotracheal tube and is not feasible in many settings. Although CPAP provides adequate respiratory support for many preterm infants, some require mechanical ventilation in an appropriately equipped intensive care unit.

Jaundice, from raised bilirubin levels, is more common in premature than term babies, and they are more vulnerable to developing brain damage from kernicterus (bilirubin deposition in the brain). Phototherapy using fluorescent or LED lights is an effective treatment in most instances, and affordable devices to deliver phototherapy are available for use in LMICs.

Beyond survival for preterm babies

Preterm babies are particularly dependent on the quality of care that they receive. This is especially notable in middle-income countries, where neonatal care has been scaled up without due attention to quality of care, and where we see higher rates of preterm survivors with hearing, visual, and neurodevelopmental impairments. The lower the gestational age of the baby at birth, the higher the likelihood of adverse outcomes. Improving the knowledge and skills of neonatal nurses and doctors is crucial. Follow-up programmes should be linked to early child development programmes. Greater emphasis on monitoring service readiness and quality of care is needed with consistent process and outcome data.

Challenges

The successful scale-up of quality facility-based neonatal care requires skilled personnel, especially nurses, robust technology, and a systems approach, which is often lacking in low-resource settings. A greater focus is required on outcomes beyond survival; it is vital to minimise the adverse consequences of prematurity, and to be able to provide the ongoing medical, social, and family support services required.

Controversies exist around the care that should be provided at limits of viability, taking into account the ethical implications and cost; better guidance will be beneficial particularly in lower-resource settings.

Future priorities

- ◆ The identification of preterm birth and assessment of gestational age is a challenge in LMICs, and more accurate simplified methods are needed. The gold standard is first trimester ultrasound dating, but this is often unavailable or unfeasible in lower-income settings. Other methods include calculations based on last menstrual period (which may be uncertain), or examination of the baby after birth using clinical scoring systems, which rely on health worker knowledge and skills and are only accurate to +/- 2 weeks.

- ◆ There is a need for standardised protocols regarding the follow up of premature babies, as well as methods for diagnosing and treating impairment in childhood, with more consistent measures and timing for comparability.

- ◆ More implementation research from LMICs is important in order to scale up high impact interventions such as neonatal resuscitation and KMC. The vast majority of published studies on neonatal care relate to high-technology care in HICs. Greater innovation of care of the premature baby is also needed, including technologies for respiratory support, non-invasive devices for detecting and managing jaundice, and safe administration of antenatal corticosteroids.

Conclusions

There is a significant burden related to prematurity worldwide. Whilst most preterm infants do not require advanced intensive care, there is a need for safe and feasible technologies in order to make rapid progress in LMICs. Inpatient care for preterm newborns requires skilled healthcare providers, especially trained neonatal nurses, a specific place of care with the appropriate equipment and medicines for infants who are unwell or very preterm, and the necessary infrastructure for family-centred care. There is a significant deficiency in research into the prevention of preterm birth, innovative and affordable technology, and monitoring of longer-term outcomes in lower-resource settings.

Case study: Grace in rural Malawi

Grace is thirty-four weeks pregnant. In addition to being underweight and working during her pregnancy, she begins to suffer from hypertension and develops symptoms of premature labour. A community health worker advises Grace to go to a health facility, where she is seen by a clinical officer who gives her a steroid injection. Baby Blessing is born by normal delivery the next day; she weighs 1.5 kg. She is breathing at birth and in good condition but, due to her size and gestational age, the midwife recommends kangaroo mother care. The nurses help Grace to express breastmilk into a clean cup. As Blessing is unable to feed by herself, a nasogastric tube is inserted so that Grace can feed Blessing. Grace has other children at home and staying at the facility is a struggle, but she is able to stay with Blessing in the kangaroo mother care room until she can feed Blessing herself and Blessing has put on weight. Grace is advised to come back to the facility if she has any problems, and has a follow-up appointment in a week's time.

Questions

1. Discuss some of the specific health problems faced by preterm newborns.

2. What is kangaroo mother care, and how effective is it in improving the health outcomes of preterm babies?

3. Discuss the areas relating to preterm birth that require further research or work.

Key publications

Blencowe H, Cousens S, Chou D, et al. (2013). Born Too Soon: The global epidemiology of 15 million preterm birth. *Reproductive Health* 10(Suppl 1): S2.
Updated statistics relating to the burden of preterm birth.

Lawn J, Davidge R, Vinod K, et al. (2013). Born Too Soon: Care for the preterm baby. *Reproductive Health* 10 (Suppl 1): S2.
An important publication on the management of preterm babies focusing on LMICs.

Bibliography

Blencowe H, Cousens S, Oestergaard M, et al. (2012). National, regional, and worldwide estimates of preterm birth rates in the year 2010 with time trends since 1990 for selected countries: a systematic analysis and implications. *Lancet* 379: 2162–72.

Blencowe H, Lee A, Cousens S, et al. (2013). Preterm associated neurodevelopmental impairment estimates at regional and global levels for 2010. Beyond Newborn survival paper 2. Pediatric research. *Nature* 74(1).

Conde-Agudelo A, Belizán J, and Diaz-Rossello J (2011). Kangaroo mother care to reduce morbidity and mortality in low birthweight infants. *Cochrane Database of Systematic Reviews* 16(3): CD002771.

Lawn J.E., Gravett M.G., Nunes T.M., Rubens C.E., and Stanton C. (2010). Global report on preterm birth and stillbirth (1 of 7): definitions, description of the burden and opportunities to improve data. *BMC Pregnancy & Childbirth*, 10(Suppl 1), S.

Lawn J, Blencowe H, Darmstadt G, and Bhutta Z (2013). Beyond newborn survival: the world you are born into determines your risk of disability-free survival. *Pediatric Research* 74: 1–3.

Lawn J, Mwansa-Kambafwile J, Horta B, Barros F, and Cousens S (2010). 'Kangaroo mother care' to prevent neonatal deaths due to preterm birth complications. *International Journal of Epidemiology* 39(Suppl 1): i144–i154.

Lissauer T, Fanaroff A, Miall L, and Fanaroff J (2016). *Neonatalogy at a Glance.* (third Edn). Wiley Blackwell: Oxford, UK.

Lissauer T, Duke T, Mellor K, and Molyneux L (2017) Nasal CPAP for neonatal respiratory support in low and middle-income countries. *Arch Dis Child Fetal Neonatal* 102: F194–6.

Moxon S, Lawn J, Dickson K, et al (2015). Inpatient care of small and sick newborns. *BMC Pregnancy & Childbirth* 15(Suppl 2): S7.

World Health Organization (2014). *Every Newborn: an Action Plan to End Preventable Deaths.* http://apps.who.int/iris/bitstream/10665/127938/1/9789241507448_eng.pdf

CHAPTER 30

Intrapartum-related events affecting the newborn

Saima Aftab, Lauren Schaeffer,
Lian Folger, and Anne CC Lee

This chapter will address the causes, burden, and interventions for intrapartum-related hypoxic events affecting the newborn, previously referred to as 'birth asphyxia'.

Key points

- Hypoxic events during childbirth are a major cause of neonatal mortality and morbidity worldwide, accounting for over 1 million neonatal deaths and 1.3 million stillbirths annually.

- Interventions may be classified into primary prevention (antenatal care and delivery), secondary prevention (neonatal resuscitation), and tertiary prevention (management of a baby with encephalopathy).

- Improving skilled birth attendance and the quality of intrapartum care can substantially improve survival and outcomes in low- and middle-income countries (LMICs).

Background

Burden

Intrapartum-related mortality and morbidity rates are highest in settings with poor access to obstetric and immediate neonatal care. In LMICs, up to half of births occur outside hospital facilities and without a skilled birth attendant (Figure 30.1).

Intrapartum stillbirth

An estimated 1.3 million babies die during childbirth each year. Approximately 98% of these intrapartum stillbirths occur in LMICs, with 75% in sub-Saharan Africa and South Asia alone (Chapter 28).

Need for resuscitation at birth

An estimated 5–10% of babies born each year require some stimulation immediately after birth to help them initiate breathing. Depressed breathing after birth may be due to a multitude of causes, including, but not restricted to, intrapartum hypoxia, respiratory distress syndrome, infection, meconium, and intracranial or neuromuscular disease. An estimated 3–6% of births require basic newborn resuscitation, including providing breaths with a bag and mask (positive pressure ventilation). Much fewer (<1% of births) may require advanced newborn resuscitation, including intubation, chest compressions, or medications.

Intrapartum-related neonatal deaths

Intrapartum-related deaths account for 26% of all newborn deaths, or approximately 691,000 deaths annually. In 2015, intrapartum-related neonatal deaths were the third leading cause of under-five child deaths.

Neurodevelopmental impairment after intrapartum-related events

In 2010, there were an estimated 1.15 million babies who developed neonatal encephalopathy (NE) associated with intrapartum events, with 96% of them in LMICs. Of those babies, 233,000 developed moderate to severe neurodevelopmental impairment and 181,000 developed milder impairments. Intrapartum-related conditions accounted for 67.9 million disability adjusted life years (DALYs) and 3.8 million years lived with disability in 2010.

Causes/risk factors

Risk factors for intrapartum-related stillbirths and/or perinatal deaths are shown in Table 30.1. The strongest predictors of poor outcomes are complications during childbirth, such as malpresentation (breech), obstructed labour, or maternal fever during labour, which carry up to eighty-five-fold increased risk of mortality. Complications in the antenatal period also carry higher risk, such as maternal hypertensive disorders, anaemia, or infections. Preconception factors are also risk factors, such as young maternal age, first pregnancy, and short maternal stature. Causes of intrapartum-related events are shown in Table 30.2. These are stratified by maternal factors (e.g. maternal disease, obstructed labour), placental factors (e.g. cord compression, placental abruption), and neonatal factors (e.g. neonatal disease, medication effect).

Interventions

Primary prevention

Primary prevention includes family planning, women's health before conception (including nutritional status and management of pre-existing diseases), antenatal recognition of at-risk pregnancies, skilled attendance at birth, and, particularly, early recognition and timely management of obstetric complications.

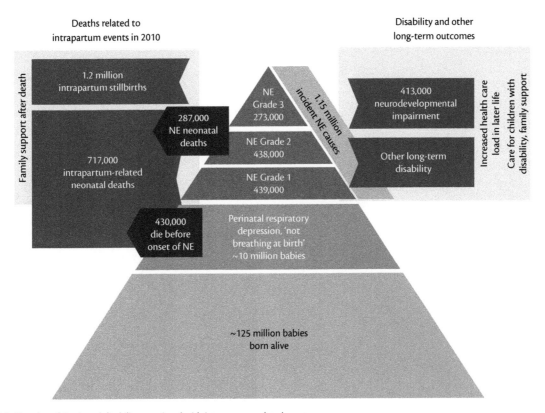

Figure 30.1 Global burden of death and disability associated with intrapartum-related events

NE = neonatal encephalopathy.

Adapted from Lee, AC. et al. Intrapartum-related neonatal encephalopathy incidence and impairment at regional and global levels for 2010 with trends from 1990. *Pediatric Research.* 74(Suppl 1), 50–72. doi:10.1038/pr.2013.206. Copyright © 2013 Nature Publishing Group. Open Access.

Antenatal screening

An important aspect of prevention of birth asphyxia, another term for intrapartum hypoxic events, is identifying pregnancies at risk (such as mulitple pregnancy, breech presentation, intrauterine growth restriction). This requires regular antenatal care and education of nurse midwives or skilled birth attendants so that timely referrals can be made to facilities with higher levels of care. The mothers also need to be educated about danger signs and when to seek care (i.e. excessive vaginal bleeding, decreased foetal movement, etc.).

Intrapartum monitoring

Monitoring of the progress of labour and identifying problems early are critical steps to prevent intrapartum hypoxic insults to the baby. Mothers with a multiple pregnancy, breech presentation, complicated labour, or a history of prior stillbirth, should be referred early to tertiary care centres where their labour can be closely monitored and they will have access to assisted vaginal delivery or Caesarean section. Nurses, midwives and skilled birth attendants should be educated and trained on early recognition of complications during labour.

In low-income settings, two feasible methods for monitoring labour include the intermittent monitoring of foetal heart rate and use of the partograph. Intermittent auscultation for foetal heart rates is one method of monitoring foetal status that is performed in low-resource settings with a Pinard stethoscope. Newer devices, such as a hand-held Doppler device, have also been used and may help identify foetal distress and the need for delivery. The partograph (or partogram) is a paper form that is designed to monitor the progress of labour when intrapartum surveillance is not possible and staffing is limited. After the onset of active labour, the form is used to routinely assess the wellbeing of the mother and newborn, and follows the progression of cervical dilation to provide identify if labour is delayed and make recommendations for intervention. While there is not conclusive evidence on the effectiveness of use of the partograph on perinatal mortality, it is commonly used in LMICs. In a large World Health Organization (WHO) study in South-East Asia (1994), use of the partograph was associated with reduced rates of prolonged labour, emergency Caesarean delivery, and stillbirth.

In high-income countries, continuous electronic foetal heart rate monitoring (EFM) and foetal pulse oximetry are used; however, they are not recommended in LMICs for reasons of feasibility and lack of evidence of effectiveness in these settings.

Emergency obstetric care

When labour is obstructed, the mother experiences other pregnancy complications, or the foetus is in distress, rapid access to skilled obstetric delivery may prevent intrapartum hypoxic injury to the foetus. Basic emergency obstetric care (BEmOC) comprises the functions that should be available at first-level facilities that provide childbirth care: parenteral antibiotics, uterotonics, and anticonvulsants; manual removal of the placenta; removal of retained products; assisted vaginal delivery; and basic neonatal resuscitation. Comprehensive emergency obstetric care (CEmOC) is the standard full package of obstetric care including Caesarean section and blood transfusion. BEmOC and CEmOC are estimated to reduce intrapartum-related neonatal mortality by 40% and 85%, respectively.

Table 30.1 Risk factors for intrapartum stillbirths/perinatal deaths

Time period	Risk factor	Range of odds ratios of stillbirth/ perinatal death
Before pregnancy (preconception)	◆ Young maternal age ◆ Maternal underweight and short stature, or overweight ◆ Parity (first pregnancy or parity >6) ◆ Poor obstetric history	1–5
During pregnancy (antenatal)	◆ Multiple pregnancy ◆ Maternal anaemia ◆ Hypertensive disorders ◆ Diabetes ◆ Maternal infectious disease (malaria, syphilis, HIV) ◆ Pre- or post-term birth	2–14
During labour and childbirth (intrapartum)	◆ Obstructed labour/dystocia ◆ Prolonged second stage of labour ◆ Meconium staining of amniotic fluid ◆ Breech position or other malpresentation ◆ Vaginal bleeding after eighth month ◆ Maternal fever during labour	2–85

Table 30.2 Causes of 'birth asphyxia'

Maternal factors	Placental factors	Neonatal factors
Maternal hypotension/ hypovolaemia	Chorioamnionitis	Infectious conditions
Maternal infections, fever during labour	Placental inflammatory conditions	Airway anomalies
Maternal seizures	Abnormal cord insertion into placenta leading to risk of bleeding	Circulatory collapse (blood loss in the baby related to organ injury or bleeding tumour/Arteriovenous malformation)
Maternal diabetes	Cord compression/ knotting	Severe pulmonary hypoplasia and hypertension (e.g. congenital diaphragmatic hernia)
Maternal hypertension and pre-eclampsia	Cord prolapse	Medication effect
Severe anaemia	Cord around baby's neck	Neurological disorders
Maternal drug use (cocaine etc.)	Placental abruption	Metabolic disorders
Obstructed labour— (shoulder dystocia, breech)	Foeto-maternal blood loss	Severe cardiac disease
Uterine rupture		

Secondary prevention

Neonatal resuscitation

Approximately 10% of births require some assistance to initiate breathing after birth. Neonatal resuscitation is a set of interventions at the time of birth which support the establishment of breathing and circulation. In order to provide timely resuscitation, there needs to be good communication between the obstetric care provider and the person resuscitating the baby. Ideally, there should be a provider trained and skilled in newborn resuscitation who is solely responsible for taking care of the baby.

The key principles of an effective resuscitation are: 1) stimulating the baby and clearing the airway; 2) ensuring thermoregulation; and 3) providing assisted breaths with a bag-mask (positive pressure ventilation) for a non-breathing baby. Basic resuscitation with bag-mask (also known as Ambu bag) is required in 3–6% of births. There is evidence of good outcomes even with room air resuscitation, so resuscitation should be provided by a bag-mask even in places where oxygen is not uniformly available. Only a very small subset (<1%) of babies will require more advanced resuscitation measures, such as cardiopulmonary rescuscitation and medications, and these are not routinely available in LMICs. Thus, neonatal resuscitation is feasible in LMICs, and now several simplified training programmes, such as the American Academy of Pediatrics' (AAP) Helping Babies Breathe programme (Figure

30.2), are available and have been used to implement neonatal resuscitation in LMICs.

As described by Lee et al. (2011), neonatal resuscitation in the facility setting may reduce intrapartum-related neonatal mortality by 30% (meta-analysis), and the impact in community/home based settings is unclear, though estimated to reach 20%.

Tertiary prevention

Tertiary prevention of birth asphyxia refers to the baby with acute complications, that is, management of the baby with neonatal encephalopathy, which is complex to address even in well-resourced health systems, and late sequelae, such as cerebral palsy.

Therapeutic hypothermia (total body cooling) is a treatment used in high-income countries to reduce mortality and risk of disability in babies with moderate to severe asphyxia with encephalopathy. It is currently not recommended in LMICs that do not have intensive care facilities.

Once the baby is stabilised, the focus should be on providing ongoing supportive care. Maintaining normal blood pressure, ventilation, normal blood sugar, and electrolyte levels are cornerstones of managing babies with birth asphyxia. It is also important to evaluate and treat for infection because it may be one of the underlying causes of birth asphyxia. Additionally, early recognition and treatment of seizures is an important part of care for the asphyxiated newborn. Phenobarbital is the recommended treatment for seizures.

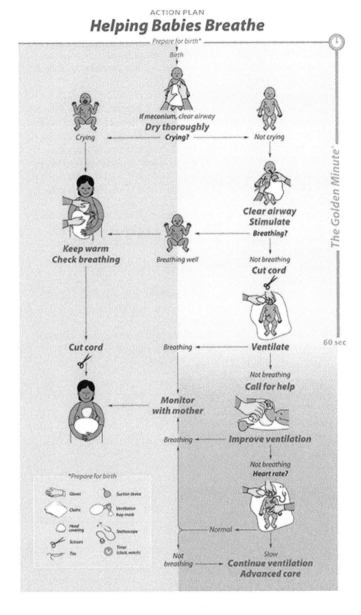

Figure 30.2 American Academy of Pediatrics Helping Babies Action Plan. Kak, L. P., et al. (eds.) (2015) *Helping Babies Breathe*. Itasca, USA: American Academy of Pediatrics. Copyright © 2015 American Academy of Pediatrics.

Challenges

A significant challenge in LMICs is how to reach babies in communities with high rates of home births and unattended deliveries. Adequate training of community health workers or traditional birth attendants (TBAs) in neonatal resuscitation is vital, as is skill retention in resuscitation training programmes.

Future priorities

◆ With such high rates of unattended deliveries, we need to improve strategies to increase the demand for and utilisation of skilled birth attendance. Community cadres of health workers should be better trained and protocols should be used to identify high-risk conditions/dangers sign to prompt referral to a facility.

◆ In order to improve neonatal resuscitation, it will be beneficial to develop low-cost, simpler equipment, training, and models for skill retention.

◆ The quality of care of intrapartum care could be increased with more widespread use of perinatal audit or checklists.

Conclusions

An estimated two million babies die during or immediately after childbirth due to intrapartum-related hypoxic insults. Improving access to and quality of intrapartum care and neonatal resuscitation may prevent an estimated 92% of these intrapartum-related deaths. Key priorities are to increase the quality, scale, and reach of these known, evidence-based interventions to those women and newborns in greatest need.

Case study: delivering a baby in Tibet with poor healthcare access

Dawa is a 17-year-old who lives in nomadic areas of the Himalayas in Tibet. Like many Tibetans, her diet is poor and she is five feet tall. She became pregnant with her first child shortly after marriage, and she never sought antenatal care as the health clinic is two days' travel and she was responsible for her yak herd. When she started having labour pains her mother-in-law came to help, but it was three days until the baby arrived. After birth the baby was limp, blue, and only weakly gasping to breathe. There was no local birth attendant, but a lama (religious leader) came and provided prayers for the infant, chanting and circumambulating around the temple. The baby passed away shortly thereafter. This was potentially an entirely preventable death that occurred due to lack of access to skilled healthcare practitioners.

Questions

1. What are the main risk factors for intrapartum-related events?

2. What are some primary and secondary prevention strategies to reduce rates of intrapartum-related events?

3. How often do babies require any resuscitation? How often do babies require advanced resuscitation measures (such as intubation or medications)?

Key publications

Lawn J, Lee A, Kinney M, et al. (2009). Two million intrapartum-related stillbirths and neonatal deaths: where, why, and what can be done? *Int J Gynaecol Obstet* 1: S5–19.

Lee A, Kozuki N, Blencowe H, et al. (2013). Intrapartum-related neonatal encephalopathy incidence and impairment at regional and global levels for 2010 with trends from 1990. *Pediatric Research* 74(Suppl 1): 50–72.
These papers provides an overview of the epidemiology of intrapartum-related stillbirths and neonatal deaths in LMICs.

Wall S, Lee A, Niermeyer S, English M, et al. (2009). Neonatal resuscitation in low-resource settings: what, who, and how to overcome challenges to scale up? *Int J Gynaecol Obstet* 107(Suppl 1): S47–64.
This paper provides a synthesis of the use of neonatal resuscitation in LMICs.

Hofmeyr G, Haws R, Bergström S, et al. (2009). Obstetric care in low-resource settings: what, who, and how to overcome challenges to scale up? *Int J Gynaecol Obstet* 1: S21–45.
This paper reviews the evidence on the effect of obstetric interventions in LMIC to prevent intrapartum-related deaths.

Bibliography

American Academy of Pediatrics. Helping Babies Survive. Available at: https://www.aap.org/en-us/advocacy-and-policy/aap-health-initiatives/helping-babies-survive/Pages/default.aspx

Bhutta Z, Das J, Bahl R, et al. (2014). Can available interventions end preventable deaths in mothers, newborn babies, and stillbirths, and at what cost? *Lancet* 384(9940): 347–70.

Byaruhanga R, Bassani D, Jagau A, Muwanguzi P, Montgomery A, and Lawn J (2015). Use of wind-up foetal Doppler versus Pinard for foetal heart rate intermittent monitoring in labour: a randomised clinical trial. *BMJ Open* 5(1): e006867.

Committee on Obstetric Practice, American College of Obstetricians and Gynecologists (2005). Committee Opinion Number 326. Inappropriate use of the terms fetal distress and birth asphyxia. *Obstet Gynecol* 106(6): 1469–70.

Lavender T, Hart A, and Smyth R (2012). Effect of partogram use on outcomes for women in spontaneous labour at term. *Cochrane Database Systematic Reviews* 8: CD005461.

Lawn J, Bahl R, Bergstrom S, et al. (2011). Setting research priorities to reduce almost one million deaths from birth asphyxia by 2015. *PLoS Med* 8(1): e1000389.

Lee A, Cousens S, Darmstadt G, et al. (2011). Care during labor and birth for the prevention of intrapartum-related neonatal deaths: a systematic review and Delphi estimation of mortality effect. *BMC Public Health* 11(Suppl 3): S10.

Lee A, Cousens S, Wall S, et al. (2011). Neonatal resuscitation and immediate newborn assessment and stimulation for the prevention of neonatal deaths: a systematic review, meta-analysis and Delphi estimation of mortality effect. *BMC Public Health* 11(Suppl 3): S12.

Liu L, Oza S, Hogan D, et al. (2017). Global, regional, and national causes of under-5 mortality in 2000–15: an updated systematic analysis with implications for the Sustainable Development Goals. *Lancet* 388(10063): 3027–35.

Rainaldi M and Perlman J (2016). Pathophysiology of birth asphyxia. *Clin Perinatol* 43(3): 409–22.

Takenouchi T, Kasdorf E, Engel M, Grunebaum A, and Perlman J (2012). Changing pattern of perinatal brain injury in term infants in recent years. *Pediatr Neurol* 46(2): 106–10.

World Health Organization (1994). Partograph in management of labour. World Health Organization Maternal Health and Safe Motherhood Programme. *Lancet* 343(8910): 1399–404.

CHAPTER 31

Neonatal infection

Anna Seale and Helen Brotherton

This chapter discusses infections in newborns, its huge burden worldwide, the importance of the diagnosis and treatment of 'possible serious bacterial infection', and the challenges of antibiotic resistance. It should be read in conjunction with Chapter 36 on infectious diseases.

Key points

◆ Infection directly accounts for a quarter of all neonatal deaths in resource-poor settings.

◆ Understanding aetiologies of infectious diseases, to target treatments and direct empiric antibiotic treatment guidelines, remains critical.

◆ Neonatal infection is diagnosed and empirically treated based on the presence of specific clinical signs of 'possible serious bacterial infection'; this is critical to addressing the high mortality associated with these serious infections.

◆ However, empiric antibiotic treatment strategies are threatened by the worldwide increase in drug resistant infections.

Background

Burden

Neonatal infection accounts for around a quarter of all neonatal deaths worldwide, and likely contributes indirectly to many others. The Global Burden of Disease Study estimates that neonatal infection accounts for around 3% of disability adjusted life years (DALYs), mostly accounted for by neonatal deaths. However, in addition to mortality, there is a considerable burden of morbidity. This includes neurodevelopmental impairment after neonatal meningitis and an unknown burden of neurodevelopmental impairment after neonatal sepsis and neonatal pneumonia (Figure 31.1).

The burden of neonatal infection on health care is considerable; there were an estimated 6.9 million neonates with clinically diagnosed 'possible serious bacterial infection' (pSBI) in South Asia, sub-Saharan Africa, and Latin America in 2012. According to international guidelines, all of these neonates should receive treatment for pSBI. However, access to clinical care can be very problematic in low-resource settings, with care seeking varying between 10% and 100%, and new World Health Organization (WHO) guidelines suggest increasing access to care through outpatient treatment, where referral to hospital for inpatient care is not possible.

Causes

A range of pathogens can cause neonatal infection: bacteria, viruses, fungi, and parasites. However, much of the focus is on serious

bacterial infection because these infections are common and, when they cause disease through infection of the bloodstream (sepsis), lung (pneumonia), or cerebrospinal fluid (meningitis), they are life-threatening. However, neonates can be cured, if treated promptly with antibiotics and given appropriate supportive care.

Newborn infection can occur before delivery, from transplacental infection, for example congenital syphilis, caused by the bacterial spirochaete *Treponema pallidum*, which is now recognised as the leading bacterial cause of congenital infection and stillbirth. It can also occur before or at delivery through ascending infection from the maternal genito-urinary tract, for example invasive Group B Streptococcal disease (GBS). After delivery, neonatal infection occurs from a variety of sources, from the environment or through person-to-person transmission, either at home or in hospital.

Neonates are at risk of healthcare associated infections (HAI) at health facility delivery and during admission to a neonatal unit. Infection rates for hospital-born neonates in low-resource settings are 3–20 times higher than rates in high-income countries. HAI are more likely to be drug resistant infections than community acquired infections, but neonates in the community are also at risk for drug resistant infection. Although data are limited, the most common bacteria causing drug resistant infections in neonates are multi-drug resistant Gram-negative bacilli (MDR-GNB), such as extended-spectrum beta-lactamases-producing *E coli* or *Klebsiella pneumoniae*.

Serious bacterial disease

Neonates who are born preterm (<37 weeks) and/or with low birthweight (<2.5 kg) are at increased risk of infection. This is due to reduced maternal antibody transfer to the newborn if delivery is preterm, and increased susceptibility due to an immature immune system and immature barriers (skin). The risk of neonatal infection is increased further by unhygienic delivery and/or early postnatal practices.

Early-onset neonatal bacterial disease (0–6 days) is frequently caused by transmission of bacteria from the maternal genito-urinary tract to the newborn, which usually presents as illness in the first 48–72 hours after birth. A range of bacteria can cause early onset disease, but *Streptococcus agalactiae* (Group B Streptococcus, GBS) and *Escherichia coli* are the most common globally. Clinical risk factors suggesting increased risk of neonatal infection, particularly GBS disease, include maternal fever (≥38°C) and prolonged rupture of the membranes (≥18 hours). Mothers who have had a previous newborn with GBS disease are at greater risk of having a newborn with GBS disease in subsequent pregnancies.

Late-onset neonatal bacterial disease (7–27 days) occurs from environmental or person-to-person transmission. In resource-limited

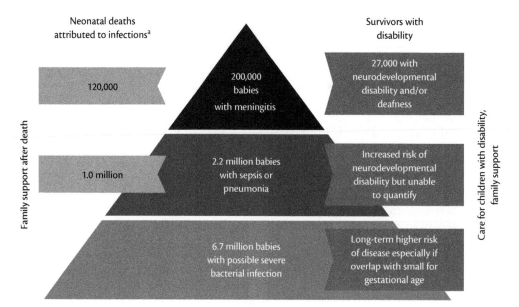

Figure 31.1 Summary of outcomes in terms of deaths and disability for neonates with sepsis, meningitis, or pneumonia born in South Asia, sub-Saharan Africa, and Latin America in 2010.

Seale, AC. et al. Neonatal severe bacterial infection impairment estimates in South Asia, sub-Saharan Africa, and Latin America for 2010. *Pediatric Research.* 74 (Suppl 1), 73–85. © 2013 Nature Publishing Group. Open Access.

settings, frequent pathogens include *Streptococcus pyogenes*, *Staphylococcus aureus*, and Gram-negative bacilli such as *Klebsiella* sp., *Pseudomonas* sp., and *Salmonellae* sp.

Other bacteria causing neonatal infection include *Bordetella pertussis*, which is often difficult to detect by culture, and neonates do not often have the characteristic whooping cough, but present with signs of pSBI, sometimes including episodes of apnoea (interruption of breathing). Neonatal tetanus is a serious, life-threatening disease; it is caused by a toxin produced by *Clostridium tetani*, the spores of which are found in soil and faeces. Risk factors for neonatal tetanus include home delivery, likely due to unhygienic delivery practices, for example cutting the cord at delivery without antisepsis measures. Maternal immunisation programmes have considerably reduced neonatal tetanus in many countries.

Viruses

Viruses cause congenital infection (infection *in utero*), which can result in congenital abnormality. Viral infections causing congenital infection include varicella zoster (VZV), rubella, cytomegalovirus (CMV), herpes simplex virus (HSV), and Zika virus. Other viruses more commonly cause illness after delivery; viral infections causing significant neonatal respiratory infection, often difficult to distinguish from bacterial pneumonia and sepsis, include respiratory syncytial virus (RSV), human meta-pneumovirus, and influenza. Other viruses such as enterovirus and HSV can cause viral meningo-encephalitis, which can be difficult to distinguish clinically from bacterial meningitis.

Fungi

Fungi, especially *Candida albicans*, can cause invasive disease, particularly in resource-rich settings where extremely preterm and very low birthweight babies survive, and antibiotic use may be prolonged.

Diagnosis

In most resource-limited settings, the diagnosis of neonatal sepsis is pragmatic, and based on the presence or absence of clinical signs. Based on these simple algorithms, treatment is given empirically for pSBI. The presence of any one of a history of difficulty feeding, convulsions, respiratory rate >60 breaths per minute, severe chest indrawing, temperature >37.5°C or <35.5°C, or movement only when stimulated, suggests pSBI. Compared to an experienced paediatrician, these clinical signs had 85% sensitivity and 75% specificity for serious bacterial infection (days 0–6) in a multi-site study. However, as Figure 31.2 illustrates, the clinical diagnosis of pSBI can include a wide variety of aetiologies.

Confirmation of serious bacterial disease (sepsis, meningitis, or pneumonia) depends on conventional microbiological culture of blood and/or cerebrospinal fluid to diagnose sepsis and/or meningitis respectively, and/or chest X-ray changes to diagnose pneumonia. However, blood cultures are insensitive, and may not detect bacterial infection. Molecular methods using nucleic acid extraction techniques are increasingly used to support diagnostics, particularly in research settings. Molecular methods can also be used to diagnose viral infections (which is otherwise by viral cell culture), but these are not usually available in clinical practice in resource-limited settings. Biomarkers for neonatal sepsis, such as C-reactive protein (CRP) and white cell count (WCC), can be used as an adjunct to support diagnoses, but they lack specificity and sensitivity for neonatal infection.

Prevention

Prevention of newborn infection is key to reducing the burden of neonatal infection. Interventions are based largely on either antisepsis or maternal vaccination. Antisepsis is important at delivery, and clean delivery kits, including antiseptics for cord care such as chlorhexidine, can prevent neonatal infection and reduce mortality

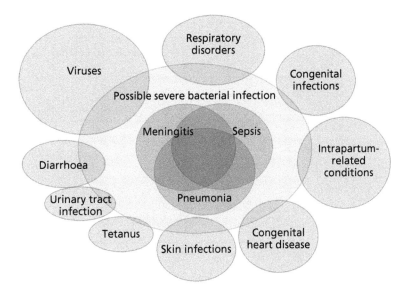

Figure 31.2 Possible serious bacterial infections.
Seale, AC. et al. Estimates of possible severe bacterial infection in neonates in sub-Saharan Africa, South Asia, and Latin America for 2012: a systematic review and meta-analysis. *The Lancet Infectious Diseases.* 14(8), 731–741. Copyright © 2014 Elsevier Ltd. Open Access.

in large clinical trials in the community. However, there is less evidence of benefit in hospital-based studies, and a large clinical trial did not find any evidence of benefit from maternal vaginal chlorhexidine wipes at delivery. Maternal vaccination is used to prevent neonatal tetanus in many countries worldwide, and in resource-rich settings, pertussis (whooping cough) vaccine and influenza vaccine are routinely provided to pregnant women to prevent these infections in mother and neonate.

Global targets

Although there are no specific neonatal infection-related international targets, reducing infection will be critical to achieving the Sustainable Development Goals (SDGs) and WHO goals on reducing neonatal mortality and stillbirth.

Interventions

It is important that all neonates with signs of pSBI are provided with supportive care as needed, and vital signs (including oxygen saturation) are measured. Strategies for management of neonatal infection, both those available and research areas for development, are summarised in Table 31.1. Respiratory support may include oxygen and/or CPAP (continuous positive airway pressure), even if there are no facilities for invasive ventilation. Fluid support may be though nasogastric tube feeding, and/or provision of intravenous fluids, whilst body temperature should be maintained through incubator or skin-to-skin care, especially for preterm and/or low birthweight babies who are more susceptible to heat loss and thus hypothermia. In the longer term, follow-up to identify and manage neurological sequelae should be included, but this may be difficult in resource-limited settings.

Neonates with signs of pSBI should be referred for hospital management. However, where this is not feasible, or refused, the WHO guidelines suggest outpatient treatment with simplified treatment courses.

Empiric treatment strategies always include antibiotic treatment where there are signs of possible serious bacterial infection. Anti-fungals and/or anti-virals are added where there is clinical suspicion of these aetiologies and/or treatment and/or diagnostics available, as this will improve outcomes. Empirical treatment for pSBI in hospital should be guided by up-to-date local, national, and international guidelines for first and second-line treatments. Increasing drug resistant infections threaten the effectiveness of standard therapies for neonatal infection, especially with extended-spectrum beta-lactamases-producing Gram negative bacilli.

There are specific management strategies for some conditions. Neonatal tetanus management should include thorough cleaning of the umbilicus, intravenous antibiotic treatment, anti-spasmodic treatment (e.g. diazepam), intravenous magnesium sulphate for stabilisation of the autonomic nervous system, and human or equine anti-tetanus immunoglobulin. The baby should be nursed in a quiet environment with nasogastric feeding once spasms are controlled, to avoid aspiration. Routine tetanus vaccination should be provided following recovery as no immunity is conferred during infection.

Challenges

There are major challenges in terms of improving and developing prevention of neonatal infection; improving diagnosis and access to care for newborns who are unwell; improving case management for newborns in terms of both effective antibiotic treatment and supportive care (support of respiration, provision of fluids, and maintenance of body temperature).

Future priorities

◆ Improvements in prevention will reduce the burden of neonatal infection, and maternal vaccines are likely to be an important contributor to this. New maternal vaccines are being developed to protect against neonatal disease, such as a Group B Streptococcal vaccine.

Table 31.1 Strategies to improve management of neonatal sepsis specifically for low-income settings

	Strategies	Additional strategies not commonly used in low-income settings/research areas
Diagnosis		
	Clinical signs and symptoms.	Could be improved by rapid diagnostics if developed.
Empiric treatment		
	As per local, national, and international guidelines. The WHO guidelines in 2013 recommend ampicillin and gentamicin as first-line treatment in hospital.	Treatment could be directed if microbiological testing and/or rapid tests if developed.
Supportive care		
Respiratory support	Appropriate delivery of oxygen and monitoring of oxygen saturation levels.	Bubble CPAP is effective and feasible at secondary and tertiary healthcare level.
Temperature control	Kangaroo mother care, incubators, hats, and regular monitoring of temperature.	
Fluids/feeds	Intravenous (IV) fluids and gastric tube feeds given appropriately for weight and age of baby.	Syringe pumps for accurate administration of IV fluids.
Blood glucose control	Testing neonatal blood sugar levels and treating hypoglycaemia.	Use of insulin infusions in intensive care settings for hyperglycaemia
Jaundice	Phototherapy, exchange transfusion for severe jaundice. Assessment of jaundice severity based on clinical features.	Regular monitoring of serum bilirubin levels to guide treatment, or a point of care test for non-invasive bilirubin levels (e.g. transcutaneous bilimeter).
Prevention		
Screening and treatment	Syphilis screening and treatment (mainly for stillbirth). Identification and treatment of neonates at 'high risk for sepsis' with maternal sepsis risk factors is performed at some tertiary health centres.	Bacteriuria screening and treatment. Screening and intrapartum antimicrobial prophylaxis for Group B Streptococcus.
Maternal immunisation	Tetanus vaccination in pregnancy.	Pertussis and influenza vaccines used in high income settings. Others are in development, e.g. Group B Streptococcus.
Anti-sepsis at delivery/ immediate postnatal period	Umbilical cord care with chlorhexidine. Avoidance of applying other substances to the cord.	
Infection control	Hand hygiene at key patient contact points. Isolation of infectious cases, barrier nursing, aseptic preparation of fluids and intravenous medications.	Antibiotic stewardship programmes; monitoring effective use of antimicrobials in hospitals.

♦ Antimicrobial resistance is a particular challenge for neonatal HAI in resource-limited settings due to a high incidence of infections, limited laboratory diagnostics to direct treatment, and limited alternative antibiotic regimens (Chapter 36). It is estimated that only 30% of neonatal HAI would be adequately treated with first-line antibiotics (ampicillin and gentamicin).

Conclusions

The burden of neonatal mortality and morbidity is high. Access to care is often limited in resource-poor settings and there is a need to both prevent disease (through antisepsis and maternal vaccination) and increase treatment, especially in community settings, to reduce the mortality burden. As laboratory diagnostics are limited, treatment is based on clinical algorithms, and sensitivity is prioritised over specificity, improving diagnosis of neonatal sepsis would help direct and target treatment. Point of care tests

for neonatal sepsis would be ideal, but have been challenging to develop to date. Reducing antimicrobial susceptibility challenges empiric treatment strategies and will increase the burden from neonatal infection.

Case study: identifying neonatal sepsis in a five-day-old baby

A mother presented to a rural district hospital in Ethiopia with her five-day-old baby boy. He was born at home, with no complications at delivery. He had been well until the previous day when she noticed he had been feeding less, then felt hot and floppy. At admission, the baby's respiratory rate was 70 breaths per minute, heart rate 120 beats per min and temperature was 37.9°C. He had severe chest recessions observed. The clinical officer advised the mother that the baby needed to be admitted to the neonatal unit, monitored, and treated for possible serious bacterial infection. He would need seven days of intravenous antibiotics, and intravenous fluids until he was able to take breast milk (by nasogastric tube or directly from the mother). He improved after twenty-four hours, and after completing the treatment course he was discharged home.

Questions

1. Discuss the risk factors and causes of possible serious bacterial infection in neonates.

2. How is neonatal infection most commonly diagnosed in resource-limited settings?

3. What threatens the effectiveness of current antibiotic treatment regimens?

Key publications

Young Infants Clinical Signs Study Group (2008). Clinical signs that predict severe illness in children under age 2 months: a multicentre study. *Lancet* 371: 135–42.
    Landmark study on the clinical signs of invasive bacterial disease in neonates.

World Health Organization (2015). *Managing Possible Serious Bacterial Infection in Young Infants When Referral is not Feasible: Guidelines.* WHO: Geneva.
    Updated guidelines on neonatal infection management in outpatient settings.

World Health Organization (2003). *Managing Newborn Problems: a Guide for Doctors, Nurses and Midwives.*
    International guidelines on the management of neonatal problems.

World Health Organization (2013). *Pocket Book of Hospital Care for Children. Guidelines for the Management of Common Childhood Illnesses.* second edition. WHO: Geneva.
    International guidelines on the management of children in hospital. WHO: Geneva.

Bibliography

Blencowe H, Vos T, Lee A, et al. (2013). Estimates of neonatal morbidities and disabilities at regional and global levels for 2010: introduction, methods overview, and relevant findings from the Global Burden of Disease study. *Pediatr Res* 74(Suppl 1): 4–16.

Herbert H, Lee A, Chandran A, Rudan I, and Baqui A (2012). Care seeking for neonatal illness in low- and middle-income countries: a systematic review. *PLoS Med* 9: e1001183.

Huynh B, Padget M, Garin B, et al. (2015) Burden of bacterial resistance among neonatal infections in low income countries: how convincing is the epidemiological evidence? *BMC Infectious diseases* 15: 127.

Lawn J, Blencowe H, Waiswa P, et al. (2016) Stillbirths: rates, risk factors, and acceleration towards 2030. *Lancet* 387: 587–603.

Liu L, Oza V, Lee A, et al. (2015). Global, regional, and national causes of child mortality in 2000–13, with projections to inform post-2015 priorities: an updated systematic analysis. *Lancet* 385: 430–40.

Muller W (2016) Treatment of perinatal viral infections to improve neurologic outcomes. *Pediatr Res* 81(1–2): 162–9.

Seale A, Mwaniki M, Newton C, and Berkley J (2009) Maternal and early onset neonatal bacterial sepsis: burden and strategies for prevention in sub-Saharan Africa. *Lancet Infectious diseases* 9: 428–38.

Seale A, Blencowe H, Zaidi A, et al. (2013). Neonatal severe bacterial infection impairment estimates in South Asia, sub-Saharan Africa, and Latin America for 2010. *Pediatr Res* 74(Suppl 1): 73–85.

Seale A, Blencowe H, Manu A, et al. (2014). Estimates of possible severe bacterial infection in neonates in sub-Saharan Africa, South Asia, and Latin America for 2012: a systematic review and meta-analysis. *Lancet Infectious diseases* 14: 731–41.

Sobanjo-Ter Meulen A, Abramson J, Mason E, et al. (2015). Path to impact: a report from the Bill and Melinda Gates Foundation convening on maternal immunization in resource-limited settings; Berlin—January 29–30. *Vaccine* 33(47): 6388–95.

Verani J, McGee L, and Schrag S (2010). *Prevention of Perinatal Group B Streptococcal Disease—Revised Guidelines from CDC, 2010.* MMWR Recomm Rep 59, 1–36.

World Health Organization (2013) *Problems of the Neonate and Young Infant.* WHO: Geneva. pp. 45–69.

Zaidi A, Huskins W, Thaver D, et al. (2005) Hospital-acquired neonatal infections in developing countries. *Lancet* 365: 1175–88.

CHAPTER 32

Congenital disorders

Sowmiya Moorthie

The term congenital disorder encompasses a wide range of conditions that arise before birth; here we concentrate on those congenital disorders that cause premature death or disability. In this chapter we describe important concepts in relation to congenital disorders, prevention activities, and key challenges to their effective delivery.

Key points

◆ Congenital disorders are of global importance due to their impact on infant mortality and long-term disability.

◆ Effective health services for congenital disorders take a holistic approach to care and prevention, involving both population health and specialist services across the lifecourse.

◆ Scaling up surgical services in low- and middle-income countries (LMICs) could significantly reduce the burden of disorders such as neural tube defects, congenital heart disease, and cleft lip and palate.

◆ Developing effective services in LMICs is compounded by the lack of data on the epidemiology, impact, and cost-effectiveness of interventions.

Background

Burden

An estimated 7.9 million children are born each year with a congenital disorder; 3% of all live births. The Global Burden of Disease study 2015 suggests that congenital anomalies account for 496,585 under-five deaths (8.53%), 96% of which occur in LMICs. Around 192,000 stillbirths are also estimated to result from congenital disorders. As rates of infant and child mortality fall, these disorders begin to contribute to increasing rates of disability; these can be both physical and mental, and lifelong.

Causes

Causes are usually divided into three groups; however, there is considerable overlap (Figure 32.1). The genetic group encompasses those that arise due to inherent biological or genetic factors, such as chromosomal disorders or inheritance of a single gene defect; examples include Down's syndrome and phenylketonuria. The environmental group comprises those that arise due to maternal exposure to environmental factors, such as an infectious agent or drug that can harm the developing foetus, for example congenital rubella syndrome or foetal alcohol spectrum disorders. Those that

are multi-factorial result from a complex interaction between genetic and environmental factors, and often the primary cause is unknown; this group is the largest and encompasses congenital disorders such as neural tube defects and orofacial clefts.

A range of determinants from individual level to wider societal factors affect the occurrence and severity of congenital disorders. These include specific risk factors such as advanced parental age, micronutrient deficiencies (iodine and folate), as well as social, ethnic, and economic factors. This is reflected in the global variation in the frequency of specific congenital disorders. In most high-income countries, many of the environmental causes of congenital disorders have been tackled, leading to a proportionally higher prevalence of those caused by genetic factors and those that are multi-factorial. This is also the case in many middle-income countries, such as the Gulf States, where infectious diseases have been combated. However, there is an increased prevalence of recessive single gene disorders as a result of customary consanguineous marriages; this is because consanguinity increases the likelihood that a couple will both carry the same recessive gene variant. In many lower-income settings, where infectious diseases persist, congenital disorders due to other causes are not yet recognised as a problem.

Surveillance

Surveillance of congenital disorders is an important public health activity. Systematic collection of data on the types, prevalence, severity, and outcomes of congenital disorders, along with analysis and interpretation of data helps to inform appropriate planning of care and prevention services and activities. Ongoing surveillance of congenital anomalies also facilitates identification of teratogenic exposures, through identification of temporal and/or geographical fluctuations in frequencies of different disorders. An example is the increase in the number of microcephaly cases identified in Brazil in 2015, which has been linked to Zika virus infection. Such surveillance activities are often conducted at the local level; however, networks such as the European Concerted Action on Congenital Anomalies and Twins (EUROCAT) and International Clearinghouse for Birth Defects Monitoring Systems (ICBDMS) enable collaboration.

The cost of comprehensive surveillance systems means that there are far fewer congenital anomaly registries in LMICs. The need for accurate diagnostic facilities also contributes to the lack of epidemiological data in many of these countries.

There are no specific international targets for reducing congenital malformations, although doing so is critical to reducing stillbirth and neonatal mortality rates.

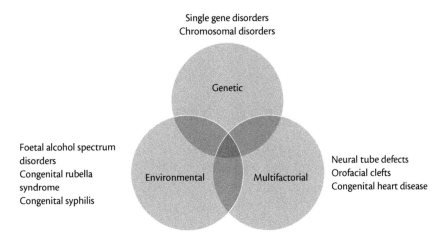

Figure 32.1 Grouping of congenital disorders.

Interventions

Prevention

It has been estimated by Christianson and Modell (2004) that 70% of congenital disorders can be prevented, or their adverse effects mitigated, through the establishment of appropriate health services. These involve activities across a range of services throughout the lifecourse including:

♦ Population, public health, and environmental health services.

♦ Family planning, women's, and reproductive healthcare services.

♦ Preconception and antenatal services.

♦ Maternity services.

♦ Newborn services, including screening and diagnosis.

♦ Paediatric services, including diagnosis, treatment, care, and management.

♦ Lifelong medical, social, and family support services for those with congenital conditions.

Prevention of many congenital disorders, in particular those with environmental causes, involves relatively low-cost interventions such as nutritional supplements (iodine and folic acid), infection control measures such as immunisation, and management of maternal health problems such as diabetes. Some genetic conditions can be partially prevented through screening. Genetic screening aims to identify carriers of recessive genetic conditions and provide information and counselling that allows them to manage their risk. If carried out during the preconception period, this may involve choosing not to marry another carrier, electing not to have children if their partner is a carrier, opting for procedures such as assisted reproduction and pre-implantation genetic diagnosis, or undergoing antenatal diagnosis to determine if the foetus is affected. In many high-income countries, specialist medical genetic services manage individuals and families suffering from conditions with a significant genetic component. Community genetic services are more common in lower-income settings where there are few specialist geneticists. Genetic counsellors and primary care doctors provide basic advice and education at the community and primary care level.

Many of these can form part of a comprehensive preconception and antenatal care programme. Additionally, many antenatal care programmes include the provision of antenatal screening and

diagnosis in order to identify babies with severe structural anomalies or babies affected with genetic conditions such as Down's syndrome. In those settings where it is legally and socially acceptable, the option of termination of pregnancy may be provided.

Management and care

Care for individuals with congenital disorders is reliant on early detection and instigation of appropriate treatment. Some congenital anomalies such as cleft lip and palate, congenital heart anomalies, and neural tube defects, can be treated by specialised surgical procedures. These services are often provided as internationally funded vertical programmes in LMICs, due to the requirement for specialised advanced care. It has been estimated that the burden of these three congenital anomalies could be halved if adequate surgical services were scaled up. Non-surgical interventions include dietary modification (for metabolic disorders), hormone therapy, or blood transfusion for haemoglobin disorders. As most congenital disorders cannot be cured completely, there is a continued need for care, including social and educational support for individuals and family members. Table 32.1 provides examples of specific services across the lifecourse.

Challenges

One of the key bottlenecks in developing policy and services for the care and prevention of congenital disorders is a lack of epidemiological data. Much of this is due to a lack of consensus and standardisation of the term 'congenital disorder'. This has hampered efforts for data comparison and comprehensive assessment of the global burden of disease due to these conditions.

Future priorities

♦ The incidence of congenital disorders cannot be precisely measured due in part to early pregnancy losses, many of which may occur before the pregnancy is confirmed. Consequently, the incidence of congenital disorders is usually described in terms of birth prevalence rather than incidence. This also acknowledges the fact that not all cases of congenital disorders may be diagnosed, such as in the case of late pregnancy losses. The denominator for calculating birth prevalence is usually all births, which excludes miscarriages and pregnancy terminations.

Table 32.1 Examples of specific interventions for congenital disorders

Service type	Intervention
Primary prevention	
Whole population programmes	Salt iodisation
	Public health programmes to reduce smoking and alcohol consumption
	Control of infectious diseases through effective education, screening, treatment, and immunisation programmes
	Environmental health services to combat industrial and agricultural pollution
	Occupational health services to minimise exposure to workplace teratogens
Interventions before pregnancy	Folic acid supplementation
	Information on risk associated with advanced maternal age
	Advice on healthy lifestyle and nutrition
	Carrier screening programmes
	Sexual health services
	Family planning
	Rubella immunisation
	Medication review for those with pre-existing conditions e.g. epilepsy
Secondary prevention	
During pregnancy	Minimising exposure to teratogens (e.g. tobacco, alcohol, and recreational drugs) through advice and interventions regarding risky behaviours
	Optimisation of diabetes control and review of medications
	Screening for rhesus blood group incompatibility, and immunoprophylaxis for rhesus-negative mothers
	Ultrasound and maternal serum screening to detect Down's syndrome, open neural tube defects, and other structural anomalies
	Services for termination of pregnancy for severe congenital disorders
During the neonatal period	Routine clinical examination after birth
	Newborn bloodspot or cord blood screening to detect a range of disorders, many of which are genetic
	Screening for common congenital conditions that are not detected by physical examination, e.g. hearing defects and congenital cataracts
	Referral to clinical specialists where congenital disorder suspected
Tertiary prevention	
Newborn with congenital disorder	Surgery for conditions such as neural tube defects, orofacial clefts, some cardiac defects
	Treatments such as dietary or enzyme replacement therapy for metabolic disorders, speech therapy for orofacial clefts, blood transfusion for haemoglobin disorders
	Infection control and pain management
	Rehabilitation and physiotherapy
	Social and psychological support to address stigmatisation and discrimination
	Special educational services for those with learning disabilities

◆ Obtaining accurate information on incidence is also dependent on accurate diagnosis. Although some congenital disorders can be identified by physical examination, other malformations and genetic disorders require clinical expertise, diagnostic facilities, and paediatric post-mortem examination.

Conclusions

Congenital disorders are an important cause of mortality and disability in both high and low-income countries; many can be prevented and treated. Access to and quality of health services have an impact on determining outcomes. Epidemiological data are lacking and require better surveillance mechanisms, clearer definitions, and more accurate and widely available diagnostic facilities.

Case study: Zika virus and microcephaly

The condition of microcephaly (head circumference <2 standard deviations below the median) has recently gained attention in the global community due to the emergence of Zika virus. Zika is transmitted by the Aedes mosquito and was first discovered in Uganda in 1947 but was thought to cause a relatively mild illness. An association with congenital microcephaly was postulated nearly seventy years later in 2015 in north-east Brazil. The association has since been proven causal and Zika virus plus the increased prevalence of microcephaly has since been declared a 'public health emergency'. The microcephaly is most likely due to stalled neuronal cell growth and cell death. It also represents one component of a constellation of symptoms, including ocular lesions and hearing loss, in congenital Zika syndrome. The full extent of the disease burden is still being established but, at the time of writing, it appears to be significant and largely confined to Latin America.

The importance of Zika virus has been established, but it is only one of a group of infectious causes of microcephaly and associated syndromes. Other important infections include cytomegalovirus, herpes simplex virus, rubella virus, and *Toxoplasma gondii*.

Questions

1. What are the main types of congenital disorder and the factors that impact on their prevalence?

2. What are the main approaches to prevention of congenital disorders?

3. What are the reasons for monitoring prevalence of congenital disorders?

Key publications

Christianson A, Howson C, and Modell B (2006). *March of Dimes Global Report on Birth Defects: The Hidden Toll of Dying and Disabled Children*. White Plains: New York, US.
    An important review of congenital and genetic disorders and approaches to preventions.

WHO (2016). Congenital Abnormalties Factsheet (2016). http://www.who.int/mediacentre/factsheets/fs370/en/
    An up-to-date overview of congenital abnormalities.

Bibliography

Alwan A, Modell B, Bittles A, Czeizel A, and Hamamy H (1997). *Community Control of Genetic and Congenital Disorders*. WHO regional office for the eastern Mediterranean: Alexandria.

Bittles A and Black M (2010). The impact of consanguinity on neonatal and infant health. *Early Hum Dev* 86: 737–41.

Botto L, Robert-Gnansia E, Siffel C, Harris J, Borman B, and Mastroiacovo P (2006). Fostering international collaboration in birth defects research and prevention: a perspective from the international clearinghouse for birth defects surveillance and research. *Am J Public Health* 96: 774–80.

Christianson A and Modell B (2004). Medical genetics in developing countries. *Annu Rev Genomics Hum Genet* 5: 219–65.

Czeizel A (2005). Birth defects are preventable. *Int J Med Sci* 2: 91–2.

Darmstadt, G, Howson C, Walraven G, et al. (2016). Prevention of congenital disorders and care of affected children: a consensus statement. *JAMA Pediatrics* 170: 790–3.

Devakumar D, Bamford A, Ferreira MU, et al. (2018). Infectious causes of microcephaly: epidemiology, pathogenesis, diagnosis, and management. *Lancet Infectious Diseases* 18: e1–13.

Dolk H (2005). Eurocat: 25 years of European surveillance of congenital anomalies. *Arch Dis Child Fetal Neonatal* 90: f355–8.

Higashi H, Barendregt J, Kassebaum N, Weiser T, Bickler S, and Vos T (2015). The burden of selected congenital anomalies amenable to surgery in low and middle-income regions: cleft lip and palate, congenital heart anomalies and neural tube defects. *Arch Dis Child* 100(3): 233–8.

Ten Kate L, Al-Gazali L, Anand S, et al. (2010). Community genetics, its definition. *J Community Genet* 1: 19–22.

World Health Organization (2006). *Management of birth defects and haemoglobin disorders: report of a joint WHO-March of dimes meeting*. WHO: Geneva.

CHAPTER 33

Low birthweight and poor foetal growth

Gabriela Cormick, Nicole Minckas, and José Belizán

This chapter will cover the physiology of foetal growth, growth restriction, types and indicators of impaired growth, and interventions during pregnancy to improve foetal growth. It should be read in conjunction with Chapter 7 (Developmental Origins of Health and Disease (DOHaD)), Chapter 24 (Maternal nutrition), Chapter 29 (Preterm births), and Chapter 37 (Child nutrition).

Key points

♦ A baby's birthweight is a significant indicator of maternal and newborn health, nutrition, and wellbeing.

♦ Between 15% and 20% of births worldwide are of low birthweight, and over 90% of them occur in low- and middle-income countries (LMICs).

♦ Chronic maternal undernutrition is linked to intrauterine growth restriction, which can lead to chronic physical and mental development impairment in the baby.

♦ Pregnancy is a crucial time to intervene in order to improve foetal growth, although interventions are required across the continuum of care from preconception through to postnatal care of a low birthweight baby.

Background

Over twenty million low birthweight (LBW) infants are born each year, with a worldwide incidence between 15% and 20% of all births. Those born in developing countries make up more than 90% of the total; half of these are born in south-central Asia.

LBW is associated with higher mortality and morbidity, both short and long-term, related to inadequate growth, impaired cognitive development and chronic diseases. It can be due to preterm birth, intrauterine growth restriction (IUGR), or the combination of both (in this chapter we will focus on IUGR; refer to Chapter 29 for preterm births). A large study by Villar and Belizan (1982) found that in countries with an incidence of LBW >10% it is primarily due to IUGR, whilst where the incidence is <10%, most are due to preterm birth.

Birthweight is a key and sensitive measure of an infant's health and of a woman's health, nutrition, and social circumstances. However, many babies are not weighed at birth, particularly in low-resource settings where a higher number of deliveries occur at home or are unattended (>40%). These are often the areas most affected by undernutrition, and challenges the accuracy of burden estimates globally.

Causes

Factors related to the baby, the mother, and the physical environment can play an important role in the duration of the gestation and the foetal growth, affecting the infant's birthweight.

The mother's health has a major impact on the baby's birthweight. This is affected by lifestyle factors such as smoking, alcohol and drug abuse, diseases such as anaemia, malaria, human immunodeficiency virus (HIV) or syphilis, complications of pregnancy such as hypertension, and undernutrition. Preterm birth often occurs spontaneously and the mechanisms are not clearly understood. Other causes are the early initiation of delivery (for medical or non-medical reasons), the induction of labour or Caesarean section, and multiple pregnancy.

Risk factors

For the same gestational age, girls weigh less than boys, firstborn infants weigh less than subsequent infants, and twins weigh less than singletons. Birthweight is significantly affected by the mother's own foetal growth, her diet from birth to pregnancy, and thus her body composition at conception. Women of short stature, living at high altitudes or of a younger age have smaller babies. Unplanned pregnancies have been shown to increase the risk of low birthweight babies. Poor maternal socioeconomic conditions are often associated with LBW as it relates to prolonged poor nutrition, higher prevalence of infection, physically demanding workload, and pregnancy complications underpinned by poverty.

Effects

LBW infants are at increased risk of physical, neurodevelopmental, and psychological sequelae, both short- and long-term. In the immediate postnatal period, they are at risk of hypothermia, hypoglycaemia, sepsis, and other complications (Chapter 29); longer term they are at high risk of developing cerebral palsy, asthma, respiratory infections, and ear infections.

Maternal chronic undernutrition (low maternal weight and height) is linked to IUGR, which can lead to physical impairment in the infant, increasing the risk of restricted growth in the next generation, and reinforcing a vicious circle of malnutrition; this is known as 'the intergenerational effect' (Figure 33.1).

There is also a significant link between foetal undernutrition and non-communicable diseases (NCDs) in adult life, including hypertension, type 2 diabetes, cardiovascular disease, and metabolic syndrome. This has been described in the DOHaD theory, which states

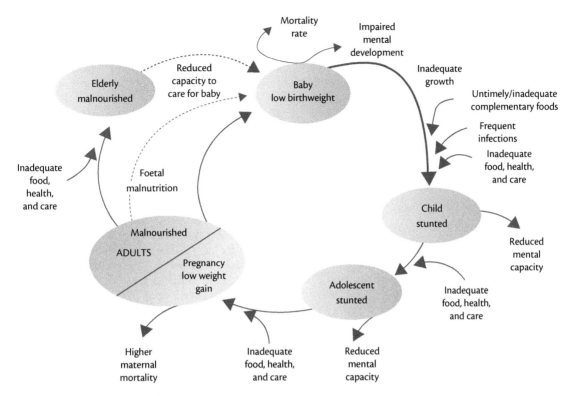

Figure 33.1 Chronic undernutrition through the lifecycle.
Adapted from Administrative Committee on Coordination/Subcommittee on Nutrition (United Nations). Fourth Report on the World Nutrition Situation. Geneva: ACC/SCN in collaboration with the International Food Policy Research Institute. Copyright © 2000 UN ACC Sub-Committee on Nutrition.

that early malnutrition, even if transient, has a significant impact on future health. Periconception is therefore a crucial time period in which to intervene (Chapter 7).

Global targets

WHO Global Targets 2025 (2014)

♦ Achieve a 30% reduction in the number of infants with a birthweight less than 2500g by the year 2025.

Interventions

Interventions focused on improving morbidity and mortality of low birthweight babies should start with prevention at preconception and pregnancy stages; focusing on maternal health and nutrition will provide the greatest impact. Interventions should continue along the continuum of care with appropriate postnatal care to manage complications and optimise weight gain, and strategies to improve child and adolescent nutrition (Chapter 37). A summary of interventions to prevent LBW are listed in Table 33.1.

Preconception and pregnancy

Optimising women's health and nutrition is key for preventing LBW. Family planning is also vital, reducing the risk by improving birth spacing, and preventing unplanned and early pregnancies. Several evidence-based comprehensive interventions level have been proven effective at country level in preventing LBW, including supporting education and empowerment of women, improving sanitary conditions, increasing access to food and tackling

micronutrient deficiencies in at-risk populations. Engagement with the health system can be encouraged through social protection systems such as conditional cash transfer programmes.

A World Health Organization (WHO) review of antenatal nutritional interventions recommends that all pregnant women should receive: 1) counselling on healthy eating and physical activity to prevent newborn macrosomia (particularly in overweight women), and 2) counseling on smoking cessation. Iron and folic acid supplementation is recommended (see Chapter 24). It is recommended that undernourished populations (defined as a low maternal body mass index (BMI) rate of greater than 20%) should receive energy and protein supplementation, for example through fortification of beverages, biscuits, and powders.

Care of the newborn

Postnatally, it is important to assess the type and cause of the low birthweight; the management of low birthweight will depend on whether it was caused by preterm birth, IUGR, or a combination of both. Babies should be monitored for hypothermia, hypoglycaemia, and polycythaemia, and examined for dysmorphic features and signs of congenital infection. Early and exclusive breastfeeding should be encouraged; although babies with IUGR and absent or reversed end-diastolic flow in the umbilical artery are at risk of necrotising enterocolitis and may not be able to tolerate oral feeding in the first 2–3 days of life (Chapter 29).

Challenges

Low birthweight is an important public health indicator; however, there are challenges with regards to reliable data. A large number

Table 33.1 Evidence-based interventions to prevent low birthweight

At country/ regional level	◆ Women's empowerment and education
	◆ Social protection systems (e.g. cash-transfer programmes) related to health-care usage
	◆ Food-distribution systems
	◆ Clean and adequate water, sanitation, and hygiene
	◆ Improvement in facility-based care, and links with community care
	◆ Universal perinatal data-collection system with electronic feedback systems
Prepregnancy	◆ Adequate nutrition for adolescent girls
	◆ Daily folic acid supplementation for at least three months prior to conception
	◆ Smoking cessation
Pregnancy and birth	◆ Counselling of dietary intake and physical exercise
	◆ Daily iron and folic acid supplements
	◆ Malaria prevention
	◆ Smoking cessation
	◆ Foetal growth monitoring
	◆ Decrease in non-medically indicated Caesarean delivery and induction
Postnatal care	◆ Adequate birth spacing

Source: data from World Health Organization. *Global Nutrition Targets 2025: Low birth weight Policy Brief.* Geneva, Switzerland: World Health Organization. Copyright © 2015 WHO.

of babies are not weighed after birth due to being born at home or without a skilled attendant, and an estimated 40% of births worldwide are not even registered. Often when a baby is weighed, it is not measured accurately, measured too long after birth, or not recorded correctly. Using data from facilities introduces bias, as babies born away from facilities may be at higher risk of undernutrition.

Monitoring of foetal growth and possible induction of labour or Caesarean section occurs in high-income countries (HICs); however, this is not feasible in many LMICs, and the consequences of early delivery in response to restricted growth can be more problematic.

Future priorities

◆ Evidence for interventions shown to be effective in preventing LBW are primarily from high-resource settings; further research is needed in LMICs.

◆ More robust data collection is crucial in order to understand the burden of disease, aetiology, and target interventions; vital registration systems need to be strengthened, as well as increased skilled birth attendance.

Conclusions

Poor foetal growth has significant consequences for infant survival and future health and development. Newborns with restricted growth due to intrauterine chronic deprivation are predominant in lower resource settings, and the effect on their physical and mental development leads to a vicious circle of underdevelopment and malnutrition. A concerted effort is required across the continuum of care to optimise the nutrition and health of women of reproductive age before and throughout pregnancy, as well as improving the postnatal management of a low birthweight baby.

Case study: low birthweight and long-term impacts

Komal, an eighteen-year-old woman from rural northern India, attends her local clinic, in labour at thirty-eight weeks' gestation and gives birth to an underweight 1.9 kg baby girl, Gita. Despite being small and initially cold after birth, Gita survives. Komal breastfeeds her baby and, as soon as she is able, introduces their mainly vegetarian diet. Gita remains generally healthy but is both short and thin for her age. During her teenage years, she moves to New Delhi, where they live in the outskirts of the city. In the city, her diet changes, with high-density fast food freely available. Gita becomes pregnant at the same age as her mother and gives birth to a 2 kg boy. He is well at birth but stops feeding soon after. Luckily, he is seen quickly in a local clinic, is given antibiotics for a presumed infection and recovers. Gita later gives birth to two more children and in her last pregnancy, she develops gestational diabetes. She then proceeds to develop type 2 diabetes five years later and suffers the consequences of this later in her life. Low birthweight has distal impacts, both into adulthood and to the next generation.

Questions

1. What are the different types and subcategories of LBW?

2. What are some of the short- and long-term consequences of LBW?

3. What evidence-based interventions have been shown to be effective in reducing the incidence of LBW?

Key publications

Bhutta Z, Daz J, Rizvi A, et al. (2013). Evidence-based interventions for improvement of maternal and child nutrition: what can be done and at what cost? *Lancet* 382(9890): 452–77.
    A recent detailed overview of high-impact interventions to improve maternal and child nutrition, and methods for delivery.

Villar J and Belizan J (1982). The relative contribution of prematurity and foetal growth retardation to low birthweight in developing and developed societies. *Am J Obstet Gynecol* 143: 793–8.
    An important and large study comparing the incidences of low birthweight associated with prematurity and IUGR worldwide.

Bibliography

Barker D (2006). Adult consequences of fetal growth restriction. *Clin Obstet Gynecol* 49: 270–83.

Belizan J, Hofmeyr J, Buekens P, and Salaria N (2013). Preterm birth, an unresolved issue. *Reprod Health* 10: 58.

Davies D, Platts P, Pritchard J, and Wilkinson P (1979). Nutritional status of light-for-date infants at birth and its influence on early postnatal growth. *Arch Dis Child* 54: 703–6.

Ota E, Tobe-Gai R, Mori R, and Farrar D (2012). Antenatal dietary advice and supplementation to increase energy and protein intake. *Cochrane Database Systematic Reviews* CD000032.

United Nations Children's Fund and World Health Organization (2004). Low Birthweight: Country, Regional, and Global Estimates. UNICEF: New York, US.

Villar J and Belizan J (1982). The relative contribution of prematurity and fetal growth retardation to low birth weight in developing and developed societies. *Am J Obstet Gynecol* 143: 793–8.

Villar J and Belizan J (1982). The timing factor in the pathophysiology of the intrauterine growth retardation syndrome. *Obstet Gynecol Surv* 37: 499–506.

Villar J, Smeriglio V, Martorell R, Brown C, and Klein R (1984). Heterogeneous growth and mental development of intrauterine growth-retarded infants during the first 3 years of life. *Pediatrics* 74: 783–91.

Villar J, Altobelli L, Kestler E, and Belizan J (1986). A health priority for developing countries: the prevention of chronic fetal malnutrition. *Bull World Health Organization* 64: 847–51.

World Health Organization (2011). *Optimal Feeding of Low Birthweight Infants in Low- and Middle-Income Countries.* WHO: Geneva.

World Health Organization (2014). *Global Nutrition Targets 2025: Low Birthweight Policy Brief.* WHO: Geneva.

World Health Organization (2016). *WHO Recommendations on Antenatal Care for a Positive Pregnancy Experience.* WHO: Geneva.

CHAPTER 34

Strategies to improve newborn health and prevent stillbirths

Samantha Sadoo, Hannah Blencowe, Cally Tann, and Joy Lawn

This chapter provides an overview of key priorities and strategies required to improve newborn mortality and morbidity, and reduce stillbirths, in the face of slow progress globally.

Key points

♦ Whilst it is important to deliver interventions across the lifecycle, the packages of care with the highest impact are those around the time of birth, and the care of small and sick newborns. Therefore, a priority is to improve skilled delivery and the quality of care in facilities.

♦ Strategies can be delivered at the community and facility level, and these should be well linked. In recent years the importance of facility-based care for newborns has been increasingly recognised.

♦ Programmatic coverage needs to be better measured; this requires every birth and death to be counted, and robust health information systems to allow tracking of interventions.

Background

Over the last few decades, remarkable progress has been made for maternal and child deaths, but neonatal mortality reduction has been about 30% slower, and stillbirth reduction even slower still. Newborn deaths were neglected in the Millennium Development Goals (MDGs), with stillbirths being entirely invisible. Global health targets have also neglected development outcomes beyond survival, increasingly affected by insults around the time of birth and neonatal care, such as early nutrition.

The Sustainable Development Goal (SDG) targets for 2015–2030 are ambitious. However, with high coverage (90%) of available interventions, three million lives could be saved per year by 2025 with great potential for a triple return on investment around the time of birth, averting maternal and newborn deaths and preventing stillbirths (Figure 34.1). Historical trends from the UK and US have shown that the largest reduction in neonatal mortality rates were achieved before neonatal intensive care (pre-1970s), with public health approaches and basic obstetric and neonatal care; this shows that progress can be made even in the poorest settings (Figure 34.2).

Interventions

Interventions for newborn health should be targeted across the reproductive, maternal, newborn, and child health (RMNCH) continuum of care, with a focus on crucial timepoints (Figure 34.3). Taking a lifecourse approach requires coordination between all levels of health care, the public and private sectors, and technical programmes, as well as collaboration amongst all stakeholders: governments, professional associations, development partners, donors, civil society, academic and research institutions, the business community, and families.

The Every Newborn Action Plan (ENAP) prioritises five strategies in order to achieve its targets for the reduction of neonatal mortality and stillbirths worldwide: strengthen and invest in care during the crucial period of labour, childbirth, and the first days of life; improve the quality of maternal and newborn care; reach every woman and newborn and reduce inequities; harness the power of parents, families, and communities for change; count every newborn and improve measurement and accountability, including birth and death registration.

Preconception

The positive impact of preconception interventions on neonatal health outcomes is well recognised, including family planning and optimising women's general health and nutrition (Chapter 26).

Pregnancy

Screening for and management of infection, particularly malaria, human immunodeficiency virus (HIV), tuberculosis, syphilis, and other sexually transmitted infections, can reduce miscarriage, neonatal mortality, preterm births, and stillbirths. Intrapartum antibiotic prophylaxis for known group B streptococcus colonisation can reduce early-onset sepsis in newborns. Prevention of infection with maternal immunisation is also important, of which tetanus has a strong evidence base. Early antenatal detection of intrauterine growth restriction with appropriate treatment and timely delivery could minimise the risks of adverse outcomes in settings with adequate facilities (Chapter 33).

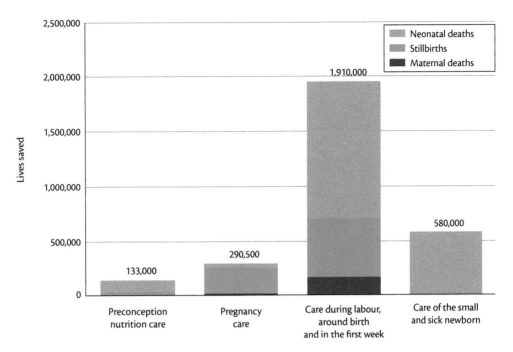

Figure 34.1 Lives that could be saved by 2025 with universal coverage of care, in seventy-five of the Countdown (highest burden) countries.
Source: data from Bhutta, ZA. Et al. Can available interventions end preventable deaths in mothers, newborn babies, and stillbirths, and at what cost?. *The Lancet*. 384(9940), 347–370. Copyright © 2014 Elsevier Ltd. All rights reserved.

Labour and birth

Care around the time of birth has the greatest potential to save newborn lives and reduce stillbirths. Obstetric care involves the monitoring of labour, the presence of skilled personnel at delivery, and the availability of assisted vaginal delivery or Caesarean section if required. The management of preterm labour includes the administration of antenatal cortico steroids to the mother to improve (primarily respiratory and neurological) outcomes in the baby, and prophylactic antibiotics for preterm premature rupture of membranes (PPROM) to reduce the risk of postnatal sepsis. For post-term births, induction/augmentation of labour can reduce meconium aspiration and perinatal deaths; however, the costs and risks associated with inducing labour do not yet support this in many low- and middle-income countries (LMICs).

Interventions for every newborn at birth involve drying and stimulation, and resuscitation for those who do not breathe after birth.

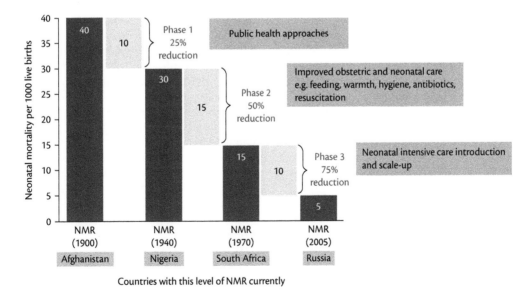

Figure 34.2 Historical phasing of reductions in neonatal mortality rates in the United Kingdom and United States during the twentieth century.
Lawn, JE. Born Too Soon: Accelerating actions for prevention and care of 15 million newborns born too soon. *Reproductive Health*, 10(1), S6. Copyright © 2013 Lawn et al; licensee BioMed Central Ltd. Open access.

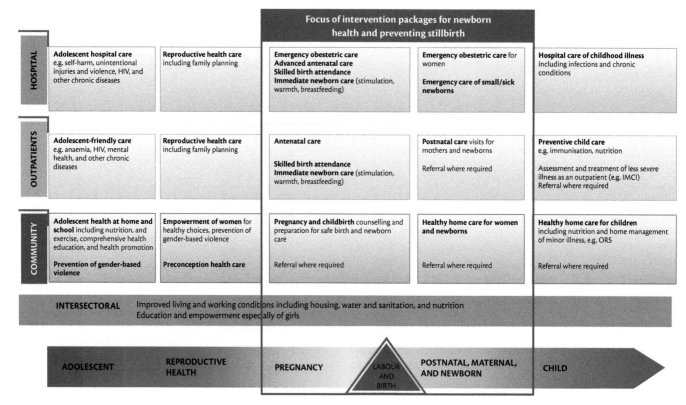

Figure 34.3 Packages of interventions across the lifecourse and the continuum of care.

Sterile cord cutting and cleansing of the umbilical cord with chlorhexidine can reduce infection and mortality. All newborns should be kept warm with skin-to-skin care, head covering, delayed bathing, and early breastfeeding should be initiated. Vitamin K should be administered to prevent haemorrhagic disease of the newborn.

Postnatal care of small and sick newborns

The main causes of neonatal deaths globally are complications from preterm birth, intrapartum-related conditions, and infections, and these should be monitored for and addressed promptly. The care of small and sick newborns can and must be improved, even in low-resource settings where advanced care may not be available. Kangaroo mother care (KMC) comprises a package of early and continuous skin-to-skin contact, breastfeeding support, supportive care in stable newborns, and potential early discharge from hospital. Small or preterm babies may need additional feeding support, for example by cup, nasogastric tube, or intravenous fluids, especially if hypoglycaemic. The timely detection and treatment of infections is crucial. They may also require oxygen and further respiratory support (Chapter 29). Supportive care, including the management of seizures in hypoxic-ischaemic encephalopathy, is important.

Community versus facility care

Both preventative and curative interventions can be delivered through a range of platforms, from community to higher level facility-based care. It is important that these are well linked, support, and complement each other.

Community care

Community care is important for improving the coverage of essential interventions and reducing inequities, reaching the most marginalised populations including those that are rural or post-conflict. 44 million births every year still occur at home, nearly all without a skilled attendant; in sub-Saharan Africa, only a third occur with a traditional birth attendant. A review of randomised trials by Lassi et al. (2010) assessing the effectiveness of community-based intervention packages, found a significant reduction in maternal morbidity (by 25%), stillbirths (19%), perinatal mortality (23%), and neonatal mortality (26%). These packages included tetanus immunisation, clean birth kits, the promotion of facility births, early initiation of breastfeeding, and health-seeking behaviours for neonatal illnesses. Community mobilisation and empowerment through support groups and women's groups have been shown to be successful, improving household behaviours and demand for services, and changing social norms and expectations regarding newborn deaths.

Whilst coverage is important, attention must be paid to the quality of training, support and supervision provided for community health workers, in order to improve outcomes. Home visits are necessary in some situations, but contact with the health system should also be promoted and health workers must have the ability to facilitate referral and transportation to facilities for emergency obstetric care if needed. There is increasing evidence for the implementation of interventions such as KMC and antibiotics for infection in communities.

Facility care

The greatest impact can be made through facility-based care during labour, birth, and the first week of life, including care for small and sick newborns. In high-income countries, facility-based neonatal care is the usual practice and historical trends clearly show the effect on neonatal mortality decline. LMICs have followed this with the establishment of neonatal units, often in the private sector or in referral hospitals in urban areas. However, they may not be adequate, sanitary, and appropriately equipped and therefore increasing births in facilities may not be sufficient to reduce neonatal deaths.

Many settings experience a consistent lack of basic supplies, or poor quality supplies. The private sector has an important role in developing, manufacturing, and distributing medicines and technologies, and reducing costs, especially in low-resource settings. Improved utilisation of information technology to manage logistics could improve needs-based forecasting of supplies.

Another major challenge is to establish and maintain a workforce that is skilled, supported, motivated, and adequate in number. Midwives are essential, as are neonatal nurses, a cadre yet to be established in many settings. Health providers in higher-level referral facilities should be multidisciplinary and include specialised obstetric, paediatric/neonatal, and anaesthetic staff, in order to effectively manage maternal and neonatal complications.

Challenges

Interventions for both mother and baby delivered at the same time, in the same place, by the same health worker will have a great impact on health outcomes. This streamlining needs to translate into the integrated design of services, the responsibilities of health workers, and funding. It is also important that neonatal and maternal health estimates converge and are interpreted together.

Whilst community-based care has been demonstrated to improve outcomes, there is an increasing recognition of the importance of facility-based care. However, the quality of services must be assured; this is important not only to reduce neonatal mortality but for preventing longer-term morbidity. For example, retinopathy of prematurity is preventable through the safer use of oxygen and monitoring, as well as adequate follow-up of preterm babies and early detection and treatment. It is important that the care of small and sick newborn babies in neonatal units is linked with community-based and outpatient follow-up care (as well as vice versa).

There is a lack of standardised global indicators for newborn health and currently few are included in national tracking systems. This leads to a lack of coverage data for maternal and newborn interventions, impeding the ability to monitor and evaluate programmes at a facility, district, and national level. Vital registration and facility information management systems need to be improved to ensure that every birth and death is registered. Perinatal audit and household surveys are also effective for collecting data. Maternal and perinatal death surveillance and audit can be a powerful approach to improving care quality, but only if the audit cycle is completed with solutions implemented and outcomes re-evaluated. There is also a need to strengthen the capacity to analyse the data and use

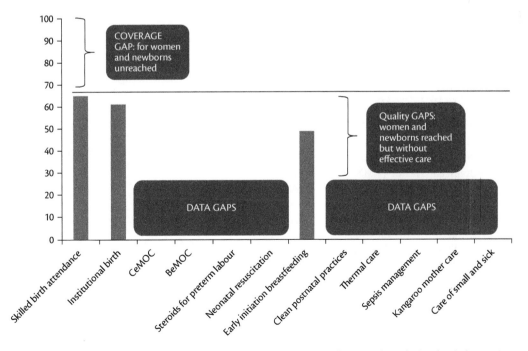

Figure 34.4 Quality gap (and data gaps): percentage coverage along the continuum of care in seventy-five Countdown (highest burden) countries.
CeMOC = Comprehensive emergency obstetric care, BeMOC = Basic emergency obstetric care.
Source: data from Lawn, JE. et al, Born Too Soon: Accelerating actions for prevention and care of 15 million newborns born too soon. *Reproductive Health*, 10(1):S6. Copyright © Lawn et al; licensee BioMed Central Ltd. 2013. Open Access.

it in decision making and implementation of strategies. Figure 34.4 shows the coverage and quality gaps for neonatal care in the Countdown to 2015 priority countries, highlighting the data gaps.

Future priorities

◆ Further research into the prevention of preterm and small for gestational age births is needed as these are still poorly understood, and they are both significant causes of neonatal mortality and morbidity. Areas of interest specifically for preterms include exploring biological causal pathways of preterm labour, new tocolytics to delay preterm birth, and cheaper, more stable surfactant with an easier mode of delivery. Other areas include early detection of high-risk women in pregnancy and labour, and improved and simplified intrapartum monitoring.

◆ In order to improve the care of small and sick newborns in facilities in LMICs, clear, standardised, and evidence-based guidelines and protocols are urgently needed, as well as further research into cost-effective innovative methods for delivering more advanced neonatal care.

Conclusions

The improvement of newborn survival is both feasible and cost-effective, and the cornerstone of the continuum of care. There is an unprecedented opportunity for progress with the establishment of the Every Newborn Action Plan, setting a framework to end preventable newborn deaths and stillbirths by 2035. To ensure that these goals are achieved, targets need to be translated into national strategies, implemented within existing health systems at local and national levels, with strong political will and leadership.

Increasing coverage must occur alongside improvements in the quality of care, with the ability to evaluate and track progress with mechanisms for accountability. Following these evidence-based strategies, we can work towards achieving a healthy start for every newborn baby, supporting their right to survive, but also to thrive and reach their full potential wherever they are born.

Case study: India taking comprehensive action to improve health care outcomes

In response to the slow progress in neonatal compared to maternal health outcomes, India implemented the Reproductive, Maternal, Newborn, Child and Adolescent Health (RMNCH+A) strategy, integrating services across the continuum of care. The newborn component comprises five main areas:

Essential newborn care: The focus has moved towards promoting facility-based births, encouraged by providing financial incentives to both pregnant women and the ASHAs (Accredited Social Health Activists), who serve as a link between the community and the health system. Demonstrating success, in 2011 India launched a scheme providing all women with a free service to deliver in public health facilities, which doubled the proportion of facility births to 83% in 2012–13. Another recent initiative has allowed assistant nurse midwives to give a pre-referral injection of gentamicin for the management of sepsis in infants <2 months of age, and prophylactic vitamin K injection at birth, part of a drive to improve the availability of emergency obstetric and essential newborn care in facilities.

Home-based newborn care: In 2011, a scheme was established supporting the training of 600,000 ASHAs to provide home-based newborn care during the first 42 days of life. They were provided with the skills to manage basic problems and refer to institutions for more advanced care if needed.

Small and sick newborn care: Neonatal units have been scaled up in district hospitals, nearly tripling in number to over 600 units in three years. These units are able to provide specialised care for newborns with severe illness and birth complications. Quality of care has been key, with appropriately skilled doctors and nurses, adherence to evidence-based protocols, and monitoring mechanisms in place for health workers. Newborn survival rates in these units are around 90%.

Adolescent health and reproductive health: ASHAs also provide reproductive health services, including counselling for birth spacing and contraception, reducing unwanted and unplanned pregnancies. India's adolescent health programme, set up in 2014, provides information and counselling on delaying marriage and early pregnancy.

Strengthening the health system: India has invested more than US$19 billion, trained more than 336,000 health workers, and added 20,000 ambulances or patient transport vehicles to the public health system.

Questions

1. What are the priority strategies set by the Every Newborn Action Plan for newborn health and stillbirths?

2. Discuss the benefits of interventions around the time of birth, and care of small and sick newborns to improve neonatal and maternal outcomes.

3. How do research priorities differ between high-income and low-income countries relating to improving newborn health?

Key publications

WHO, UNICEF (2014). *Every Newborn: an Action Plan to End Preventable Deaths.* World Health Organization: Geneva.
    This provides a roadmap of the actions required to end preventable newborn mortality and stillbirth.

Healthy Newborn Network. Available at: http://www.healthynewbornnetwork.org/
    This is an online community that discusses key global issues surrounding newborn health.

Bibliography

Bhutta Z, Das J, and Bahl R (2014). Can available interventions end preventable deaths in mothers, newborn babies, and stillbirths, and at what cost? *Lancet* 384(9940): 347–70.

Dickson K, Simen-Kapeu A, Kinney M, et al. (2014). Health-systems bottlenecks and strategies to accelerate scale-up in countries. *Lancet* 384(9941): 438–54.

Dickson K, Kinney M, Moxon S, et al. (2015). Scaling up quality care for mothers and newborns around the time of birth: an overview of methods and analyses of intervention-specific bottlenecks and solutions. *BMC Pregnancy & Childbirth* 15(Suppl 2): S1.

Lassi Z, Haider B, and Bhutta Z (2010). Community-based intervention packages for reducing maternal and neonatal morbidity and mortality and improving neonatal outcomes. *Cochrane Database Systematic Reviews* 10(11): CD007754.

Lawn J, Kinney M, and Belizan J (2013). Born Too Soon: accelerating actions for prevention and care of 15 million newborns born too soon. *Reproductive Health* 10(1): S6.

Lawn J, Blencowe H, Oza, S, et al. (2014). Every Newborn: progress, priorities, and potential beyond survival. *Lancet* 384: 189–205.

Mason E, McDougall L, Lawn J, et al. (2014). From evidence to action to deliver a healthy start for the next generation. *Lancet* 384(9941): 455–67.

Roos N, Tunçalp Ö, and Kerber K (2016). Learning from every stillbirth and neonatal death. *Lancet* 388(10046): 741–3.

SECTION 7

Child health

CHAPTER 35

Introduction to child health

Dan Magnus, Sebastian Taylor, and Bhanu Williams

In this chapter the main indicators for global child health and the global distribution and causes of child mortality will be discussed.

Key points

- There were 5.4 million deaths among children aged less than five years in 2017.
- Leading causes of death in children under five years (excluding causes in the neonatal period) were pneumonia, diarrhoea, malaria, and congenital anomalies.
- Mortality and morbidity are shifting from infectious to non-communicable diseases.
- Global under-five mortality rate has fallen from 91 per 1000 live births in 1990 to 39 per 1000 in 2017, but this masks wide inter-country variation (e.g. Sierra Leone 111 per 1000 and UK 4 per 1000).

Background

Globally, there were 5.4 million deaths among children aged less than five years in 2017. Approximately half of these deaths were in sub-Saharan Africa and one-third in South-East Asia. There are also large numbers of children living in states of less than full health and with disability. The leading causes of disability-adjusted life years (DALYs) affecting younger children include lower respiratory infection, neonatal preterm birth, diarrhoeal diseases, neonatal encephalopathy, and road injuries.

Indicators of child health

No single indicator can completely describe the health of a population's children; the best picture of child health in any given population will be gained by using a combination of indicators (Table 35.1). Under-five mortality rate is the most widely used measure of child health. The proportion of children who are underweight and overweight will give useful information on population level nutritional status. Immunisation coverage, access to clean water, maternal education, and family income all have a significant effect on child health and are markers of the health system overall and wider health determinants. Some other factors are rarely measured, such as educational attainment and mental and emotional health, but are important for the overall wellbeing of a child. Access to health care is important and amount spent on health per capita, government health expenditure, 'out of pocket' health expenditure, and health care coverage are all useful in assessing this. Rates for individual countries will mask wide differences within countries, with poorer children usually having worse health outcomes than their richer peers. All of these data should be disaggregated by age, gender, migrant status, rural/urban habitation, and socioeconomic group in order to unmask inequity in access to health care and health outcomes.

The global development agenda is now dominated by the Sustainable Development Goals (SDGs), of which one, SDG 3, aims to 'ensure healthy lives and promote wellbeing for all at all ages'.

Global targets

Sustainable Development Goals (2015)

Goal 3 (Health)

- By 2030, end preventable deaths of newborns and children under five years of age, with all countries aiming to reduce neonatal mortality to at least as low as 12 per 1000 live births and under-five mortality to at least as low as 25 per 1000 live births.
- By 2030, reduce by one-third premature mortality from non-communicable diseases through prevention and treatment, and promote mental health and wellbeing.
- By 2020, halve the number of global deaths and injuries from road traffic accidents.
- Support the research and development of vaccines and medicines for the communicable and non-communicable diseases that primarily affect developing countries, provide access to affordable essential medicines and vaccines.
- Achieve universal health coverage, including financial risk protection, access to quality essential health care services and access to safe, effective, quality, and affordable essential medicines and vaccines for all.

Global causes, distribution, and trends in child mortality

Across the world, the number of children dying before reaching their fifth birthday has roughly halved since 1990. This is largely due to reduced deaths from pneumonia, diarrhoea, and measles, secondary to concerted efforts at prevention through improved immunisation coverage and case management at community level. But in this time the proportion of all under-five deaths attributable to neonatal mortality has risen to 46% and there continues to be great disparity in the health outcomes for children between and within countries.

Causes and distribution of child deaths

The leading causes of death among children younger than five years globally in 2015 were pneumonia, preterm birth complications,

Table 35.1 Child health indicators

UN population division region	Under-five mortality rate	Infant mortality rate	Neonatal mortality rate
Sub-Saharan Africa	84	57	29
Africa	76	52	27
Asia	34	28	19
Europe	6	5	3
Latin America/Caribbean	18	15	9
North America	6	6	4
Oceania	24	19	11
World	43	32	19

Source: Data from UNICEF, Statistics and Monitoring; Core indicators in depth. Copyright © 2017 UNICEF. Available at https://www.unicef.org/statistics/index_24296.html

intrapartum-related events (such as neonatal encephalopathy following birth trauma and asphyxia), malaria, and diarrhoeal deaths (Figure 35.1). In children aged 5–9 years, diarrhoeal disease, lower respiratory tract infections, road injuries, gastrointestinal infections (notably typhoid and paratyphoid), and malaria accounted for 181,000 deaths or 39% of deaths.

The overwhelming majority of children dying from malaria (97%) and human immunodeficiency virus (HIV) (90%) are in sub-Saharan Africa. Pneumonia and preterm birth complications are also leading causes of death in this region. The rates of under-five mortality remain highest in sub-Saharan Africa and South Asia. (Figure 35.2). However, in terms of absolute numbers, over half of all child deaths occur in just five countries: India,

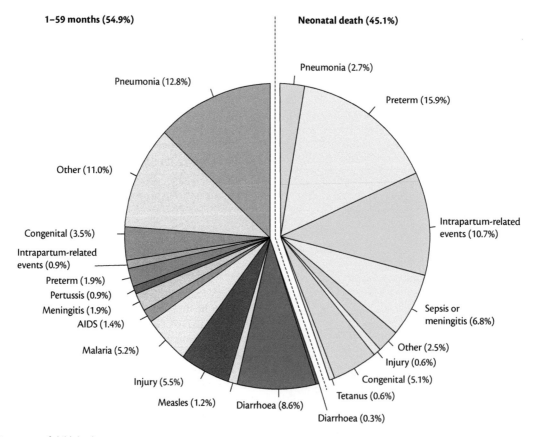

Figure 35.1 Major causes of child deaths.

Reproduced from Liu, L. et al. Global, regional, and national causes of under-5 mortality in 2000–15: an updated systematic analysis with implications for the Sustainable Development Goals. *The Lancet* 388(10063): 3027–3035. Copyright © 2016 The Author(s). Published by Elsevier Ltd. This is an Open Access article under the CC BY license.

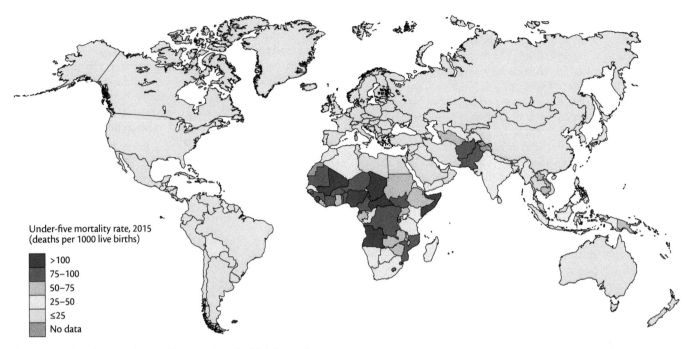

Figure 35.2 Under five mortality rate (deaths per 1000 live births) in 2015, by country.
Reproduced with permission from United Nations Inter-agency Group for Child Mortality Estimation (UN IGME). Levels & Trends in Child Mortality: Report 2017. New York, USA: United Nations Children's Fund. Copyright © 2017 UN IGME.

Nigeria, Democratic Republic of Congo (DRC), Pakistan, and China.

Reductions in child mortality and trends

There have been substantial global improvements in child mortality over the last fifty years and reductions since 2000 in under-five mortality rates continue to accelerate in many countries, especially those in sub-Saharan Africa. The quick and sustained decrease in child deaths in some developing countries is likely to be attributable to the agenda surrounding the Millennium Declaration and associated increased global aid and expenditure on health.

Reductions in child mortality and improvements in child health globally may be attributable to a number of factors, including reducing poverty, enhancement in community-oriented and primary health care services, and improved maternal education. These improvements, in turn, may be attributable to major health and child health initiatives, within the scope of the Millennium Development Goals (MDGs), including the Global Fund for AIDS, TB, and Malaria, the Global Alliance for Vaccines and Immunisation (GAVI), as well as the global movement for Every Woman, Every Child. These initiatives have been supported with increasing quantities of health finance, including through bilateral and multilateral donors, the international finance institutions (in particular the World Bank), and the rapid growth of global health philanthropy, most substantially reflected in the Bill and Melinda Gates Foundation.

The transition point between the MDGs and the SDGs sets out a pathway for health to 2030. Continued and sustainable improvements in global child health will depend on a number of non-clinical factors, including maximising economic growth potential, especially in low-income countries in sub-Saharan Africa and South Asia. This will need to be through strengthening governmental capacity to build domestic tax-based revenue streams and growing long-term financing capacity to improve key social determinants of health, as well as health systems and care. Also important will be policy-setting sovereignty to allow national and sub-national government actors, working with non-government partners, to address issues of socioeconomic inequality and health inequity.

Child morbidity and disability

In addition to the focus on child mortality, there is also a need to look at child morbidity and disability. DALYs are used for this as they combine the years of life lost from mortality with years of life lived with disability or in a state of less than full health. Approximately a third (31%) of total global DALYs are attributable to communicable, maternal, neonatal, and nutritional causes, but there is variation between regions, with nearly two-thirds (62%) of DALYs from these causes in the World Health Organization (WHO) African region. In the last fifteen years there have been impressive global reductions in DALYs from conditions affecting children, largely as a consequence of decreases in years of life lost due to mortality. In 2015, 28% of total DALYs globally were borne by children under the age of fifteen years (this number was 41% in 2000) and of these, 87% were caused by premature death, with 13% attributable to ill health and disability.

The leading causes of DALYs affecting younger children include lower respiratory infection, neonatal preterm birth, diarrhoeal diseases, neonatal encephalopathy, and road injuries. Many of the health problems seen in adolescence start during the first decade, emphasising the need for programming across the lifecourse.

Social determinants of health

Societally, well-known and evidenced health determinants continue to present a major challenge to improving child health. Social determinants of health are a key feature of health action in countries at all stages of economic development and wealth. Low-income countries in particular continue to struggle to finance major infrastructural and institutional investments in universal, accessible, quality public services, in systemic poverty reduction and social protection, in access to basic health commodities, and clean water, adequate sanitation, and clean air. In the absence of more effective integrated action on health determinants upstream, continuing and likely increasing pressure will fall on healthcare interventions further downstream.

Challenges

Accurate ascertainment of cause of death is challenging in countries without comprehensive registration systems for birth and death, and where data on maternal and child morbidity and mortality is unreliable, inconsistent, and does not cover large segments of the population. The Global Burden of Disease Study used data from vital registration systems, cancer surveillance systems, verbal autopsy (questioning family members about symptoms prior to the patient's death to retrospectively decide upon a likely diagnosis), police records and surveys of hospital, census and mortuary data.

Future priorities

- While there has been excellent progress in reducing mortality and morbidity from diarrhoea, pneumonia, and measles, there has been slower progress in reducing neonatal and child deaths from congenital causes, prematurity, sepsis, and injury. The latter causes respond less well to vertical programmes and require health systems strengthening including training of health workers, hitherto neglected in favour of 'quick wins' under the MDG agenda.

- Despite great improvements in global child health, there is still much to be done and without further accelerated progress, many countries in West and Central Africa, in particular, will still have high levels of under-five mortality in 2030. Estimates by Liu et al. (2015) based on current trends suggest that 4.4 million children younger than five years will still die in 2030, with 60% of these deaths in sub-Saharan Africa. There needs to be a clear international and country level health policy focus on interventions for the poorest children in order to reduce inequity. Requiring governments to disaggregate mortality data by household income decile could help to support this.

- Improved breastfeeding practices, implementation of the WHO expanded programme of immunisation, case management of pneumonia and diarrhoea, malaria prevention with insecticide-treated bed nets, and scale-up of prevention of mother-to-child transmission of HIV are all medical programme interventions that have been important in improving child health globally, but could still reduce child deaths further with greater access and coverage. Reducing poverty, improving access to clean piped water, sanitation, and improving female education are important non-medical approaches to improving child health.

- In addition to the disease-specific strategies for improving child health that have been highly visible in recent years, there are several examples of significant child health challenges in low-income countries that will require additional attention and priority in the future. These include: focusing on and addressing the problem of stillbirths and preterm birth complications and developing strategies for reducing and treating congenital abnormalities; strengthening systems for diagnosing and treating childhood cancers and sickle cell disease; improving data, prevention, and treatment strategies for reducing childhood injuries and trauma; reducing morbidity, supporting children with disabilities and improving early childhood development; transitioning from child to adult services, for example for adolescents with HIV; and developing paediatric health services and universal health coverage for children.

Conclusions

There have been substantial and sustained improvements in global child health and mortality over the last twenty years, largely thanks to improved prevention and management of childhood diarrhoea, pneumonia, malaria, and measles. However, in 2017, 46% of all under-five deaths occurred in the neonatal period and the rates of under-five mortality and absolute numbers of deaths continue to be a significant challenge in sub-Saharan Africa and South Asia. Addressing current and future threats to child health will require national and international level programme approaches to deal with key child health threats such as prematurity, pneumonia, and injuries, as well as health system strengthening, strategies for improving the social determinants of health, and investments in supporting research and data systems.

Case study: rapid reduction in under-five mortality in Malawi

Malawi is a landlocked country in Africa with a population of 16.3 million people. It ranked 173 out of 188 countries on the Human Development Index in 2014, has a life expectancy at birth of 62.8 and 5.8% of the population are estimated to be Internet users. The leading causes of under-five child mortality are malaria (14%), pneumonia (13%), HIV (12%), and diarrhoea (7%), with 34% of deaths occurring in the neonatal period. And yet its progress in reducing child mortality has been impressive. The under-five mortality rate in Malawi fell from 247 per 1000 in 1990 to 64 per 1000 in 2015 representing an annual rate of reduction in child mortality of 5.4% (1990–2013). The substantial improvements in child mortality in Malawi have been attributed to reductions in malnutrition (specifically wasting and stunting), decrease in fertility rate, increased facility birth care, better HIV prevention and treatment strategies including prevention of mother to child transmission, coverage with insecticide-treated bednets to prevent malaria, and improved recognition and treatment of diarrhoea, pneumonia, and malaria. Much of this success has come from increases in donor funding and government health expenditure on reproductive, maternal, newborn, and child health, alongside national and community level policy, programme, and financial investments and strategies for improving child health.

Questions

1. What are the leading global causes of child mortality in children aged under five years?

2. Can you define (a) under-five mortality rate; (b) infant mortality rate; (c) neonatal mortality rate?

3. Name five targets related to child health outlined in Sustainable Development Goal 3 and how they might be achieved.

Key publication

Liu L, Oza S, Hogan D, et al. (2015). Global, regional, and national causes of child mortality in 2000–13, with projections to inform post-2015 priorities: an updated systematic analysis. *Lancet* 385(9966): 430–40.

Epidemiology of child mortality, in the context of priority setting in the SDG era.

Bibliography

Kanyuka M, Ndawala J, Mleme T, et al. (2016). Malawi and Millennium Development Goal 4: a Countdown to 2015 country case study. *Lancet Global Health* 4(3): e201–14.

United Nations Inter-Agency Group for Child Mortality Estimation (2015). Levels and trends in child mortality. http://www.unicef.org/media/files/IGME_Report_Final2.pdf

Wang H, Liddell C, Coates M, et al. (2014). Global, regional, and national levels of neonatal, infant, and under-5 mortality during 1990–2013: a systematic analysis for the Global Burden of Disease Study 2013. *Lancet* 384(9947): 957–79.

CHAPTER 36

Child infection

Mark Lee, Bhanu Williams, and Anu Goenka

This chapter will address the role of infectious diseases in child mortality and morbidity. It should be read in conjunction with Chapter 31 (Newborn infection) and Chapter 15 (Adolescent infection).

Key points

- Infectious diseases such as pneumonia, diarrhoea, and malaria remain the biggest killers of children outside the neonatal period.
- Effective evidence-based interventions exist to reduce mortality and morbidity from childhood infectious diseases.
- Infection control programmes have been undermined by inadequate implementation, particularly for children living in poverty.

Background

In the under-five age group, outside the neonatal period, the largest causes of mortality are almost exclusively infectious diseases including pneumonia (13%), diarrhoea (9%), malaria (7%), measles (2%), and human immunodeficiency virus and acquired immune deficiency syndrome (HIV/AIDS) (2%). Among children aged 5–9 years, pneumonia, diarrhoeal disease and malaria were among the top five leading causes of death, as well as morbidity measured by disability adjusted life years (DALYs). Some infections are associated with disproportionately higher morbidity compared with mortality: tuberculosis, HIV/AIDS, meningitis, and typhoid fever.

Children living in poverty are more likely to develop severe infections, and to die as a result. For example, diarrhoea is most common in countries with poor access to safe drinking water and sanitation. Half of the child deaths globally from diarrhoea occurred in India, Pakistan, Nigeria, Democratic Republic of Congo, and Ethiopia. The link between poverty and child deaths from infectious diseases is multi-factorial. One key factor is maternal education, where higher levels are associated with a significantly decreased risk of child death from an infectious disease. Other factors that are closely interrelated include vaccine access/uptake, food security, feeding practices, safe drinking water and sanitation, as well as access to skilled health care. Malnourished children (and those who are HIV-infected) are immunosuppressed and are left more vulnerable to both common and more unusual opportunistic pathogens.

Global targets

Sustainable Development Goals (SDGs) (2015)

Goal 3 (Health)

- By 2030, end preventable deaths of newborns and children under five years of age, with all countries aiming to reduce

neonatal mortality to at least as low as 12 per 1000 live births and under-five mortality to at least as low as 25 per 1000 live births.
- By 2030, end the epidemics of AIDS, tuberculosis, malaria, and neglected tropical diseases, and combat hepatitis, water-borne diseases, and other communicable diseases.

Major infectious diseases causing child death

The overall reduction in child deaths in 1990–2015 has, in large part, been driven by a reduction in the absolute number of under-five deaths attributable to the commonest infections, for example 70% reduction in deaths due to pneumonia and diarrhoea, and 36% reduction in deaths due to malaria. However, infectious diseases remain a major cause of child mortality, with just eight infections (Table 36.1) contributing to 58% of under-five deaths outside the neonatal period in 2015, compared with 69% in 1990. Pneumonia and diarrhoea still account for as many as two million deaths a year, with the majority occurring in the first year of life. Although tuberculosis was associated with significantly less mortality (100,000 child deaths in 2015), the real figure is likely to be higher owing to the difficulties in achieving an accurate diagnosis.

Interventions

Evidence-based interventions (Table 36.1) have helped reduce the mortality and morbidity from infectious diseases. The success of these interventions has largely been determined by their coverage, particularly among the world's poorest children. For severe cases of malaria, a Cochrane review by Sinclair et al. (2012), which included multicentre studies from Asia and sub-Saharan Africa, showed that artesunate, instead of quinine, significantly reduced mortality in children, saving an extra 26 lives for every 1000 children treated. However, approximately 80% of the 80 million sub-Saharan African children with malaria did not receive appropriate antimalarials in 2015.

For HIV, the World Health Organization (WHO) recommends that all newly diagnosed children should start antiretroviral treatment. The evidence is strongest in infants; a randomised control trial by Violari et al. (2008) demonstrated a 75% reduction in mortality for those started on antiretroviral treatment at diagnosis, compared with those started only when their disease progressed. However, inadequate implementation of paediatric HIV programmes has meant that only 49% of HIV-exposed infants were tested for HIV in 2014, and only 30% of HIV-infected children received antiretroviral treatment.

Table 36.1 Major infectious diseases causing child death

	Major pathogens	Transmission	Clinical presentation	Complications	Key prevention interventions	Key management interventions	Key targets and policy documents
Pneumonia	Bacteria: *Streptococcus pneumoniae*, *Haemophilus influenzae* Viruses: influenza, human rhinoviruses, coronaviruses, respiratory syncytial virus, human metapneumovirus, adenovirus, parainfluenza	Airborne, droplet	Respiratory distress, fever, cough, poor feeding, lethargy, cyanosis	Respiratory failure Sepsis Empyema Pleural effusion	Vaccination (PCV, Hib vaccine, influenza vaccine, Measles vaccine, pertussis vaccine) Reduction in indoor air pollution	Oral antibiotics for moderate Intravenous antibiotics for severe Oxygen therapy	End preventable deaths by 2025 (WHO) WHO Global Action Plan for Pneumonia and Diarrhoea (2013) WHO/UNICEF Integrated Management of Childhood Illness
Diarrhoea	Viruses: Rotavirus Bacteria: *Escherichia coli*, *Vibrio cholerae* *Shigella dysenteriae* Protozoa: *Cryptosporidium* spp., *Giardia lamblia*	Faeco-oral	Vomiting, diarrhoea, fever, lethargy, blood in the stool (pathogen dependant)	Dehydration, electrolyte imbalances, hypovolaemic shock, malnutrition	Exclusive breastfeeding for first 6 months Access to safe drinking water Sanitation Hand hygiene Vaccination (rotavirus) Vitamin A supplementation	ORS plus zinc supplements, intravenous fluids if severe dehydration, antibiotics if dysentery	
Malaria	Protozoa: *Plasmodium falciparum*, *Plasmodium vivax*, *Plasmodium malariae*, *Plasmodium ovale*, *Plasmodium knowlesi*	Vector-borne: female anopheles mosquito	Fever, deep breathing, lethargy/coma, seizures, pallor	Cerebral malaria, respiratory distress, anaemia, jaundice, renal impairment, hypoglycaemia, acidosis	Long-lasting insecticide treated nets Indoor residual spraying Removal of mosquito breeding sites Seasonal malaria chemo-prevention for under fives Vaccines currently in development (e.g. RTS,S/AS01)	Use of rapid diagnostic tests Oral artemisinin-based combination therapy	Reduce malaria attributable deaths by 90% by 2030 (WHO) WHO's Global Technical Strategy for Malaria 2016–2030 (2015)
TB	*Mycobacterium tuberculosis*	Airborne, droplet	Persistent non-remitting cough >2 weeks, reduced playfulness, persistent fever, poor growth, lethargy	Dissemination to: CNS, lymph nodes, pleural cavity, bones, abdomen, pericardium Malnutrition	BCG vaccine Effective adult TB control programme (reduces transmission to children) Isoniazid preventive therapy (IPT) for contacts (<5 years old and/or HIV) Integration of TB and HIV services	Acquisition of gastric washings or induced sputum Access to liquid culture and resistance testing Rapid PCR (GeneXpert) Adherence support (DOTS) Registration with national TB control programme	Reduce TB attributable deaths by 90% by 2030 (WHO) WHO Roadmap for Tuberculosis: Towards Zero Deaths (2013)

(continued)

Table 36.1 Continued

	Major pathogens	Transmission	Clinical presentation	Complications	Key prevention interventions	Key management interventions	Key targets and policy documents
HIV	HIV-1 HIV-2	Vertical: mother to child Horizontal: sexual Blood products Intravenous drug use	Weight loss, recurrent infections, persistent diarrhoea, chronic otitis media, oral thrush, generalised lymphadenopathy PJP in infants	AIDS, malnutrition, severe opportunistic infection, malignancy	Effective adult control programme PMTCT PITC	Access to HIV testing (antibody and PCR) ART programme Co-trimoxazole prophylaxis (to prevent PJP) Nutritional support Psychosocial support	90-90-90 target: by 2030, 90% of all people living with HIV will know their status, 90% will receive ART, and 90% of all receiving ART will have viral suppression (UNAIDS) UNAIDS Global AIDS Update (2016)
Meningitis	Bacteria: *Neisseria meningitidis, Streptococcus pneumoniae, Haemophilus influenzae, Mycobacterium tuberculosis*	Close contact via respiratory and throat secretions	Fever, irritability, poor feeding, lethargy, neck stiffness, photophobia, bulging fontanelle, headache, seizures, coma	Hydrocephalus, stroke, chronic neurodisability, deafness	Vaccination (PCV, Hib vaccine, BCG vaccine and meningococcal vaccines covering serogroups A, B, C, ACWY) Contact tracing and prophylaxis	Lumbar puncture for confirmation of diagnosis IV antibiotics, neurorehabilitation	Different strategies and targets for different pathogens
Measles	Measles virus	Airborne, droplet	Fever, coryza, conjunctivitis, maculopapular rash	Acute malnutrition, pneumoni, diarrhoea, otitis media, croup, vitamin A deficiency (blindness)	Measles vaccine Vitamin A supplementation Outbreak identification and control	Vitamin A, supportive care, nutritional support, Treat complications	Elimination from five WHO regions by 2020 (WHO) Global Vaccine Action Plan 2011–2020 (WHO)
Whooping cough	*Bordetella pertussis*	Airborne, droplet	Coryza, paroxysmal cough, inspiratory 'whoop'	In young infants: apnoea, respiratory failure, pulmonary hypertension, very high white blood cell count	Maternal vaccination at 28 weeks' gestation Infant vaccination Antibiotics to reduce transmission	Supportive treatments may reduce mortality in young infants (oxygen, ventilatory support)	Achieve 90% coverage with 3 doses of diphtheria-tetanus-pertussis- containing vaccines Global Vaccine Action Plan 2011–2020 (WHO)

AIDS: Acquired Immunodeficiency Syndrome; ART: antiretroviral therapy; ORS: oral rehydration solution; BCG: Bacillus Calmette-Guérin; CNS: central nervous system; Hib: directly observed treatment short-course; Hib: *Haemophilus influenzae* type b; MTCT: maternal to child transmission; ORS: oral rehydration solution; PCR: polymerase chain reaction; PCV: pneumococcal conjugate vaccine; PITC: provider initiated testing and counselling; PJP: *Pneumocystis jirovecii* pneumonia; PMTCT: prevention of maternal to child transmission; UNAIDS: Joint United Nations Programme on HIV/AIDS.

A key tool in reducing deaths from infectious diseases is vaccination. Global deployment of the measles vaccine was responsible for 23% of the overall reduction in child mortality between 1990 and 2008. Despite these gains, approximately twenty million children per year still do not receive their first dose of measles vaccine, which resulted in more than 100,000 child deaths in 2014. Unsubstantiated concerns about the safety of measles vaccines have reduced their uptake in many industrialised countries, resulting in unvaccinated susceptible cohorts that have fuelled outbreaks. In many low-income countries (LICs), outbreaks have been predominantly related to the logistical and financial challenges in ensuring universal access to vaccination.

Children often present to primary healthcare facilities with several unmet health needs that span infection(s), nutrition, vaccination, and neurodevelopment. To better meet these needs, the Integrated Management of Childhood Illness (IMCI) was developed by the WHO and United Nations Children's Fund (UNICEF) in the early 1990s. IMCI is a comprehensive approach that supports healthcare workers in assessing a sick child for multiple common conditions in the same consultation, while addressing wider health issues such as the provision of feeding advice, vitamin A supplementation, and deworming. This community case management approach is complemented by health system strengthening. IMCI is adapted to reflect local epidemiology, for example dengue fever is highlighted as an important cause of fever or shock in the Indian adaptation of IMCI, and most of the African countries have included HIV in IMCI. Successful implementation of integrated prevention and control programmes has the potential to make significant gains, for example by effective deployment of the interventions in Table 36.2, it is estimated that 95% of deaths due to diarrhoea and 67% of deaths due to pneumonia could be prevented.

Neglected tropical diseases

The WHO Neglected Tropical Diseases (NTDs) are a group of seventeen chronic infections that disproportionately affect the world's most impoverished communities and cause significant morbidity (Table 36.3). Approximately 1.5 billion individuals are affected by NTDs, and one-third of these are children. NTDs often result in chronic debilitating illnesses that are accompanied by social stigma. In 2010, NTDs were collectively responsible for

approximately forty-eight million DALYs, a burden of morbidity comparable to tuberculosis (forty-nine million DALYs). Eleven of the seventeen NTDs are currently being targeted by the WHO for elimination/eradication by 2020 (Table 36.3), and several of these affect children disproportionately.

A successful control programme has almost eradicated dracunculiasis (Guinea worm infection). This has been achieved through coordinated efforts to prevent exposure to the pathogen (safe drinking water, vector control, and health education), as well as surveillance to prevent spread (case detection and containment). In contrast, ongoing efforts are struggling to control soil transmitted helminth (STH) infections. The STHs are nematode worms whose transmission occurs following ingestion of soil contaminated with human faeces, or skin penetration. Disease control is challenging, principally owing to the large reservoir of infection (around a quarter of the world's population are infected). STH infections cause impaired physical and cognitive development by contributing to macronutrient and micronutrient deficiencies, for example the adult hookworm resides in the small bowel, drawing blood from the intestinal mucosa, causing iron-deficiency anaemia. Deworming programmes deliver annual antihelminthic therapy (such as single dose albendazole) to all children at immunisation clinics and schools.

Challenges

Antimicrobial resistance (AMR) is the ability of a microbe to resist effects of medication previously used to treat them. An estimated 700,000 people died in 2014 due to infections caused by bacteria resistant to antibiotics. AMR is prevalent in low- and middle-income countries (LMICs), where one review by Le Doare et al. (2015), which included data from over 70,000 children with bloodstream infections, showed median resistance rates of *Klebsiella pneumoniae* to cephalosporin treatment was 84% in Asia and 50% in Africa. Neonatal infections due to resistant organisms are thought to cause almost 60,000 deaths every year in India. Resistance to newer antimicrobial treatments is also emerging, such as artemisinin for malaria in South-East Asia. We are entering the 'post-antibiotic era' in which some infections are resistant to all existing antimicrobials, such as colistin resistant *Escherichia coli*, and totally drug-resistant

Table 36.2 Evidence-based interventions that reduce diarrhoea and pneumonia

Interventions that reduce diarrhoea	Interventions that reduce both diarrhoea and pneumonia	Interventions that reduce pneumonia
Vitamin A supplementation	Breastfeeding promotion and support	Vaccination—PCV, Hib, pertussis
Vaccination—rotavirus	Adequate complementary feeding	Reduce household air pollution
Safe drinking water and sanitation	Measles vaccination	Antibiotics for pneumonia
Low osmolality ORS and zinc	Handwashing with soap	Oxygen therapy
	Prevention and treatment of HIV	
	Improved care seeking behaviour and referral	
	Improved case management at community and health facility levels	
	Continued feeding	

Hib: *Haemophilus influenzae* type b; ORS: oral rehydration solution; PCV: pneumococcal conjugate vaccine.

Source: data from World Health Organization and UNICEF. *Ending preventable child deaths from pneumonia and diarrhoea by 2025: The integrated Global Action Plan for Pneumonia and Diarrhoea*. Geneva, Switzerland: World Health Organization. Copyright © 2013 WHO/UNICEF.

Table 36.3 The WHO neglected tropical diseases

Buruli ulcer	Human African trypanosomiasis*	Rabies
Chagas disease*		Schistosomiasis*
Dengue and Chikungunya	Leishmaniasis*	Soil-transmitted
Dracunculiasis (guinea-worm disease)*	Leprosy (Hansen's disease)*	helminthiases
		Taeniasis/Cysticercosis
Echinococcosis	Lymphatic filariasis*	Trachoma*
Foodborne trematodiases	Onchocerciasis (river blindness)*	Yaws (endemic treponematoses)*

*Targeted for elimination/eradication by the WHO.

TB. The global epidemic of AMR is being driven by a number of factors, many of which can be addressed with evidence-based interventions (Table 36.4). Antibiotic stewardship programmes coordinate implementation of such interventions with the aim of reducing the impact of AMR on clinical outcomes.

Emerging infections

Emerging infections are caused by microbes that were previously unknown, as well as microbes that have re-emerged following a period of decline or are now being found in new geographical areas. International air travel has contributed to the increased incidence of emerging infections. Climate change has also resulted

Table 36.4 Drivers of increasing global antimicrobial resistance (AMR) and evidence-based interventions

	AMR driver	Intervention
Population	Vaccine hesitancy	Public education
	Purchase of antimicrobials without prescription	Improved access to health care
		Government legislation
	Poor adherence to antimicrobial treatment	Adherence support interventions
	Increased migration	Global surveillance systems and new-entrant screening programmes
Health care	Poor hand hygiene	Clinical audit and care bundles of infection control interventions
	Poor adherence to infection control measures	
	Inappropriate prescription of antimicrobials	Education of clinicians
		Development of near-patient diagnostics
Government	Poor AMR surveillance systems	Nationally co-ordinated AMR surveillance
	Non-therapeutic use of antimicrobials in agriculture	Government legislation
	Lack of legislation re: quality/sale of antimicrobials	
	Diminishing antibiotic pipeline of new drugs	Investment in novel drug/vaccine research

in the migration of disease vectors into new regions, such as the outbreak of Chikungunya virus in North-East Italy as a result of the spread of the Tiger mosquito (*Aedes albopictus*) into more temperate climate areas. Increasing urbanisation, along with poverty and wars, has resulted in larger cohabiting populations that facilitate transmission. The 2014 Ebola outbreak in West Africa is an example of how these factors aligned to propagate an unprecedented epidemic by a virus that had previously caused relatively minor isolated outbreaks in rural areas. Other recent epidemics (Table 36.5) highlight the need for a coordinated and rapid response between monitoring agencies such as the WHO, non-governmental organisations (NGOs), governments, and the local population. Continued investment in improving healthcare infrastructure in LICs is also of paramount importance in reducing the impact of future outbreaks.

Future priorities

♦ To ensure the continued progress in reducing the burden of childhood infectious diseases, there must be a co-ordinated global effort to increase investment in evidence-based infection prevention and control programmes. The success of these programmes is heavily dependent on reducing societal inequality, increasing female literacy, and a commitment to improve infrastructure and access to health care.

♦ Future priorities also include directing investment toward programmes that reduce the burden of neglected tropical diseases, antimicrobial resistance, and emerging infections.

Conclusions

Tackling infectious diseases was very successful in the Millennium Development Goal (MDG) era, both in terms of reductions in mortality, and increasing prioritisation. However, certain populations have been left behind, and certain diseases, particularly the neglected tropical diseases, require more focus. At the same time, it is important we remain aware of the dangers of inappropriate antibiotic prescription and the possibility of emerging infections that require a rapid, coordinated global effort to address.

Case study: a potentially preventable death from an infection in Zambia

Thandi is a nine-month-old girl living in rural Zambia with a short history of fever, cough, coryza, rash, and diarrhoea. She is taken to a primary healthcare clinic 25 km from her home by her thirteen-year-old sister. Her mother died two months ago from an undiagnosed chronic breathing problem. Thandi is clearly malnourished. Her health card has been lost, which contained her growth charts and vaccination status. She is assessed by a nurse who prescribes co-trimoxazole for pneumonia, and standard oral rehydration solution (ORS) sachets for diarrhoea. Thandi returns home and although her coryza and cough begin to settle down, her diarrhoea continues. She is taken back to the healthcare clinic two days later, where she is immediately noted to be severely dehydrated. The nurse attempts to resuscitate Thandi, but sadly her efforts are unsuccessful and Thandi dies. Thandi's death was preventable and a complex interplay of potential factors was responsible for her presentation (Figure 36.1).

Table 36.5 Significant outbreaks caused by emerging infections

Infection	Year of last significant outbreak	Year discovered	Country of origin	Transmission (enzootic/natural reservoir/host)	Geographical distribution	Significant clinical features
Zika virus	2015	1947	Uganda	*Aedes* spp. Mosquito (enzootic – non-human primates)	South-East Asia, Africa, French Polynesia, North, Central and South America	Congenital infection with microcephaly Guillain-Barré syndrome Case fatality: unknown
Ebola virus	2014	1976	Zaire (DRC)	Direct contact with bodily fluids (natural reservoir, bats)	West, Central and East Africa	Fever, diarrhoea, bleeding, Case fatality: 25–90% median 50%
MERS-CoV	2012	2012	Saudi Arabia	?Person-to-person (?enzootic/?natural reservoir, dromedary camels)	Middle East, North Africa, South Korea	Influenza-like illness, pneumonia Case fatality: 30–40%
Swine influenza (H1N1)	2009	1918	Unknown	Airborne/droplet (enzootic, pigs)	Worldwide, >100 countries	Influenza-like illness Case fatality: 0.03% (2009 pandemic)
Avian influenza (H5N1)	2008	1997	Hong Kong	Airborne/droplet (enzootic, poultry/wild birds)	South-East Asia, Mongolia, Russia, Kazakhstan	Influenza-like illness, pneumonia Case fatality: 61–89%
SARS-CoV	2003	2002	China	Airborne/droplet (enzootic ?animal)	South-East Asia, Canada	Influenza-like illness, pneumonia Case fatality: 10%

DRC: Democratic Republic of Congo; MERS: Middle East respiratory syndrome; SARS: severe acute respiratory syndrome.

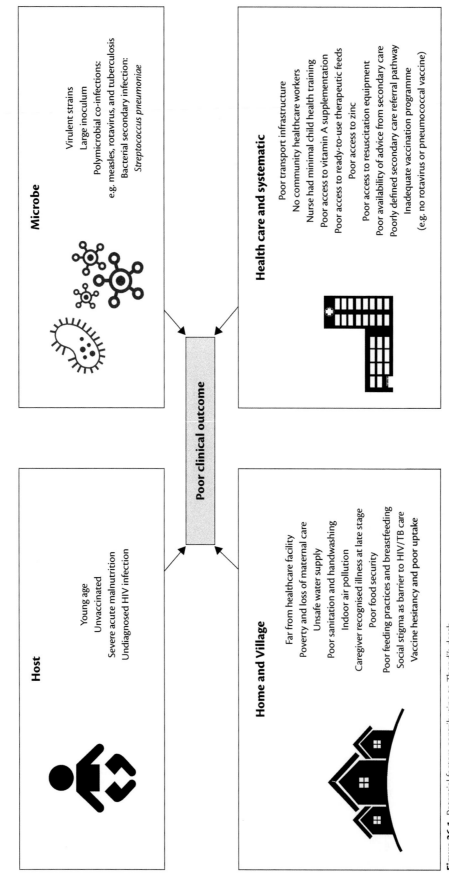

Host

Young age
Unvaccinated
Severe acute malnutrition
Undiagnosed HIV infection

Microbe

Virulent strains
Large inoculum
Polymicrobial co-infections:
e.g. measles, rotavirus, and tuberculosis
Bacterial secondary infection:
Streptococcus pneumoniae

Poor clinical outcome

Home and Village

Far from healthcare facility
Poverty and loss of maternal care
Unsafe water supply
Poor sanitation and handwashing
Indoor air pollution
Caregiver recognised illness at late stage
Poor food security
Poor feeding practices and breastfeeding
Social stigma as barrier to HIV/TB care
Vaccine hesitancy and poor uptake

Health care and systematic

Poor transport infrastructure
No community healthcare workers
Nurse had minimal child health training
Poor access to vitamin A supplementation
Poor access to ready-to-use therapeutic feeds
Poor access to zinc
Poor access to resuscitation equipment
Poor availability of advice from secondary care
Poorly defined secondary care referral pathway
Inadequate vaccination programme
(e.g. no rotavirus or pneumococcal vaccine)

Figure 36.1 Potential factors contributing to Thandi's death.

Questions

1. What are the barriers to achieving universal vaccination?

2. What factors contributed to the Ebola epidemic in West Africa?

3. Where should governments be focusing their resources to tackle antimicrobial resistance?

Key publications

GBD 2015 Mortality and Causes of Death Collaborators (2016). Global, regional, and national life expectancy, all-cause mortality, and cause-specific mortality for 249 causes of death, 1980–2015: a systematic analysis for the Global Burden of Disease Study 2015. *Lancet* 388(10053): 1459–544.
Outlines the contribution of infectious disease to the global burden of disease.

Walker C, et al. (2013). Global burden of childhood pneumonia and diarrhoea. *Lancet Series on Childhood Pneumonia and Diarrhoea* 381: 1405–16. Comprehensive overview of two of the most important infectious diseases. Available at: https://www.thelancet.com/series/childhood-pneumonia-and-diarrhoea

UNAIDS (2016). *Global AIDS Update 2016*. Available at: http://www.unaids.org/en/resources/documents/2016/Global-AIDS-update-2016
Comprehensive overview on AIDs.

World Health Organization (2015). *World Malaria Report 2015*. http://www.who.int/malaria/publications/world-malaria-report-2015/report/en/
Comprehensive overview on malaria.

World Health Organization (2016). *Global Tuberculosis Report*. http://www.who.int/tb/publications/global_report/en/
Comprehensive overview on TB.

Bibliography

Beigel J, Farrar J, Han A, et al. (2005). Avian influenza A (H5N1) infection in humans. *New Eng J Med* 353(13): 1374–85.

Chopra M, Mason E, Borrazzo J, et al. (2013). Ending of preventable deaths from pneumonia and diarrhoea: an achievable goal. *Lancet Series on Childhood Pneumonia and Diarrhoea* 381(9876): 1499–506.

Kyu H, Pinho C, Wagner J, et al. (2016). Global and national burden of diseases and injuries among children and adolescents between 1990 and 2013. *JAMA Pediatrics* 170(3): 267.

Le Doare K, Bielicki J, Heath P, and Sharland M (2014). Systematic review of antibiotic resistance rates among Gram-negative bacteria in children with sepsis in resource-limited countries. *Journal of the Pediatric Infectious Diseases Society* 4(1): 11–20.

Mayo-Wilson E, Imdad A, Herzer K, Yakoob M, and Bhutta Z (2011). Vitamin A supplements for preventing mortality, illness, and blindness in children aged under 5: systematic review and meta-analysis. *BMJ* 343(1): d5094.

Rezza G (2014). Dengue and chikungunya: long-distance spread and outbreaks in naïve areas. *Pathogens and Global Health* 108(8): 349–55.

Sinclair D, Donegan S, Isba R, and Lalloo D (2012). Artesunate versus quinine for treating severe malaria. *Cochrane Database of Systematic Reviews* 6: CD005967.

Uyeki T (2009). Human infection with highly pathogenic avian influenza A (H5N1) virus: review of clinical issues. *Clinical Infectious Diseases* 49(2): 279–90.

Violari A, Cotton M, Gibb D, et al. (2008). Early antiretroviral therapy and mortality among HIV-infected infants. *New Eng J Med* 359(21): 2233–44.

Wikan N and Smith D (2016). Zika virus: history of a newly emerging arbovirus. *Lancet Infectious Diseases* 16(7): e119–26.

World Health Organization (2012). *Global Vaccine Action Plan 2011–2020*. Available at: http://www.who.int/immunization/global_vaccine_action_plan/GVAP_doc_2011_2020/en/.

World Health Organization (2013). *Ending Preventable Child Deaths from Pneumonia and Diarrhoea by 2025. The integrated Global Action Plan for Pneumonia and Diarrhoea (GAPPD)*. Available at: http://www.who.int/maternal_child_adolescent/documents/global_action_plan_pneumonia_diarrhoea/en/.

World Health Organization (2013). *Roadmap for Childhood TB: Toward Zero Deaths*. Available at: http://www.who.int/tb/publications/tb-childhoodroadmap/en/.

World Health Organization (2016). *Global Malaria Report 2016*. Available at: http://www.who.int/malaria/publications/world-malaria-report-2016/report/en/.

World Health Organization (2016). *Integrated Management of Childhood Illness: Towards a Grand Convergence For Child Survival and Health: a Strategic Review of Options for the Future Building on Lessons Learnt From IMNCI*. Available at: http://www.who.int/maternal_child_adolescent/documents/strategic-review-child-health-imnci/en/.

CHAPTER 37

Child nutrition

Marly Cardoso and Jonathan Wells

This chapter addresses the global burden of childhood under and over-nutrition, highlighting the main public health interventions for improving child nutrition. It should be read in conjunction with Chapter 7 (Developmental Origins of Health and Disease (DOHaD)) and Chapter 24 (Maternal nutrition).

Key points

- Breastfeeding is both an effective and cost-effective way to improve child health.

- Optimal infant feeding may have long-term benefits, helping adults to become taller, stronger, healthier, and more intelligent.

- Food-based interventions to promote healthy diet should emphasise meals made from unprocessed or minimally processed foods derived from sustainable food systems and established food cultures.

Background

The 'first 1000 days of life', covering conception to age two, is recognised as a critical period for the growth and development of young children. Convincing evidence suggests that good nutrition in early life can help adults become taller, stronger, healthier, and more intelligent and, thus, more economically productive, with many benefits for the next generation as well.

Data from 2016 (available at http/data.unicef.org) shows that 154.8 million (95% CI: 142.7–166.9 million) (23%) children under five years old suffered from stunted growth, most of whom live in sub-Saharan Africa and South Asia. Also, 51.7 million (95% CI: 44.5–58.9 million) children were wasted, of whom 16.9 million (95% CI: 13.3–20.5 million) had severe acute malnutrition (SAM), that is, a weight-for-height z-score <-3 or associated oedema. Most incidents of stunting occur before two years of age when there is increased demand for adequate nutrition to fuel rapid foetal/infant growth. Conversely, an increase of about eleven million overweight children younger than five years has been observed over the past fifteen years globally, and is an important contributor to adult obesity, diabetes, and other chronic non-communicable diseases (NCDs). Worldwide in 2016, 40.6 million children (95% CI: 33.5–47.7 million) (6%) under the age of five years were overweight or obese. Although the prevalence of overweight in high-income countries is more than double that in low- and middle-income countries (LMICs), most affected children (76% of the total) live in developing areas.

Iron deficiency anaemia is one of the most common preventable nutritional problems among young children. In 2011, the highest global prevalence of anaemia was in preschool children (42.6%, 95% CI: 37–47). Vitamin A and iodine deficiency each affect up to one-third of children under five years. The United Nations Children's Fund (UNICEF) conceptual framework on the determinants of undernutrition in childhood was first designed in 1990 and has been updated in different publications as shown in Figure 37.1. The framework revolves around basic factors (social, economic, environmental, and political), underlying factors (household food security, adequate care and feeding practices, access to health services, and residing in a healthy environment), and immediate causes of malnutrition (inadequate food intake and disease).

The *Lancet Nutrition Series*, the Global Nutrition Report, and the post-Millennium Development Goals set by the World Health Assembly highlight the need to address the global burden of childhood under-nutrition and overweight and to scale up nutrition action through proven nutrition-specific interventions (Table 37.1). Nutrition-sensitive interventions and programmes in agriculture, social safety nets, early child development, education, and water and sanitation have the potential to enhance the scale and effectiveness of nutrition-specific interventions. The effect of cash transfer programmes on breastfeeding practices, immunisation coverage, diarrhoea management, healthcare use, and other preventive strategies have the potential to promote increased coverage of several important child health interventions, but the quality of evidence available on how to deliver them at scale sustainably is low.

Obesity and related NCDs are becoming increasingly common in children from most global regions, especially in Latin America. The Pan-American Health Organization (PAHO) responded by approving a five-year plan of action on childhood obesity (2014–2019) designed to halt further increase of obesity in children and adolescents. PAHO identifies the current environment as one that causes overweight and obesity, where diet as well as trade and agriculture policies are the main determinants of food supply quality and thus of dietary patterns. Its recommendations include fiscal policies and other incentives for increased production and consumption of healthy food; the regulation of marketing of unhealthy food; better labelling of processed food and drink products; and improvement of school food and increased physical activity among schoolchildren. The recommendations build on public policies already initiated in Latin America, such as the Mexican tax on sugary drinks and energy-dense snacks; regulation of food marketing to children in several countries; and the Brazilian food and meal-based dietary guidelines based on the NOVA food classification system. This system describes four food groups according to the nature, purpose, and extent of its processing: 1) Unprocessed foods—foods that have not undergone any industrial processing; 2) Processed culinary—substances

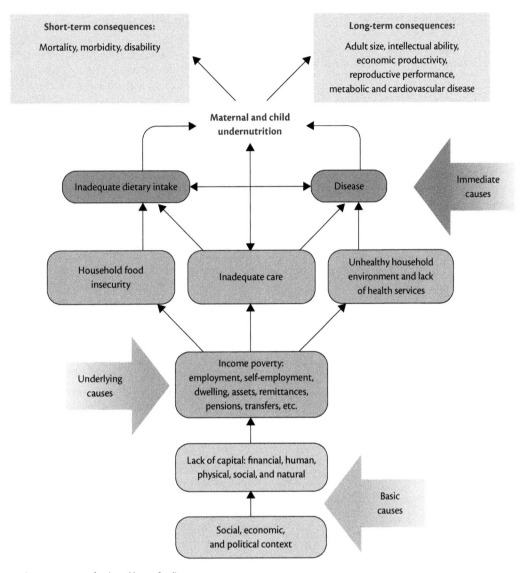

Figure 37.1 Causes and consequences of reduced breastfeeding rates.

extracted and purified by industry from food constituents (such as fats, oils, salt, and sugars); 3) Processed foods—manufactured by adding fats, oils, sugars, salt, and other culinary ingredients to minimally processed foods, including simple breads and cheeses, salted and cured meats/seafood, preserved fruits, legumes, and vegetables; 4) Ultra-processed food and drink products—industrial formulations.

Global targets

WHO Global Nutrition Targets 2025 (2014)

- Achieve a 30% reduction in low birthweight (<2500 grams).
- Achieve a 40% reduction in the number of children under five years who are stunted.
- Ensure that there is no increase in childhood overweight.
- Reduce childhood wasting to less than 5%.

Interventions

Healthy diets are generally based on fresh, handmade meals derived from sustainable food systems and established food cultures, whereas diets largely composed of ready-to-consume ultra-processed products of the globalised industrial food system are not. Examples of ultra-processed products include crisps and many other types of fatty, salty, or sugary packaged snack products. Nutritionally imbalanced products, such as energy-dense, ultra-processed items, are considered the main dietary cause of micronutrient deficiencies, excessive weight gain, and chronic diseases.

Breast and complementary feeding

Promotion, protection, and support of breastfeeding are recognised as the most important evidence-based interventions, especially in countries with the double burden of under-nutrition and overweight. Globally, exclusive breastfeeding rates increased

Table 37.1 Selected evidence-based interventions for under and over-nutrition in childhood

Nutritional problem	Interventions	Recommendations
Severe acute malnutrition	Treatment of infections, fluid management, and ready-to-use therapeutic foods throughout community-based delivery platforms.	Further evidence is needed for effective strategies of prevention and management in infants less than 6 months.
Wasting/stunting	Breastfeeding promotion, support and protection actions. Promotion of dietary diversity and healthy complementary feeding. Micronutrient supplementation (at least iron, vitamin A, and zinc).	Further research on innovations and strategies for scaling up coverage of nutrition interventions in working women, especially in underprivileged communities.
Iron deficiency anaemia and vitamin A deficiency from 6 months to 11 years of age	Delayed cord clamping after birth. Exclusive breastfeeding for six months. Home fortification of complementary feeding with multiple micronutrients in powder.	In malaria endemic areas, the WHO recommends administration of iron supplements through malaria prevention and treatment programmes.
Overweight	Dietary patterns based on meals made from unprocessed or minimally processed food. Physical activity promotion.	PAHO identifies the current environment as one that causes overweight and obesity.

from 14% in 1985 to 38% in 1995, but decreased subsequently in most regions.

The World Health Organization (WHO) recommends exclusive breastfeeding from birth to six months, the introduction of healthy complementary foods at six months, and continued breastfeeding until at least two years of age. In addition to meeting the newborn's nutritional needs, breast milk includes many essential bioactive components, such as antimicrobial and anti-inflammatory factors, enzymes, and growth factors.

Inappropriate complementary feeding practices, such as early onset of weaning and inadequate nutritional content of weaning foods, related to cultural practices, food insecurity, or lack of maternity leave for working women, have been identified as contributing to undernutrition, growth faltering, diarrhoea, increased rate of infections, micronutrient deficiency, poor cognitive development, and increased mortality among children.

Educational interventions can be used to improve complementary feeding practices. Counselling sessions, lectures, cooking workshops, and educational videotape interventions integrated into home visits have improved such outcomes as infant growth and feeding practices, and mothers' knowledge. Nutrition education through group discussions is also effective in preventing malnutrition and growth faltering in children under two years.

Severe acute malnutrition

The WHO recommends inpatient treatment for children with complicated severe acute malnutrition (SAM) (including medical complications, such as severe oedema or poor appetite), with stabilisation and appropriate treatment of infections, fluid management, and dietary therapy, and also supports community-based care. Children with uncomplicated SAM, not requiring admission, and who are managed as outpatients, should be given a course of oral antibiotics such as amoxicillin. Substantial programmatic evidence supports the use of ready-to-use therapeutic foods (RUTF) for uncomplicated SAM in community settings. However, the quality of programme design and implementation seems to be crucial to the improvement of outcomes for children with SAM.

Micronutrients

Vitamin supplements given to babies as part of recommended public health interventions are not considered part of complementary feeding. Interventions to prevent or treat micronutrient malnutrition typically include exclusive breastfeeding during the first six months; dietary diversification to include foods with highly absorbable vitamins and minerals; and control of parasitic infections.

In 2016, a WHO technical publication examined strategies to prevent/control anaemia in childhood, suggesting the addition of multiple micronutrients in powder (MNP) to semi-solid foods as a home-based strategy for health promotion. In populations where the prevalence of anaemia in young children is 20% or higher, MNP containing at least iron, vitamin A, and zinc is recommended to improve iron status and reduce anaemia among infants and children 6–23 months of age. Evidence relating to MNP reported in a Cochrane systematic review by De-Regil et al. (2013) showed that home fortification is effective in preventing iron deficiency and iron deficiency anaemia. This should be integrated with health care and education, starting at 6–8 months of age with the transition from breastfeeding to complementary feeding, to benefit linear growth and micronutrient status.

Obesity

A Cochrane review by Waters et al. (2011) examined the effects of different obesity prevention interventions on changes in body mass index in children, suggesting a significant beneficial effect across age groups. They found the following to be promising policies and strategies:

◆ School curriculum that includes healthy eating, physical activity, and body image.

◆ Increased sessions for physical activity and the development of fundamental movement skills throughout the school week.

◆ Improvements in nutritional quality of the food supply in schools.

◆ Environments and cultural practices that support children eating healthier foods and being active throughout each day.

◆ Support for teachers and other staff to implement health promotion strategies and activities (e.g. professional development, capacity building activities).

◆ Parent support and home activities that encourage children to be more active, eat more nutritious foods and spend less time on screen-based activities.

Overall, the interventions that combined physical activity and diet were more effective than either delivered alone. However, significant effects were observed for children aged 6–12 years with non-significant effects in younger children and adolescents. Interventions are summarised in Table 37.1.

Challenges

The concept of a 'window of opportunity' is essential for designing intervention strategies. However, how to promote healthy growth in the first 2–3 years, without provoking excess weight gain and adiposity, is a major challenge for public health policymakers. Existing data from LMICs suggest that faster growth during infancy tends to benefit human capital, whereas by early childhood it promotes rapid weight gain and overweight.

Future priorities

◆ The evidence of effectiveness of obesity prevention interventions and implementation are considered weak.

◆ More studies using the NOVA food classification system and methodology are needed to supplement existing findings, particularly those producing data comparable across countries.

◆ Strategies such as the PAHO Plan of Action findings and recommendations for the Americas could serve as a guide for other regions.

Conclusions

Improvements in women's, children's, and adolescents' health care globally, including effective strategies to promote, support, and protect exclusive breastfeeding practices, with sustainable access to healthy food, are necessary to reduce short and long-term health complications related to the childhood dual burden of under and over-nutrition.

Case study: factors associated with stunting and obesity in Amazonian children

In 2007, a population-based study in Acrelandia, West Brazilian Amazonia, found a prevalence of stunting of 7.1% and overweight of 20.6% among children aged under five years. Stunting was associated with the lowest maternal height tertile, low birthweight, diarrhoea, and geohelminth infections. Overweight was associated with Caesarean delivery, birthweight ≥3500 g and iron deficiency. Among children younger than twenty-five months, almost two-thirds had stopped breastfeeding before six months of age, and three quarters had previously been bottle-fed. Such associations encompass a double burden of disease that can affect the development from the early stages of life. From an early age, this population has a low intake of fruit and vegetables and substantial consumption of unhealthy foods, such as processed foods high in sodium, preservatives, sugars, and fats. Changes in diet quality are characteristic of the nutritional transition faced by countries undergoing rapid economic development. While national programmes are in place to help prevent micronutrient deficiencies and promote healthy eating habits, what remains challenging is how to promote infant growth and development with morbidity

and nutritional deficiency prevention without producing excessive weight gain and adiposity.

Questions

1. Why do you think exclusive breastfeeding for six months is not a universal practice?

2. What is the double burden of child malnutrition and why does it occur?

3. How can we successfully address both underweight/stunting and overweight at the same time?

Key publications

Black R, Victora C, Walker S, et al. (2013). Maternal and childhood undernutrition and overweight in low-income and middle-income countries. *Lancet Maternal and Childhood Nutrition Series* 382: 427–51.
Comprehensive review of the evidence for maternal and child undernutrition, and also examines the growing problems of overweight and obesity for women and children, and their consequences in low-income and middle-income countries.

Victora C, Bahl R, Barros A, et al. (2016). Breastfeeding in the 21st century: epidemiology, mechanisms and lifelong effect. *Lancet Breastfeeding Series* 387: 475–90.
Review of evidence for benefits of breastfeeding.

World Health Oranization (2014). *Comprehensive Implementation Plan on Maternal, Infant and Young Child Nutrition.*
This action plan illustrates a series of priority actions that should be jointly implemented by WHO member states and international partners to achieve by the year 2025.

Bibliography

Adair L, Fall C, Osmond C, et al. for the COHORTS group (2013). Associations of linear growth and relative weight gain during early life with adult health and human capital in countries of low and middle income: findings from five birth cohort studies. *Lancet* 382: 525–34.

Cardoso M, Augusto R, Bortolini G, et al. and ENFAC Working Group (2016). Effect of providing multiple micronutrientes in powder through primary healthcare on anemia in young Brazilian children: a multicenter pragmatic controlled trial. *PLoS One* 11: e0151097.

Cobayashi F, Augusto R, Lourenço B, Muniz P, and Cardoso M (2014). Factors associated with stunting and overweight in Amazonian children: a population-based, cross-sectional study. *Public Health Nutr* 17: 551–60.

De-Regil L, Suchdev P, Vist G, Walleser S, and Peña-Rosas J (2013). Home fortification of foods with multiple micronutrient powders for health and nutrition in children under two years of age (Review). *Cochrane Review Journal* 8: 112–201.

Fall C, Borja J, Osmond C, et al. and the COHORTS group (2011). *Int J Epidemiol* 40: 47–62.

Kearns A, Castro M, Lourenço B, Augusto R, Cardoso M, and ACTION Study Team (2016). Factors associated with age at breastfeeding cessation in Amazonian infants: applying a proximal-distal framework. *Matern Chil Health J* 20: 1539–48.

Ministry of Health (Brazil) (2014). Dietary guidelines for the Brazilian population. Brasília: Ministry of Health. Available from: nupensusp. wix.com/nupens#!__english

Pan American Health Organization (2014). Plan of action for the prevention of obesity in children and adolescents. 53rd Directing Council,

66th Session of the Regional Committee of WHO for the Americas, Washington, DC, 29 September–3 October 2014. PAHO: Washington, DC. Available from: http://www.paho.org/hq/index.php?option=com_docman&task=doc_view&Itemid=270&gid=28890&lang=en

Tzioumis E and Adair L (2014). Childhood dual burden of under and over-nutrition in low- and middle-income countries: a critical review. *Food Nutr Bull* 35: 230–43.

United Nations Children's Fund, the World Health Organization and World Bank Group (2016). *Levels and trends in child malnutrition.* UNICEF/WHO/World Bank Group Joint Child Malnutrition Estimates: Key findings of the 2016 edition. Available from: http://www.who.int/nutgrowthdb/estimates2015/en/

Waters E, de Silva-Sanigorski A, Hall B, et al. (2011). Interventions for preventing obesity in children. *Cochrane Database Systematic Reviews* 12: CD001871.

Wells J (2016). *The Metabolic Ghetto: an Evolutionary Perspective on Nutrition, Power Relations and Chronic Disease.* Cambridge University Press: Cambridge, UK.

World Health Organization (2001). *Iron Deficiency Anaemia: Assessment, Prevention, and Control. a Guide for Programme Managers.* World Health Organization: Geneva.

World Health Organization (2011). *Use of Multiple Micronutrient Powders for Home Fortification of Foods Consumed by Infants and Children 6–23 Months of Age.* World Health Organization: Geneva.

World Health Organization (2015). *The Global Prevalence of Anaemia in 2011.* World Health Organization: Geneva.

World Health Organization Guideline (2016). *Use of Multiple Micronutrient Powders for Point-of-use Fortification of Foods Consumed by Infants and Young Children aged 6–23 Months and Children aged 2–12 Yyears.* World Health Organization: Geneva.

CHAPTER 38

Child development and disability

Richard Rosch, Michelle Heys, and Hannah Kuper

In this chapter, we highlight current issues and key concepts in child development and childhood disability.

Key points

♦ Children with developmental delays are at risk of disability and vice versa.

♦ Emerging evidence-based interventions has focused on how cognitive stimulation and adequate childhood nutrition can improve developmental outcomes.

♦ Low- and middle-income countries (LMICs) often experience the highest prevalence of disability and have the fewest available resources with which to support affected children.

♦ The optimisation of developmental outcomes for children and young people, especially in LMICs, will ensure several Sustainable Development Goals (SDGs) are achieved. SDGs relate not only to improving development directly, but also to improving factors like poverty and overall health, which are both linked to disability.

Background

Child development is the process of emotional, physical, psychosocial, and cognitive changes occurring from birth to the end of adolescence. According to Black et al. (2016), an estimated 250 million children (43%) surviving to age five in LMICs are at risk of not meeting their developmental potential. Furthermore, within LMICs, children from poorer backgrounds are more likely to experience developmental delays; those children do less well at school, earn less as adults, are at higher risk of cognitive and health problems, and have lower social capital, thus perpetuating a cycle of poverty and inequity.

Children with disabilities are those who do not participate in society on an equal basis with others because of an impairment (e.g. physical, mental, intellectual, or sensory), together with unfavourable personal or environmental factors (e.g. inaccessible buildings). The international classification of functioning, disability, and health (Figure 38.1) by the World Health Organization (2016) is a model capturing these interacting domains.

Globally, the World Health Organization (WHO) estimates that at least 93 million children aged 0–14 are living with disability, most of whom are in LMICs. The prevalence of types of impairment is difficult to quantify, but communication, mobility, and visual impairments are amongst the most common.

Global targets

Sustainable Development Goals (2015)

Goal 4 (Education)

♦ Build and upgrade education facilities that are child, disability, and gender sensitive.

♦ By 2030, ensure that all girls and boys have access to quality early childhood development (ECD), care, and pre-primary education.

Goal 10 (Inequality)

♦ By 2030, empower and promote the social, economic, and political inclusion of all, irrespective of age, sex, disability, race, ethnicity, origin, religion or economic, or any other status.

Goal 17 (Global partnership)

♦ By 2020, enhance capacity-building support to developing countries … to increase significantly the availability of high-quality, timely, and reliable data disaggregated by income, gender, age, race, ethnicity, migratory status, disability, geographic location.

Optimising early child development also links indirectly to other SDGs like alleviating poverty (Goal 1), and ensuring healthy lives (Goal 3).

Assessing development and disability

Measuring development

Developmental assessment is often based on recording a child's achievements in specific, linked domains (e.g. sensorimotor, cognitive-language, social-emotional). Tools are available to evaluate development quantitatively: for example the Griffiths developmental assessment tool (Griffiths and Huntley, 1996). These are based on standardised questionnaires and observations, and validated on a representative sample. However, many have limited generalisability (e.g. validated in a high-income country only). There is increased interest in developing more inclusive tools for use in LMICs, for example the Malawi Developmental Assessment Tool developed by Gladstone et al. (2010) in 2010.

Evaluating disability

The presence of an impairment can be measured clinically (e.g. audiometry to assess hearing). To investigate disability, standardised questionnaires can assess functioning and participation, for example the UNICEF-Washington Group Child Functioning Module. These may overlap with methods to assess childhood development, and so children with disabilities will likely be also flagged as experiencing delays in their development.

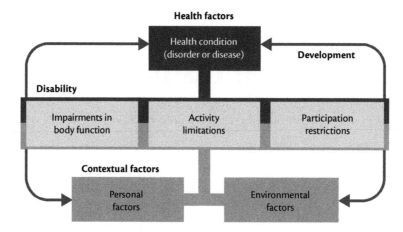

Figure 38.1 International Classification of Functioning, Disability and Health Model of disability.
Adapted with permission from World Health Organization. How to use the ICF: A practical manual for using the International Classification of Functioning, Disability and Health (ICF); Exposure draft for comment. Geneva: World Health Organization. Copyright © 2013 World Health Organization.

Atypical development

Whilst the timing of acquired skills may vary during development, a typically developing child follows a predictable sequence (e.g. standing before walking). Atypical development can fall into three main categories: delay in all skills, delay in a subset of skills, or an atypical pattern of development. This may either be due to conditions affecting the individual ('intrinsic' causes, e.g. genetic conditions), or additional risk factors ('extrinsic' causes, e.g. psychosocial context). Factors interact, leaving children with 'intrinsic' causes for developmental delay more at risk of further 'extrinsic' restrictions. Examples of this can include a child with a neurological condition or visual impairment ('intrinsic') who does not experience a stimulating environment, due to sensory deprivation or neglect ('extrinsic'), thus experiencing further avoidable developmental delay.

Some avoidable risk factors have emerged as common causes for atypical development: for example inadequate early cognitive stimulation, dietary deficiencies, infectious diseases, maternal mental health, and poverty. Risk factors rarely occur in isolation and are often clustered (e.g. poverty, dietary deficiencies, and infectious disease) resulting in cumulative risk.

Development in the context of disability

Children with disabilities are less likely to attend school and often experience social exclusion and bullying. Children in low socioeconomic circumstances are at higher risk of disability, and caring for a child with a disability can further increase poverty (e.g. due to lost work opportunities).

Development may be delayed in children with disabilities for two reasons. First, the underlying health condition may also result in delays in development (e.g. delay in motor development in children with spasticity). Second, the interaction of their disability with their environment may impact on their development (e.g. lack of appropriate educational opportunities for children with visual impairment). These interactions make children with disability vulnerable to developmental delay, but many of these additional developmental restrictions can be mitigated with appropriate interventions.

Interventions

Interventions to optimise child development and outcomes for children with a disability should consider exposures from preconception through to adolescence. Addressing a combination of risk factors for poor development has proven most effective in improving early child development. In a randomised trial by Nahar et al. (2012) in severely malnourished children in Bangladesh, psychosocial stimulation and food supplementation in combination provided additive benefits for cognitive development. Opportunities for intervention arise at three interlinked levels: the individual/family, the neighbourhood, and the wider socio-political context. Yet the limited availability of integrated interventions across these levels, particularly for children with specific needs arising from a disability, means that opportunities are missed to improve developmental outcomes.

Challenges

Data on child development and childhood disability from LMICs, are extremely limited. Yet high-quality information is essential for understanding underlying causes and for planning possible interventions. There are a few notable, recent exceptions, such as the Multiple Indicator Cluster Survey, illustrating that evidence derived from typically developing populations of children is increasing. In contrast, evidence addressing clinical and psychosocial issues for children with atypical development or disability are still much needed. Qualitative studies have shown limited understanding and a stark lack of services and support for children with atypical development in rural low resource settings in particular. There is ongoing controversy about how to best deliver appropriate and inclusive education and support for children with disability. A 'twin-track' approach may offer targeted disability-specific services (e.g. physiotherapy) while ensuring social inclusion with peers.

Future priorities

♦ Establishing meaningful and inclusive measurements of child development throughout childhood and adolescence at both population and individual level.

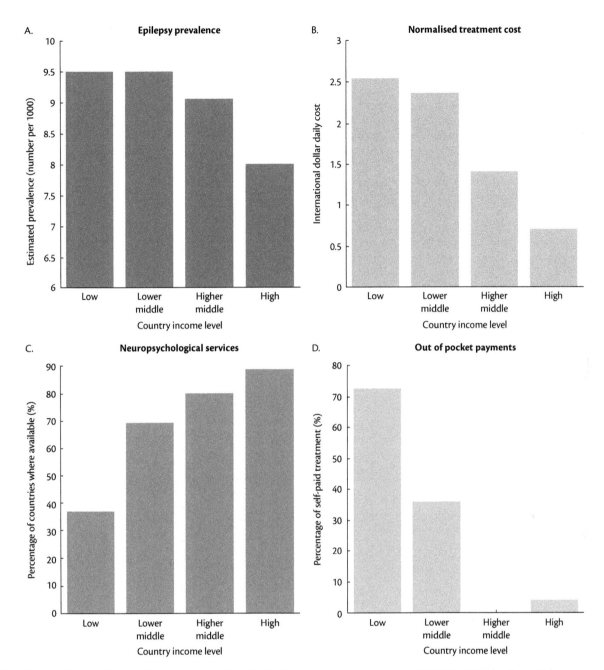

Figure 38.2 Global epilepsy prevalence, health care and cost are inequitably distributed: reported prevalence in LMIC is 15–20% higher than in high-income countries (A), specialist services are less commonly available in LMICs (B), median treatment cost (here for carbamazepine) estimated in 'international dollars' is highest in LMICs (C), most costs are paid directly out of pocket in LMICs.

Source: data from World Health Organization, International League Against Epilepsy, International Bureau for Epilepsy. (2005) *Atlas: Epilepsy care in the world*. Geneva: World Health Oragnization. © 2005 WHO.

◆ Identification and quantification of risk and protective factors, particularly in LMICs.

◆ Effective and integrated public health strategies to modify risk factors.

◆ Translation and implementation of evidence-based interventions promoting child development at scale using lifecourse and multi-sectoral approaches.

◆ Integrative, multi-agency approaches to maximise developmental opportunities for all children.

Conclusions

Time-critical developmental processes occur during childhood, and the presence of disability can have a dramatic effect on the individual child and their families.

Models of child development and childhood disability allow the assessment of developmental trajectories and the impact of disability across different functional domains. Yet the assessment tools and interventions that have emerged from this evolving understanding are too often not relevant or have not been applied to LMICs, where atypical development and disability are most prevalent.

Aside from achieving good quality data to inform the development of potential interventions, it is the global socioeconomic context of children affected by atypical development and disability that remains the major challenge. Globally, areas with the highest prevalence remain the most underfunded, posing the highest degree of economic burden and stress on individual patients and their families. We need to urgently address such an unequal burden as this further limits the potential for developmental achievement of the children affected.

Case study: an overview of epilepsy and its overlap with developmental issues

Childhood epilepsy is common among children with developmental delay, due to shared aetiologies and risk factors (e.g. brain injuries and infections); it can also itself cause disability. Epilepsy refers to a group of primary neurological disorders with a particularly high incidence in childhood and a high prevalence in LMICs. It is associated with *transient* impairments during seizures, but also subtle yet pervasive cognitive difficulties and social restrictions that have an impact on development. Antiepileptic medication can control seizures in the majority of patients, yet there is a large treatment gap globally. Even effective treatment of seizures may not reduce epilepsy-associated disability.

Epilepsy care is distributed unequally and the socioeconomic impact is larger in LMICs (Figure 38.2). Associated stigma and social exclusion may be potentiated by cultural beliefs about epilepsy. These factors result in a disproportionate impact of epilepsy on the lives of patients in LMICs.

Three interacting groups of effects specific to epilepsy are believed to influence its associated disability and the psychosocial impact:

1. Neurological status (including seizure control, associated brain lesions, aetiology).

2. Medication effects (side effect of specific medications, appropriate dosing).

3. Psychosocial variables (stigma, fear of seizures, social support, socioeconomic impact).

There are thus several ways in which the developmental and disabling impact of childhood epilepsy can be reduced, for example advances in the surgical treatment may reduce the neurological impact of a brain lesion and reduce the need for long-term medication. Furthermore, interventions targeting knowledge and perceptions around epilepsy can reduce stigma experienced by patients. More work is needed to ensure inclusion of children with epilepsy in education, and to provide families and caregivers with strategies to further maximise development of children living with epilepsy.

This case study demonstrates the complex nature of developmental problems associated with just one disease. The mechanism of disability is multifactorial, and the management options are diverse and highly context specific.

Questions

1. What is the difference between impairment and disability?

2. Why might a child with disabilities experience developmental delay?

3. How might a condition like epilepsy impact on a child's development?

Key publications

World Health Organization (2008). *World Report on Disability*. World Health Organization: Geneva.
Comprehensive and readable overview of many global issues related to disability, including some global demographics, and chapters on education and enabling environments.

Britto P, Lye S, Proulx K, et al. (2017). Nurturing care: promoting early childhood development. *Lancet* 389(10064): 91–102.
Review of multi-sectoral intervention packages to promote early childhood development in the context of the United Nations Sustainable Development Goals.

Gladstone M, Lancaster G, Umar E, et al. (2010). The Malawi Developmental Assessment Tool (MDAT): the creation, validation, and reliability of a tool to assess child development in rural African settings. *PLoS Med* 7: e1000273.
Good example of context-appropriate tool generated for the assessment of child development in a LMIC.

UNICEF (2013). *The State of the World's Children 2013*. Children with disabilities. UNICEF: New York, US.
Comprehensive report on childhood disability. Includes a suggested agenda for action at the end.

International Centre for Evidence in Disability (2013). *Getting to Know Cerebral Palsy. Working With Parent Groups—a Training Resource for Facilitators, Parents, Caregivers, and Persons with Cerebral Palsy*. LSHTM: London, UK.
Example of an integrated intervention manual, addressing needs of people living with cerebral palsy and their families

Bibliography

Baker G (2002). The psychosocial burden of epilepsy. *Epilepsia* 43: 26–30.

Batura N, Hill Z, Haghparast-Bidgoli H, et al. (2015). Highlighting the evidence gap: how cost-effective are interventions to improve early childhood nutrition and development? *Health Policy Plan* 30: 813–821.

Black M, Walker S, Fernald L, et al. (2016). Early childhood development coming of age: science through the lifecourse. *Lancet*.

Bornstein M, Britto P, Nonoyama-Tarumi Y, et al. (2012). Child development in developing countries: introduction and methods. *Child Dev* 83: 16–31.

Brabcova D, Lovasova V, Kohout J, Zarubova J, and Komarek V (2013). Improving the knowledge of epilepsy and reducing epilepsy-related stigma among children using educational video and educational drama—a comparison of the effectiveness of both interventions. *Seizure* 22: 179–84.

Grantham-McGregor S, Cheung Y, Cueto A, et al. (2007). Developmental potential in the first 5 years for children in developing countries. *Lancet* 369: 60–70.

Griffiths R and Huntley M (1996). *The Griffiths Mental Development Scales-Revised Manual: From Birth to 2 Years*. Association for Research in Infant and Child Development (ARCID).

Heys M, Alexander A, Medeiros E, et al. (2016). Understanding parents and professionals' knowledge and awareness of autism in Nepal. *Autism*.

McCoy D, Peet E, Ezzati M, et al. (2016). Early childhood developmental status in low- and middle-income countries: national, regional, and global prevalence estimates using predictive modeling. *PLOS Med* 13: e1002034.

Nahar B, Hossain M, Hamadani J, et al. (2012). Effects of a community-based approach of food and psychosocial stimulation on growth and development of severely malnourished children in Bangladesh: a randomised trial. *Eur. J. Clin. Nutr* 66: 701–9.

Newton C and Garcia H (2012). Epilepsy in poor regions of the world. *Lancet* 380: 1193–201.

Nores M and Barnett W (2010). Benefits of early childhood interventions across the world: (under) investing in the very young. *Econ Educ Rev* 29: 271–82.

UNICEF/Washington Group on Disability Statistics Child Functioning Module (2016). Available at: http://data.unicef.org/topic/child-disability/child-functioning-module/

World Health Organization (2016). *International Classification of Functioning, Disability and Health* (ICF). (2016). at http://www.who.int/classifications/icf/en/

CHAPTER 39

Non-communicable diseases in childhood

Jessica Mvula, Takondwa Chimowa, Elizabeth Molyneux, and Bernadette O'Hare

This chapter covers the common non-communicable diseases (NCDs) that present in childhood, including asthma, cancer, diabetes, rheumatic fever, and sickle cell disease. We also discuss NCD exposures which occur during pregnancy and childhood.

Key points

♦ Childhood is the time when lifestyle choices are developed which lead to NCDs in adulthood and the focus should be on the prevention of these.

♦ As countries undergo the epidemiological transition the burden of NCDs will increase relative to infectious diseases.

♦ Governments should use tax policies to re-price sugary foods, tobacco, and alcohol, and use the revenue to promote healthy lifestyles, fund the determinants of health, and strengthen health systems.

Background

NCDs are non-infectious, non-transmissible, and cause 60% of global premature mortality, 80% of which occurs in low- and middle-income countries (LMICs). Childhood deaths from NCDs vary by region but the proportion of deaths due to childhood NCDs in most LMICs is small, as infectious and neonatal causes still predominate. In 2008, Black et al. (2010) estimated that NCDs caused 2% of the deaths in children in Africa, whereas they cause 14% in Europe and the US. The most common NCDs experienced by children fall into two main groups. The first are those where the prevalence could be reduced with improved living conditions, diet, and health care, such as rheumatic heart disease (RHD), diabetes mellitus type II (T2DM), asthma, and obesity. The second are those that are not preventable with current knowledge, but screening (sickle cell disease (SCD)) and treatment is possible (diabetes mellitus type 1 (T1DM) and most cancers), but are not widely available in LMICs.

NCDs of childhood pose a financial and emotional burden on families. Health care costs quickly drain resources and cause poverty. Young adults with chronic childhood illness are less likely to complete higher education, find employment, and often experience low self-esteem and rejection by peers.

The NCDs commonly associated with adulthood account for most global deaths and are mainly due to cardiovascular diseases (heart attacks and stroke), cancers, chronic respiratory diseases, and diabetes. The modifiable lifestyle factors, including tobacco use, alcohol abuse, unhealthy diet, and lack of physical activity are established in childhood and adolescence; therefore a lifecourse approach to the prevention of NCDs is required.

Global targets

Sustainable Developmental Goals (2015)

Goal 3 (Health)

♦ By 2030, reduce by one-third premature mortality from non-communicable diseases through prevention and treatment and promote mental health and wellbeing.

The Global Asthma Network (2014)

♦ Reduce severe asthma by 50% by 2025

The World Health Organization (WHO) Global Action Plan for the prevention of NCDs (2013)

♦ A 25% relative reduction in the risk of premature death from cardiovascular disease, cancer, diabetes, or chronic respiratory disease by 2020.

♦ A 10% relative reduction in the prevalence of insufficient physical activity by 2020.

♦ A 30% relative reduction in prevalence of current tobacco use by persons aged 15+ by 2020.

Common NCDs of childhood

Asthma

Asthma is a disease typified by recurrent episodes of reversible lower airway obstruction, which vary in severity and frequency, between and within individuals. Around 235 million people suffer from asthma. One in six of the world's children have had asthma symptoms in the last year, but prevalence varies widely among countries, from >20% in South America, Europe, US, and Australia to <5% in India, Asia Pacific, and East Europe. Asthma results from multiple genetic and environmental influences and there has been an increase in asthma prevalence in LMICs over the last twenty-five years. Explanations include increased exposure to a 'western' lifestyle, such as processed food, and indoor and outdoor allergens. The most common triggers include pollen, house dust mite, dog, cat, and cockroach allergen, open fire cooking, and cigarette smoke. Exposure to farm animals and manure early in life and exclusive breastfeeding appears to decrease the risk of asthma. Children with asthma present with wheeze, cough, and shortness of breath. Avoiding triggers and ensuring children and/or families can use devices correctly and have an asthma action plan is critical.

Cancer

Cancer is the uncontrolled growth of cells, which can affect any part of the body and may invade surrounding tissue and/or metastasise to distant sites. The incidence of cancer in children in high-income countries (HICs) is 140/million children <15 years and in LMICs the range is from 45–65/million. This difference may be due to different environmental exposure or biological susceptibility, but is more likely to be due to under-reporting. A fraction of the expected numbers of children with cancer are diagnosed in LMICs and cancer registration is minimal. Children often present late and the signs and symptoms of malignancies often mimic other childhood illness, which is difficult to differentiate due to limited diagnostic capacity. The treatment can begin only after histological confirmation and when the extent of disease is defined or staged, limiting access to treatment. Treatment may include surgery, radiotherapy, and chemotherapy, and may follow a graduated approach according to resources available. Two thirds of infection-attributable cancers occur in LMICs and vaccines such as hepatitis B and human papillomavirus vaccine are critical to reducing liver and cervical cancer respectively.

Diabetes

Diabetes mellitus occurs when the body does not produce enough insulin (T1DM) or is resistant to insulin (T2DM). Two thirds of new diabetes diagnoses in children are T1DM. Incidence varies from 65 per 100,000 in Finland to 0.1 per 100,000 in China. Age of presentation in children is bimodal, with peaks at 4–6 years and 10–14 years. The incidence of T1DM has been increasing worldwide for several decades. In Europe, annual increases of 2–4% have been reported and this is more marked in children younger than five years. T1DM results from the autoimmune destruction of pancreatic cells in genetically susceptible individuals. Environmental associations include viral infections, immunisation, and early exposure to cow's milk, but causation has not been demonstrated.

Children with T1DM present in two main ways: with polydipsia (abnormally increased thirst), polyuria (abnormally large volume of urine), and weight loss, or with diabetic ketoacidosis (DKA) (a crisis that occurs when a lack of insulin leads to very high blood sugar levels and the breakdown of fat as a fuel source). The mean duration of symptoms prior to the presentation is ten days in HICs but is likely to be much longer in LMICs. Children in LMICs are more likely to present with DKA due to limited access to health care.

The global epidemiology of T2DM is changing; because of lifestyle changes, it now presents in young adults, adolescents, and even children. Eating and physical activity habits are formed early in life and this is the critical time to intervene. The most commonly used diagnostic criteria is a random blood glucose in a child with symptoms of hyperglycaemia; other criteria include an elevated random blood glucose and fasting blood glucose levels. The WHO have called for a whole government approach to the prevention of T2DM, including the health impact of policies in trade, agriculture, finance, transport, education, and urban planning.

Rheumatic heart disease

Acute rheumatic fever is an abnormal response to a group A streptococcal infection, usually of the throat, 2–4 weeks after infection. This response may damage heart valves and lead to chronic RHD. Predisposing factors include poverty, crowding, and delay in treating infections with antibiotics. The prevalence of RHD is 40/1000 in schoolage children in LMICs; it is extremely rare in high-income countries. The presentation is usually with symptoms of heart failure. Prophylaxis with long-acting penicillin reduces the recurrence of episodes of acute rheumatic fever and valve disease. Nearly all patients in LMICs use intramuscular penicillin for prophylaxis, while upper middle-income countries use oral and parenteral antibiotics in equal proportions. Adherence is higher for parenteral penicillin when administered every four weeks (82%) versus every two weeks (68%). Heart failure is treated symptomatically and regular follow-up is required, with consideration of valve replacement. Valve repair is uncommonly available in LMICs.

Sickle cell disease

Sickle cell disease (SCD) is a common genetic condition where the mutant gene is inherited from both parents. If a person has one gene they are said to be carriers and have sickle cell trait, which is common in Africa because the trait confers some resistance to malaria. In SCD the red cell is abnormally shaped and less soluble, which results in decreased blood flow to organs and red blood cells that rupture easily, resulting in anaemia. Africa is home to 85% of persons with SCD and 200,000 babies are born with SCD each year. A patient presents with symptoms due to poor blood flow to organs (such as strokes and acute chest syndrome) and anaemia. Individuals with SCD suffer from repeated ischaemic episodes, resulting in functional hyposplenism and recurrent infections. Screening can detect carriers before marriage or pregnancy, or at birth, but is not widely available in LMICs. The main cause of death is infection and malaria, and median survival is thought to be less than five years in Africa. Activities for the management of SCD should be based at the primary healthcare level, with emphasis on recording the family history and thus detecting the genetic risk, and ensuring the provider has adequate links into secondary and tertiary care.

Avoiding NCD exposure

For NCDs of childhood in many countries, the structural barriers of weak health systems, combined with the fact that they account for a small proportion of overall mortality, limits the political will to prioritise them. However, for asthma, increasing public education about exposure to smoking and indoor air pollution and the incorporation of asthma prevention and treatment into the curriculum of community health workers would reduce its impact. Health system strengthening and the provision of social support using domestic resources is likely to be much more effective than a vertical single-disease approach.

On the other hand, for NCDs that have their origins in childhood (almost all), there is an opportunity to avoid larger burdens of disease later in life. In settings of limited resources, LMICs should focus on the prevention of NCD exposures before and during pregnancy, and in early life (exercise, what children inhale and ingest). Table 39.1 shows examples of actions to reduce NCD exposures. However, considerable political will is needed to regulate companies which stand to make a profit from sales of tobacco, alcohol, and sugar laden foods, and from the pharmacological treatment to counter their effects, rather than preventative lifestyle changes.

Challenges

NCDs which affect children are very poorly managed in LMICs. Challenges include weak health systems and poverty. Lack of access to essential asthma drugs is common, and many countries do not include essential asthma medications on their national list.

Barriers to care for children with cancer include a delay in diagnosis at family and health clinic level, poor pathology services, and cost of treatment. Long hospital stays and the demands of home often lead to families abandoning treatment. Child mortality in LMICs is still high from infectious causes, therefore cancer, which only causes a small fraction of overall mortality, receives little attention from policymakers and funding organisations. However, the WHO's essential drug list now includes cancer drugs, and palliative care is increasingly available.

Diagnosis of DM is extremely challenging; only one in three LMICs report that their primary healthcare facilities have the basic technology for diagnosis and management. Equally, insulin, oral hypoglycaemic agents, self-monitoring devices, and strips are unavailable for the majority.

The main barrier to a reduction in deaths from RHD is poverty. The cost of end-stage intervention is much higher than preventative programmes and surgery is challenging in LMICs due to the infrastructure required for cardiac surgery and for the post-surgical care.

Challenges for prevention of SCD include absences of a carrier and neonatal screening programme, insufficient analgesia, insufficient blood supply, and poor access to treatment (hydroxyurea).

Table 39.1 NCD exposures before and during pregnancy and childhood that cause disease (arrow indicates an increase or decrease in risk of outcomes)

		Preconception and Pregnancy	Infancy and childhood	Adulthood
Policies to curtail	Cigarette smoke passive and maternal	↑ADHD	↑LRTI, asthma	↑CVA, IHD, COPD, cancer (mouth, throat, larynx, oesophagus, lung, stomach, pancreas, kidney, and cervix)
	Indoor air pollution from solid fuel	↑LBW and stillbirth	↑Pneumonia, asthma	↑CVA, IHD, COPD, lung cancer
	Outdoor air pollution		↑Pneumonia	↑CVA, IHD, COPD, lung cancer
	Alcohol abuse	↑ADHD, Foetal alcohol spectrum disorder		↑Alcoholism, hypertension, CVA, liver disease, diabetes, cancer (mouth, pharynx, larynx, oesophagus, liver, colorectal, and breast)
	Processed food Sugary drinks		↑Obesity, diabetes mellitus	↑Obesity, diabetes mellitus, hypertension, CVA, cancer of the oesophagus, colorectum, breast, endometrium, and kidney
	Malnutrition	↑LBW	↑Obesity, diabetes mellitus	↑Obesity, DM, hypertension, CVA
Policies to promote	Breastfeeding		↓ Asthma	↓Obesity, hypertension, dyslipidaemia, T2DM
	Physical activity		Improves cognition	↓Obesity, diabetes mellitus, hypertension, CVA, depression
	Vaccines—HPV and hepatitis B			↓Liver and cervical cancers

ADHD = attention deficit hyperactivity disorder; COPD = chronic obstructive pulmonary disease; CVA = cerebrovascular accident; DM = diabetes mellitus; IHD = ischaemic heart disease; HPV = human papilloma virus; LBW = low birthweight

Source: data from Mick, E. et al. Case-control study of attention-deficit hyperactivity disorder and maternal smoking, alcohol use, and drug use during pregnancy. *Journal of the American Academy of Child & Adolescent Psychiatry*. 41(4): 378–85. © Copyright 2002, Elsevier Inc. All rights reserved; Bruce, N. et al. Indoor air pollution in developing countries: a major environmental and public health challenge. *World Health Organization Bulletin*. 78(9), 1078–1092. © Copyright 2009, WHO; World Health Organization. (2017) *WHO Cancer Resolution: Cancer prevention and control in the context of an integrated approach*. Geneva, Switzerland: WHO. © Copyright 2017, WHO; Pope, D.P. et al. Risk of Low Birth Weight and Stillbirth Associated With Indoor Air Pollution From Solid Fuel Use in Developing Countries. Epidemiological Reviews, 32(1): 70–81. © Copyright 2010, Oxford University Press; World Health Organization. (2016). *Household air pollution and health*. Fact Sheet N°292. Geneva, Switzerland: WHO. © Copyright 2016, WHO. Available at: http://www.who.int/mediacentre/factsheets/fs292/en/ ;Parry, C.D. et al. Alcohol consumption and non-communicable diseases: Epidemiology and policy implications. *Addiction*, 106(10),1718–1724. © Copyright 2011, John Wiley & Sons, Inc. All rights reserved; Proimos J, Klein JD. Noncommunicable Diseases in Children and Adolescents. *Pediatrics*. 2012;130(3):379–81. © Copyright 2012, American Academy of Pediatrics; Dogaru, CM. et al. Systematic Reviews and Meta-and Pooled Analyses Breastfeeding and Childhood Asthma. *American Journal of Epidemiology*, 179 (10), 179(10):1153-67. © Copyright 2013, Oxford University Press; Kelishadi, R. & Farajian, S., 2014. The protective effects of breastfeeding on chronic non-communicable diseases in adulthood: A review of evidence. *Advanced Biomedical Research*, 3:3. © Copyright 2014, Advanced Biomedical Research. Published by Wolters Kluwer.

Future priorities

◆ NCDs such as ischaemic heart disease and diabetes need to be recognised as having their origins in childhood, and this should be reflected in both research, policy and intervention strategies.

◆ With respect to NCDs of later childhood and adulthood, the main challenges are the sale of unhealthy commodities such as tobacco, alcohol, and high sugar food in LMICs.

◆ Governments need to use tax policy to limit the sale of harmful commodities and to generate revenue to strengthen health systems and fund the determinants of health such as water and sanitation.

Conclusions

Current resources for the management of NCDs of childhood in LMICs are extremely limited. The use of tax policy to re-price harmful products and generate revenue to strengthen health systems and promote healthy lifestyles must be the priority.

Case study: the struggle of diagnosis in resource poor setting

Jonas, a ten-year-old boy, is brought to his community health worker because he is losing weight and passing a lot of urine. His village health worker treats him for worms. The family return a week later as his condition has deteriorated. He is referred to the local hospital but there is no petrol in the ambulance, so his family have to raise enough money to get a bus to the hospital. When he arrives at the hospital he is complaining of abdominal pain and is very dehydrated and breathing fast. He is taken to theatre for suspected appendicitis. It is noted during his operation that his appendix is normal and after his operation his condition deteriorates. He is more dehydrated and increasingly drowsy. One of the nurses notes his breath smells sweet and wonders about diabetes. There is a gluconometer but there are no sticks. He is referred to the central hospital but on arrival he is comatose, his blood sugar is unrecordably high. Intravenous fluids and insulin are commenced but the insulin is out of date and there is no infusion pump. The fluids go in much faster than prescribed. He dies three hours later, the cause is likely to be cerebral oedema due to hyperglycaemia; a post-mortem is not carried out as there is no pathologist available.

Questions

1. What public health policies/actions might reduce the incidence and prevalence of asthma?

2. What are the main barriers to good outcomes for childhood cancer in LMICs?

3. What are the barriers to good glycaemia control for a child with T1DM in an LMICs?

Key publications

Proimos J and Klein J (2012). Noncommunicable diseases in children and adolescents. *Pediatrics* 130(3): 379–81.
The authors highlight the importance of a lifecourse approach to the prevention of NCDs, the habits which result in these are often established in childhood.

Moodie R, Stuckler D, Monteiro C, et al. (2013). Profits and pandemics: prevention of harmful effects of tobacco, alcohol, and ultra-processed food and drink industries. *Lancet* 381(9867): 670–9.
The authors highlights the role of industry in the NCD epidemic which is unfolding.

Bibliography

Atkinson M, Eisenbarth G, and Michels A (2014). Type 1 diabetes. *Lancet* 383(9911): 69–82.

Black R, Cousens S, Johnson H, et al. (2010). Global, regional, and national causes of child mortality in 2008: a systematic analysis. *Lancet*, 375(9730), 1969–87. Available at: http://www.ncbi.nlm.nih.gov/pubmed/20466419.

Global Asthma Network (2014). *The Global Asthma Report 2014.* Global Asthma Network.

Hunger S, Sung L, and Howard S (2009). Treatment strategies and regimens of graduated intensity for childhood acute lymphoblastic leukemia in low-income countries: a proposal. *Pediatric Blood & Cancer* 52(5): 559–65.

Israels T, Ribeiro R, Molyneux E, et al. (2010). Strategies to improve care for children with cancer in sub-Saharan Africa. *European Journal of Cancer* 46(11): 1960–6. Available at: http://linkinghub.elsevier.com/retrieve/pii/S0959804910002583.

McCoy D (2017). Framing the tax and health nexus: a neglected aspect of public health concern. *Health Economics, Policy and the Law* 12(2): 79–194.

NCD Alliance (2011). *NCD Alliance Briefing Paper on Children and NCDs in Every Policy: Recommendations for a Lifecourse Approach to NCDs.* pp.1–4.

World Health Organization (2006). Sickle cell anaemia. *Fifty-ninth World Health Assembly*, A59/9(April), pp.1–5.

World Health Organization (2013). *Global Action Plan for the Prevention and Control of Noncommunicable Diseases 2013–2020.* p. 102. Available at: http://apps.who.int/iris/bitstream/10665/94384/1/9789241506236_eng.pdf

World Health Organization (2014). *The Global Asthma Report 2014.* Available at: http://www.globalasthmareport.org/management/medicines.php

World Health Organization (2016). *Global Report on Diabetes.* p. 88. Available at: http://apps.who.int/iris/bitstream/handle/10665/204871/9789241565257_eng.pdf

Zühlke L, Engle M, Karthikeyan K, et al. (2014). Characteristics, complications, and gaps in evidence-based interventions in rheumatic heart disease: the Global Rheumatic Heart Disease Registry (the REMEDY study), *Eur Heart J* 36(18): 1115–22a.

CHAPTER 40

Children in difficult circumstances

Therese Hesketh and Zhou Xudong

This chapter introduces the concept of children in difficult circumstances, the importance of the United Nations Convention on the Rights of the Child, and draws on two examples: child labour and sexual abuse and exploitation.

Key points

- Difficult circumstances are caused by poverty, disruption of family and support systems, deficiencies in the education system, and ineffective enforcement of legislation.

- Difficult circumstances during childhood are likely to have detrimental effects for development, educational attainment, health, and lifelong prospects.

- In most countries, legislation around the protection of children from the effects of difficult circumstances is based on the UN Convention of the Rights of the Child (UNCRC, 1989).

Background

The types of situation included as 'difficult circumstances' vary widely according to the social, cultural, political, and economic condition of a country or setting. Table 40.1 shows important categories. There is clearly considerable overlap between these groups, and being in one group makes a child vulnerable to other forms of difficult circumstance or exploitation, so there is a potential downward spiral once a child faces difficult circumstances. For example, a child orphan is more likely to end up in child labour or on the streets.

Difficult circumstances have detrimental effects on education, health, and lifelong prospects. However, we should not assume that difficult circumstances are always harmful. Children respond very differently to adverse circumstances. Some can gain strength and resilience as a result of adverse situations. For many, the circumstances will be the norm in their experience, for example many children in poor communities would expect to work throughout childhood alongside their peers. In addition, the impacts of difficult circumstances can be mitigated where children feel loved and cared for by significant adults, and in settings where there are good child protection services.

How many children live in difficult circumstances?

We know that large numbers of children are living in difficult circumstances, but we can only make rough estimates for a number of reasons:

- The definitions are not always clear. For example, a teenage girl caring for younger siblings at home may or may not be classified as a child worker.

- Information collection systems are usually very poor.

- Many of the activities of children in difficult circumstances are illegal and hence hidden.

- Governments are not motivated to reveal real figures for fear of criticism.

Where figures are available they are rarely disaggregated by age and sex. For example, in some settings it may be acceptable for a sixteen-year-old to work on a sugar plantation during the school holidays, but not a six-year-old. Information sources are improving, partly driven by United Nations Children's Fund (UNICEF), which now requests that governments collect data on birth registration, child labour, child marriage, female genital mutilation/cutting, and violence (including sexual violence and violent discipline).

Some official estimates for numbers of children in difficult circumstances, mainly sourced from UN organisations, are shown in Table 40.2.

What are the causes of difficult circumstances?

The causes are multifactorial and will vary by situation and country. The major causes can be grouped into four categories. First, poverty, for example almost all child work is driven by underlying economic necessity at the individual level. Second, disruption of family and support systems. This may be because of conflict, migration for work, or incarceration of a parent. Third, deficiencies in the education system. There may be inaccessible, unaffordable, or poor quality schooling. Finally, ineffective enforcement of legislation.

Table 40.1 A categorisation of child labour according to circumstance; adapted from UNESCAP 2003

Work	Children living and working on the street
	Children involved in hazardous and worst forms of labour
War and other forms of organised violence	Child soldiers
	Refugees and displaced children
Sexual abuse and exploitation	Sexually abused children
	Sex workers, including those involved in prostitution and pornography
	Child marriage
Children without parental care (loss or incapacity of family and primary caregivers)	Orphans (loss of one *or* both parents)
	Separation from parents because of abduction, trafficking, displacement
	Children of parents with disability, mental illness (including substance abuse) or learning difficulties
	Children of imprisoned mothers
	Child carers
	'Left behind children' of migrant workers
Deficient laws and juvenile justice system	Children in prison or detention in their own right, or because their mother is detained (usually young children)

Source: data from United Nations Economic and Social Commission for Asia and the Pacific (UNESCAP). Social context of children in especially difficult circumstances. Bangkok, India: UNESCAP. Avilable at: http://lastradainternational.org/lsidocs/2(1).pdf

Table 40.2 Latest global estimates for some categories of children in difficult circumstances (child defined as less than eighteen years old, unless stated otherwise)

Category	Global estimate (millions)	Notes
Children in work	120	Defined as 5–14 years
Children living on the street	10	This does not include children who work on the street but return home at night
Orphans	26	Defined as loss of both parents*
Child soldiers	0.3	
Children in prostitution	5	
Children detained in prison	1	Excludes children accompanying their mothers in prison.
Child marriage	700	Defined as women alive today who married under age 18
Child refugees	8	Defined as fleeing persecution and violence Excludes economic migrants

*The higher number of orphans (up to 150 million) is often quoted, which includes single orphanhood, that is, loss of one parent.

This means children do not get protection even though illegal activities are taking place.

Legislation

In most countries, legislation around the protection of children from the effects of difficult circumstances is based on the UN Convention of the Rights of the Child (UNCRC, 1989). This has been a highly influential document in defining rights of all children (under the age of 18) around the world. All but one country (the US) has ratified the Convention and many countries have incorporated some of the content into national legislature.

Many governments cannot guarantee these rights, partly because of resource constraints and partly because of lack of political will to address these issues. Most countries still do not have a formal system of child protection. However, all signatory countries report to the UN Committee on the Rights of the Child and need to demonstrate progress towards meeting the obligations and standards in the UNCRC.

The range of types of children in difficult circumstances is very wide. This chapter will focus on two examples, both of which account for large numbers of children globally: child labour and child sexual abuse and exploitation.

Child labour

Child labour has been defined by The International Labour Organization (ILO) in 2008 as work which 'deprives children of their childhood, their potential and their dignity, which interferes with their education and which is harmful to physical and mental development'. Globally there has been a steady decline in child labour over the last two decades, but progress remains slow. At current rates, more than a hundred million children will still be in child labour by 2020.

Until recently, the international community focused on the abolition of all child labour. But it is now generally agreed that children's or adolescents' participation in work which does not affect their health and personal development, or interfere with their schooling, can be very positive, actually contributing to a child's development. So the ILO has further defined two categories of child labour which should be targeted for abolition.

The first is hazardous labour. This is work that 'jeopardises the physical, mental, or moral wellbeing of a child, either because of its nature, or because of the conditions in which it is carried out'. The second is, broadly speaking, all of the worst forms of child labour. This includes all forms of slavery, such as the sale and trafficking of children, debt bondage and forced labour, forced recruitment for armed conflict, child prostitution and pornography, and illicit activities, especially drug trafficking.

There is considerable debate about the role of child labour in poor communities. It is widely acknowledged that child labour reinforces intergenerational cycles of poverty. Working as a child leads to loss of education now and to loss of earnings in the long term. However, over half of child workers are also involved in some form of education, and work enables them to afford to attend school. For example, in many sub-Saharan African countries schooling takes place in the morning, so children often work in the afternoon, sometimes helping to pay for the costs of their education.

Table 40.3 Potential health hazards of child labour

General	Exhaustion
	Exploitation and abuse
	Impact on education, especially in the long term
	Injuries
Specific by type of work	
Agricultural work	Pesticide toxicity
	Parasitic diseases
	Heat stroke
Manufacturing	Hearing loss because of excessive workplace noise
	Exposure to toxins/solvents
Domestic service	Physical and sexual abuse
Street work	Road traffic accidents
	Violence
	Substance abuse
Mining/construction	Respiratory illness
	Musculoskeletal problems

Child work tends to be concentrated in certain sectors, including agriculture (around 70% of all child work), manufacturing, construction, quarrying and mining, and service (especially shops, hotels, restaurants, and domestic service). There are around fifteen million child domestic workers in non-family homes, mostly girls, who by the nature of the work are hidden, and may face particular hazards. A further thirty million children, mostly girls, do unpaid housework and childcare in their own homes, and are not counted in the child labour statistics. The potential hazards of the common forms of child labour are shown in Table 40.3.

Interventions to reduce child labour have centred around four broad areas. First, encouraging communities to change the cultural acceptance of child labour. Second, supporting programmes to provide an alternative income to families. These programmes involve giving money to families on the condition that the child does not work, but attends school instead. Such programmes have been especially successful in Latin America, but they are expensive. Third, improving access to free, good quality education. Even in countries where education is officially free there are often hidden costs which deter children from attending school. Finally, strengthening of child protection systems. This is very complex and in many countries there is still no system of child protection.

Child sexual abuse and exploitation

This is defined as sexual contact between a child and an adult (or older child) when the child is being used as an object of gratification for adult sexual needs or desires. Sexual abuse takes place in all countries and across all classes of society, unlike most other forms of difficult circumstance. It is only in the last two or three decades that the enormity of the problem of child sexual abuse has been widely acknowledged and measures have been taken to try to address it.

Sexual abuse is divided into three categories:

◆ Non-contact abuse—this includes exposure, verbal abuse, and grooming. Unwanted sexting would also fit into this category.

◆ Non-penetrative contact—this refers to inappropriate touching and fondling.

◆ Penetrative abuse—this includes digital, partial or full intercourse, or use of objects.

Accurate figures are very difficult to get, not least because much sexual abuse is perpetrated by family members or adults in the household, and is highly secretive, with children often told not to tell others. Despite this, there are global estimates: 150 million girls and seventy million boys under eighteen have experienced forced sexual intercourse or some other form of sexual violence. Other estimates by Pereda et al. (2009) based on studies conducted in student populations suggest that in most populations 10–20% of girls, and less than 10% of boys have experienced some kind of sexual abuse as a child. It should be noted, that some of this child sexual abuse occurs within the context of marriage. While it affects both boys and girls, girls are much more likely to marry early, often to older men, and sexual abuse and intimate partner violence are more likely to occur in these marriages. More than 700 million women alive today were married as children; over a third of these were married before the age of fifteen.

Sexual exploitation is generally divided into two categories. First, pornography. The advent of the Internet and digital photography has hugely increased the volume of child pornography globally over the last few years. Most worrying is the growing involvement of children in more extreme forms of pornography. Second, commercial sex work. UNICEF estimates that around two million girls aged under eighteen are involved in prostitution.

These forms of sex work are known to be linked to coercion and trafficking, and involve some of the most vulnerable children in the world. The UNCRC has an additional protocol specifically on the sale of children for prostitution and pornography.

Developing successful interventions to reduce sexual abuse and exploitation are among the most challenging, because of the secrecy of much of the activity in this area. Child pornography is a good example. Much child pornography, available globally on the Internet, is produced in countries where legal systems are inadequate. From 2000, one of the global responses has been to target users of child pornography, in an attempt to reduce demand and profitability. The related police investigation in the UK, Operation Ore, resulted in 1451 convictions. In the wider investigation, 390,000 individuals were found to have accessed child pornography across sixty countries, with large numbers convicted.

Challenges

The challenges in addressing children in difficult circumstances are huge and naturally will vary depending on the type of difficult circumstance and the local context. It is often very difficult to even find these children, let alone remove them from harm. This is true even for child labour which may be regarded as one of the easier issues to address. Children in the most extreme forms of child labour are usually the most hidden. In addition, measures to improve the condition of children in hazardous work are impeded because workplace regulations often apply only to employees in the formal sector and most children work in the informal sector. Because children are not officially permitted to work, there is often no legislation to protect them from more hazardous tasks.

Future priorities

◆ It is crucial to develop a better understanding of the scale of the various types of children in difficult circumstances at a local level. Only in this way can targeted interventions be developed.

◆ Few low- and middle-income countries (LMICs) have formal child protection systems in place. Governments, with the support of children's organisations such as UNICEF, need to consider child protection measures appropriate for their particular context.

Conclusions

As child survival rates improve in many of the poorest LMICs, numbers of children living in difficult circumstances will remain high. Many millions of children are still unable to fulfil their developmental potential because of their difficult circumstances, and many are left with long-term health and psychosocial problems. The development of locally appropriate systems of child protection should be a government priority for all nations.

Case study: using conditional cash transfers to reduce child labour and increase school attendance

In Cambodia, from 1999 a programme of conditional cash transfers was introduced in an attempt to reduce child labour. This involved compensating families for the loss of child labour income to incentivise school attendance. Children aged between ten and fifteen were targeted. School registration increased, the number of hours worked decreased (with the decrease higher in boys than girls), and the benefits were greater for poorer families. However, the overall results were not as dramatic as hoped, for example the increase in school registration did not always equate with attendance, and attendance overall only increased marginally. This shows the complexity of the determinants of child labour: it is not driven simply by economic factors. The child labour rate has, however, decreased over the past decade as a result of socioeconomic improvements. Thus, addressing underlying poverty is fundamental to reducing levels of child labour in LMICs.

Questions

1. Why is it so difficult to get accurate figures for children in difficult circumstances?

2. What are the main underlying causes of difficult circumstances in children?

3. What can be done to reduce child labour?

Key publications

The UN Convention on the Rights of the Child
https://www.unicef.org.uk/what-we-do/un-convention-child-rights/
This should be compulsory reading for all child health professionals working in any country.

Reuther E and Osofsky J (2013). Resilence after trauma in early development. In *Encyclopedia on Early Child development.* http://www.child-encyclopedia.com/resilience/according-experts/resilience-after-trauma-early-development.
This explains the important role of resilience in children, including those in difficult circumstances, and is very well referenced.

Fassa A, Parker D, and Scanlon T (2010). *Child Labour: a Public Health Perspective.* Oxford University Press: Oxford, New York.
An excellent text which explores the complexities and controversies in child labour through a public health lens.

Bibliography

Fassa A (2003). *Health benefits of eliminating child labour.* IPEC/ILO: Geneva.

Hesketh T, Gamlin J, and Woodhead M (2006). Child labour: policy and the importance of health. *Arch Dis Child* 91(9): 721–3.

International Labour Organization (2002). *Investing in Every Child, an Economic Study of the Costs and Benefits of Eliminating Child Labour.* ILO: Geneva.

Pereda N, Guilera G, Forns M, and Gómez-Benito J (2009). The international epidemiology of child sexual abuse: a continuation of Finkelhor. *Child Abuse and Neglect* 33(6): 331–42.

UN (2006). Report on Violence Against Children www.unviolencestudy.org

CHAPTER 41

Child injury, maltreatment, and safeguarding

Geoff Debelle, Qingfeng Li, and Delan Devakumar

This chapter will define child maltreatment in terms of children's rights, examine its burden and consequences and actions to prevent, recognise, and respond to it, including support for survivors. It should be read in conjunction with Chapter 16 (Adolescent injuries).

Key points

- ◆ Child maltreatment and intentional injuries are major public health challenges of this century, incurring huge costs for both individuals and society.

- ◆ In many resource-constrained countries, material poverty, natural disasters, and armed conflict leave large numbers of displaced children at risk of exploitation by traffickers.

- ◆ A child rights and public health approach are key to its prevention, recognition, and response.

Background

Violence is an abuse of power and includes acts of commission and omission. Collective violence results in children who are displaced, orphaned or abandoned, being forced to become child soldiers, 'street kids', or victims of domestic or sexual exploitation. While there has rightly been increased attention on the brutality of collective violence, much violence against children occurs every day in the 'invisible sanctuaries' of the home and schools. Despite a common conceptual and operational definition, estimates of the global prevalence of violence against children are unreliable and vary hugely. Around six children per 100,000 population die from violence and maltreatment. Rates vary from 0.8/100,000 in well-resourced countries to over 30/100,000 in some low- and middle-income countries. The Global Burden of Disease (2015) found that fatalities from intentional injuries are slightly higher among males than females (24,000 vs 22,000 respectively) in the <10-year-old age group. Deaths in children from injuries are most commonly due to drowning, road injuries, foreign bodies, mechanical forces, and fires/heat. This is in contrast to adolescents, where deaths are predominantly due to suicide and community violence (gang-related knife and firearm attacks). Child homicide rates are highest in countries in Latin America but the greatest number of deaths was in Nigeria. Homicides are more common in 15–19-year-olds than in younger age groups combined. Additionally, there is an even larger number of non-fatal intentional injuries that may lead to permanent disabilities and require long-term medical treatments.

Child maltreatment should be considered within a wider context of violence such as self-directed violence (self-harm and suicide), interpersonal violence (intimate partner violence, family violence and community violence), and collective violence (social, economic, and political violence). Emotional abuse, for example, can involve bullying (including cyberbullying) and seeing or hearing the ill-treatment of another, such as a child witnessing intimate partner violence. Globally, estimates of non-fatal child maltreatment from survivor self-reports are strikingly higher than from informant studies from agencies. The combined global prevalence rate for all forms of maltreatment from informants in one meta-analysis was 4/1000 live births, compared with 76/1000 from self-report studies. In both fatal and non-fatal child maltreatment, rates are higher in countries affected by war, famine, social inequality, and economic transition, and in communities with marginalised indigenous and disabled groups. In some countries, females are at higher risk of infanticide (such as in parts of India and China), sexual abuse, forced early marriage, harmful gender-based practices such as 'cutting', and neglect, whereas males are at greater risk of harsh and degrading punishment and being forced into combat. Children who witness intimate partner violence are at risk of other forms of maltreatment.

The United Nations Convention on the Rights of the Child

This is a legal instrument that is the cornerstone of a child's rights agenda. Ratified by most counties in the early 1990s, it sets universally appropriate and humane obligations towards children and sets standards for the protection of children against maltreatment, exploitation and discrimination (Articles 3, 6, 19, 32, 34, and 36) and implores us to listen to the voice of the child (Article 12). It represents a strong international consensus and provides professionals, non-governmental organisations, and others with the means to advocate for children and to hold governments accountable.

Global targets
Sustainable Development Goals (SDGs) (2015)

Goal 5 (Gender equality)

- ◆ Eliminate all forms of violence against all women and girls in the public and private spheres, including trafficking and exploitation.

United Nations (UN) world report on violence against children (2006)

◆ Ensure that all currently lawfully accepted violence against children, including all corporal punishment, all harmful traditional practices, and all sexual violence, is prohibited and also effectively eliminated through awareness raising and public education.

◆ Support the development of a multi-faceted and systematic framework to respond to violence against children, fully integrated within national planning processes.

Risk factors

A number of risk factors have been identified, but gaps remain in elucidating causal pathways, with some factors neither necessary nor sufficient for child maltreatment. The 'ecological model' conceptualises child maltreatment as determined by dynamic and multiple transactions between individual relationships, community, and society. The risk factors within these domains are listed in Table 41.1.

Long-term consequences

Growing evidence shows that child maltreatment is associated with a wide range of long-term physical and mental health outcomes that result in a substantial burden on the individual and society (Table 41.2). The term 'adverse childhood experiences' has been coined to describe the wide array of factors that can affect early child development and wellbeing. These have been linked to long-term risk of mental and physical ill health. Cumulative trauma, particularly when associated with parental social isolation, maternal childhood abuse, and childhood disordered attachment, can alter the trajectory of a child's neurodevelopment, manifesting as neurochemical and structural magnetic resonance imaging (MRI) brain changes. Early privation and neglect have been associated with a distinctive form of 'attention deficit hyperactivity disorder' characterised by inattention, and autistic-like traits and social disinhibition. The effect of early life stresses on later illness may be mediated by epigenetic mechanisms.

Intergenerational transmission

Exposure to violence and maltreatment in one generation can have lasting effects in the next, through both social and biological mechanisms. Learned behaviours, for example, can transmit from parent to child. Violence affecting the mother, both at an individual level and a societal level, can lead to health consequences in the child through the mediating impact of altered stress responses in utero and in the young child. This can increase the risk of long-term non-communicable diseases in the child and potentially reduce life expectancy.

Interventions

Resilience

Early childhood adversity does not necessarily predict poor outcome; a large proportion of children do recover from short-lived trauma. It is therefore necessary to move away from a deterministic framework to one of resilience that mirrors the ecological model for child maltreatment (Table 41.1).

Table 41.1 Risk factors for child maltreatment and the social ecology of resilience

Domain	Risk factors	Adaptive systems
Individual	History of cumulative trauma in their own childhood No name or property rights	Self-efficacy Adaptive coping style
Relationship	Disconnectedness between parent and child Poor emotional responsiveness to child Intimate partner violence 'Absent father' Drug and alcohol misuse Severe mental health condition in one or both parents Early child marriage	Family cohesion Social support—material support and mentoring Positive parenting/enhancing the role of fathers in parenting
Community	Lack of social cohesion/social capital Social isolation Poor housing Chronic unemployment	Strengthening neighbourhood/village social cohesion Provision of affordable housing/shelter Safer communities Preventing intimate partner violence/ provision of 'safe houses' Positive peer/school/faith networks/provision of refuge for children at risk of cutting Employment opportunities
Society	Attitudes towards corporal punishment Poverty Social equalities Cultural dissonance and marginalisation Gender-based violence Humanitarian crises, including war and famine Abandonment Trafficking and exploitation	A child's rights approach is embedded, including rejection of physical punishment as a form of discipline Strengthen birth registrations Positive cultural practices and kinship adoption Promote 'rites of passage' and rituals that are not harmful Reduce social inequalities and poverty

Primary prevention

The early identification of vulnerable children and families is one of the many tasks for health professionals working with the difficulties of high caseloads, patchy universal services, resource constraints, and loss of community cohesion. There is no risk factor or combination of risk factors that can reliably and accurately predict maltreatment and this makes the task even more fraught.

A public health approach that enhances resilience by delivering evidence-based parenting programmes, supporting fathers, and providing material and social support through mentoring and

Table 41.2 Long-term consequences of child maltreatment

Low educational achievement
Internalising behaviour problems:
◆ Anxiety
◆ Depression
◆ PTSD
Externalising behaviour problems:
◆ Aggression
◆ Conduct disorder
◆ Violence and criminality
◆ Obtrusive sexual behaviour and risk taking
Self-harm and suicide
Domestic and sexual exploitation
Alcohol and substance misuse/risk of foetal alcohol syndrome in offspring
Physical health problems, for example:
◆ Increased cardiac risk
◆ Obesity

Table 41.3 Signs of suspected inflicted injury

Bruising	Bruising in any location in a premobile infant
	Bruising to ear, cheeks, neck, buttocks, abdomen, arms, and hands
	Multiple bruises
	Bruises in clusters
	Bruises showing positive or negative imprint of hand/implement
Bite marks	Human bite mark—annular lesion made up of two arcs facing each other
Burns	Forced immersion scald into hot water (symmetrical, uniform thickness and clear tide mark)
	Contact burns (cigarette, iron)
	Burns to unusual locations (e.g. genitalia)
Fractures	Limb fracture in a young infant (humerus, femur)
	Multiple fractures
	Occult rib and metaphyseal fractures in infants
Head injury	Skull fractures in infants (equal probability for inflicted and non-inflicted injury)
	'Abusive head trauma': acute encephalopathy, multifocal subdural haemorrhage, and severe, bilateral retinal haemorrhage
Sexual abuse	Disclosure
	Sexually-transmitted infection in a prepubertal child
	Signs of genital trauma (e.g. complete hymenal transection)

home visiting, provides a strong buffer against child maltreatment. Governments need to raise community awareness of child maltreatment and ensure that resources are available and used effectively to produce good outcomes for the child and family.

Secondary prevention

Over the past decade, the evidence base has increased for the characteristics of inflicted injury and sexual abuse (Table 41.3). Despite this, diagnostic uncertainty can lead to indecision. Health professionals therefore need access to advice, support, supervision, and peer review. Education and learning must also incorporate local knowledge of the indigenous culture and social mores.

The immediate response is referral to a body with statutory authority to intervene and ensure the child's safety, while reducing secondary victimisation. Child advocacy centres such as 'one-stop centres', established in many countries, have been beacons of good practice (see case study).

Tertiary prevention

It is never too late to intervene with children and adolescents who have suffered cumulative trauma, as the brain has sufficient plasticity and resilience to overcome this in early childhood. Evidence-based therapeutic intervention, using 'non-talking therapies' such as mindfulness, trauma-focused therapy, and family therapy have achieved good outcomes, especially for survivors of sexual abuse and war.

Challenges

The greatest challenge facing communities is prevention. The shift from being a child that is at risk to one that is resilient is important. A public health response, based on a 'strengthening families' model is key. Child rights should underly all interventions. Current data

sources are generally unreliable due to the inconsistency in tools, under-reporting and the hidden nature of violence.

Future priorities

◆ Vital registration systems should be established to provide quality data on the incidence and causes of intentional injuries. Due to the sensitivity of intentional injuries among children, the collection of information on intentional injuries among children under ten years old requires a complicated, multi-sectoral effort that includes medical and legal concerns.

◆ There is an urgent need to develop reliable, accurate, and culturally appropriate tools to predict and prevent child maltreatment. While we know much about the characteristics of inflicted injury, high-quality prospective studies comparing inflicted and non-inflicted injury with respect to history, presentation, and time to seek medical attention need to be undertaken.

◆ Prevention strategies should be expanded for intentional injuries, including rigorous validation and appropriate adaption.

Conclusions

Violence perpetrated against children, within and outside households, is a global scourge that has lasting consequences for survivors and institutions. There must be a comprehensive, well-resourced child's rights and public health response to prevention, detection, and intervention. Non-governmental organizations (NGOs) must challenge governments on United Nations Convention on the Rights of the Child (UNCRC) violations and hold perpetrators accountable. Every child matters and safeguarding them is everyone's business.

Case study: setting up a centre for disclosure of abuse in Malawi

A one-stop centre was established at the Queen Elizabeth Central Hospital in Blantyre, Malawi, in response to the growing number of children and young people presenting with acute rape or disclosing abuse. In an eight-month period, 228 survivors were seen at the centre, with fear of human immunodeficiency virus (HIV), seeking justice, and confirmation of alleged rape being the predominant reasons for use. The majority were satisfied with the holistic service which they received, but lack of transport was a constraint. This can provide a model for a comprehensive and coordinated service for survivors.

Source: Yabwile Mulambia. Dissertation Submitted for Master of Medicine, University of Malawi.

Questions

1. How does abuse in early life affect the health of a child?

2. Name three violations of the UNCRC in your region

3. What is available in your region to support families in difficulty?

Key publications

Pinheiro P (2006). *World Report on Violence Against Children: Independent Report for the UN*. United Nations: Geneva.

World Health Organization and the International Society for Prevention of Child Abuse and Neglect (2006). *Preventing Child Maltreatment: a Guide to Taking Action and Generating Evidence*. WHO: Geneva.
These documents give a wide-ranging and detailed account of the global phenomenon of violence against children and how a robust governmental and non-governmental response can tackle it.

United Nations Children's Fund (2013). *Female Genital Mutilation/Cutting: a Statistical Overview and Exploration of the Dynamics of Change*. UNICEF: New York.
This is a key document for understanding the context and complexity surrounding 'cutting' and how activists within the practising communities and other groups are seeking to eradicate this harmful, culturally sanctioned practice.

CORE Info. *Cardiff Child Protection Systematic Reviews*. Available at http://www.core-info.cardiff.ac.uk.
This provides access to up-to-date, comprehensive systematic reviews on the signs of child maltreatment from authorities in the field.

Bibliography

Belsk J (1980). Child maltreatment. An ecological integration. *American Psychologist*, 35, 320–35.

Berlin L, Appleyard K, and Dodge K (2011). Intergenerational continuity in child maltreatment: mediating mechanisms and implications for practice. *Child Development* 82: 162–76.

Chaffin M, Bonner B, and Hill R (2001). Family preservation and family support programs: child maltreatment outcomes across client risk levels and program types. *Child Abuse & Neglect* 25: 269–89.

Finkelhor D and Lannen P (2015). Dilemmas for international mobilization around child abuse. *Child Abuse & Neglect* 50: 128–40.

Gilbert R, Kemp A, Thoburn J, et al. (2009). Recognising and responding to child maltreatment. *Lancet* 373: 167–80.

Global Burden of Disease (2015). Mortality and causes of death collaborators. Global, regional, and national life expectancy, all-cause mortality, and cause-specific mortality for 249 causes of death, 1980–2015: a systematic analysis for the global burden of disease study. *Lancet* 388:1459–544.

Global Burden of Disease Pediatrics Collaboration (2016). Global and national burden of diseases and injuries among children and adolescents between 1990 and 2013. Findings From the Global Burden of Disease 2013 Study. *JAMA Pediatrics* 170(3): 267–87.

Hodges M, Godbout N, Briere J, Lanktree C, Gilbert A, and Kletzka N (2013). Cumulative trauma and symptom complexity in children: a path analysis. *Child Abuse & Neglect* 37: 891–8.

Korbin J (1991). Cross-cultural perspectives and research directions for the 21st century. *Child Abuse & Neglect* 15 (suppl 1): 67–77.

McCory E, DeBrito S, and Viding E (2010). Research review: the neurobiology and genetics of maltreatment and adversity. *Journal of Child Psychology & Psychiatry* 51: 1079–95.

Maguire-Jac K and Showalter K (2016). The protective effect of neighborhood social cohesion in child abuse and neglect. *Child Abuse & Neglect* 52: 29–37.

Molyneux E, Kennedy N, Dano A, and Mulambia Y (2013). Sexual abuse of children in low-income settings: time for action. *Paediatrics & International Child Health* 33: 239–46.

Munro E, Taylor J, and Bradbury-Jones C (2014). Understanding the causal pathways to child maltreatment: implications for health and social care policy and practice. *Child Abuse Review* 23: 61–74.

Reading R, Bissell S, Goldhagen J, et al. (2009). Promotion of children's rights and prevention. *Lancet* 373: 332–43.

Stoltenborgh M, Bakermans-Kranenburg M, Lenneke R, Marinus H, and van Ijzendoorn H (2015). The prevalence of child maltreatment across the globe: review of a series of meta-analyses. *Child Abuse Review* 24: 37–50.

Tinajero A, Cohen N, and Ametorwo S (2015). No data, no problem, no action: parenting programs in low income countries. Making the social-emotional outcomes more visible. *Child: Health Care and Development* 42: 117–24.

Ungar M, Ghazinour M, and Richter J (2013). What is resilience within the social ecology of human development? *Journal of Child Psychology & Psychiatry* 54: 348–66.

CHAPTER 42

Strategies to improve child health

Fred Martineau

This chapter examines the key priorities facing child health practitioners and policymakers to build on recent improvements in global child health and wellbeing. It analyses what has underpinned these successes, why shortcomings persist, and how best to address them.

Key points

- Scaling up established health interventions, particularly in primary care, while addressing fundamental social determinants has substantially reduced child mortality in many countries.

- This 'success' is, however, partial and unfairly distributed. The most important child health priorities today are to:

  - Understand and address between and within-country child health inequities.

  - Ensure that every child not only survives but also attains their full state of development and wellbeing.

- Addressing these priorities requires locally adapted strategic frameworks that co-produce child health policy with patients and communities.

Background

There is much to celebrate about recent progress in child health. Global under-five mortality has reduced by 52% from 1990 to 2015, with fifty-eight countries achieving a two thirds reduction. Child health improvements are broadly attributable to two approaches: scaling up key health interventions and improving underlying social determinants. These are not separate agendas—both are co-dependent and mutually reinforcing. Effectively scaling up essential child health interventions has proved capable of overcoming poverty and inequality.

Yet the global child health agenda remains incomplete. Global reductions in child deaths conceal wide variations in individual countries' success in reducing child mortality. Many regions and countries have made worryingly little progress in addressing child health disparities, in particular sub-Saharan Africa, where under-five mortality is still twenty-three times higher than in West Europe. Furthermore, child health is not just about survival. Child mortality reductions now need to be matched by long lasting improvements in child development and wellbeing.

Global Strategy for Women's, Children's, and Adolescents' Health

An integral component of the Sustainable Development Goals (SDGs), the Global Strategy's key objectives and child health targets (Table 42.1) address a number of key limitations of previous global initiatives such as the Millennium Development Goals (MDGs), including:

1. Pursuing equity between countries by setting an absolute rather than relative child survival target for every country.

2. Prioritising child wellbeing and development equally with survival.

3. Explicitly recognising the interdependence of health with social, economic, and political determinants through an integrated, multi-sector approach.

The Global Strategy sets out key 'action areas' and cross-cutting 'guiding principles' that will enable global child health initiatives to truly 'survive, thrive, and transform' across the continuum of care.

Interventions

As emphasised throughout this book, child health strategies should be positioned within a lifecourse approach (Figure 42.1). Maternal nutrition, education, and newborn care are particularly crucial to child health—and vice versa.

Primary health care

In contrast to maternal or neonatal health, most child mortality and morbidity can be effectively prevented or treated in primary care—including community outreach. Intervention packages with the most potential to save lives are:

- Infant and young child feeding, especially during the first 1000 days: enabling exclusive breastfeeding for six months; continued breastfeeding, and complementary feeding from six months onwards.

- Responsive caregiving and stimulation to enable carers to provide play and communication activities using household items, and to strengthen responsive care, using, for example, the UNICEF/WHO Care for Child Development package.

- Immunisation through universal coverage of the extended programme for immunisations, plus periodic vitamin A supplementation where appropriate.

Table 42.1 Global strategy: objectives and key child health targets

Survive—end preventable deaths

◆ Reduce under-five mortality to below 25 per 1000 live births in every country.

Thrive—ensure health and wellbeing

◆ End all forms of malnutrition and address the nutritional needs of children.

◆ Ensure all girls and boys have access to good quality early childhood development.

◆ Achieve universal health coverage, including financial risk protection and access to quality essential services, medicines, and vaccines.

Transform—expand enabling environments

◆ Eradicate extreme poverty.

◆ Ensure all girls and boys complete free, equitable, and good-quality primary and secondary education.

◆ Eliminate all harmful practices, discrimination, and violence against women and girls.

◆ Achieve universal and equitable access to safe drinking water, sanitation, and hygiene.

Action areas

◆ Country leadership

◆ Financing for health

◆ Health system resilience

◆ Individual potential

◆ Community engagement

◆ Multi-sector action

◆ Humanitarian and fragile settings

◆ Research and innovation

◆ Accountability

Guiding principles

Country-led, universal, sustainable, rights-based, gender-responsive, evidence-informed, partnership-driven, people-centred, community-owned, accountable, and aligned with development effectiveness and humanitarian norms.

Source: data from Independent Expert Review Group (iERG). Every Woman, Every Child, Every Adolescent: Achievements and Prospects - Executive Summary. © 2015 Every Woman Every Child.

◆ Integrated management of acute illnesses: using Integrated Management of Childhood Illnesses (IMCI) and Integrated Community Case Management of Childhood Illness (iCCM) approaches to target pneumonia, diarrhoea, sepsis, malnutrition, and (where endemic) malaria.

There is clear, established evidence for affordable community and clinical interventions in each of these areas, as outlined in Chapters 36 and 37. Where these interventions have been effectively rolled out at scale, child mortality has consistently dropped. Yet coverage remains incomplete, particularly amongst the most vulnerable and marginalised populations (Figure 42.2). For example, child survival rates in the poorest economic quintile are half that of the richest.

The evidence base supporting child development and wellbeing interventions in resource-poor settings emphasises the importance of responsive and nurturing care, the treatment and rehabilitation of disabilities, maternal mental health, and adequate social protection to reduce and protect against poverty.

The strategic priority today is to understand and address the reasons for implementation gaps. In particular, child health initiatives need to engage more effectively with local contexts by not just asking 'what works' clinically but 'what works here' programmatically, through implementation and social science research into local situational understandings of health, social, and political systems.

Hospital care

Primary care services cannot function in isolation. Mutually supportive links with both inpatient services and communities are needed to deliver comprehensive, quality, and trusted primary care services. Children whose illnesses or injuries are not manageable in primary care—malaria or severe acute malnutrition with complications, or road traffic accidents, for example—need timely referral to secondary care.

Even in secondary care, clinical care priorities should focus on the quality delivery of relatively simple interventions to manage severe illnesses and injuries, especially in the first twenty-four hours of admission. Prompt emergency assessment and treatment by skilled staff trained and equipped to safely provide intravenous fluids, antibiotics, and blood transfusions save more lives than high-technology intensive care equipment. Again, service fragmentation should be avoided by strengthening hospital care using an integrated approach. In addition, as countries go through the epidemiological transition, increasing numbers of children will suffer from more complex chronic conditions that are better managed at higher-level facilities.

Functional links between primary and secondary care are also important for health staff. Effective referral pathways avoid frustration with limited local capacity and reduce time spent away from other essential primary health activities. Such links also strengthen supportive supervision and continuing professional education that build staff motivation and quality.

Community and intersectoral priorities

Strong, equitable governance mechanisms between health workers and the communities they serve are crucial to fostering a responsive and accessible health system. Communities are also central to addressing wider social, economic, and political health determinants, maintaining the economic and social stability that is fundamental to child health and wellbeing.

Key child health determinants include:

◆ Local and planetary environments that are conducive to child health and development, in particular access to water, sanitation, and hygiene.

◆ Sustainable livelihoods.

◆ Food security and nutrition, including breastfeeding.

◆ Education, both as a direct component of child wellbeing and for children as future parents and health workers.

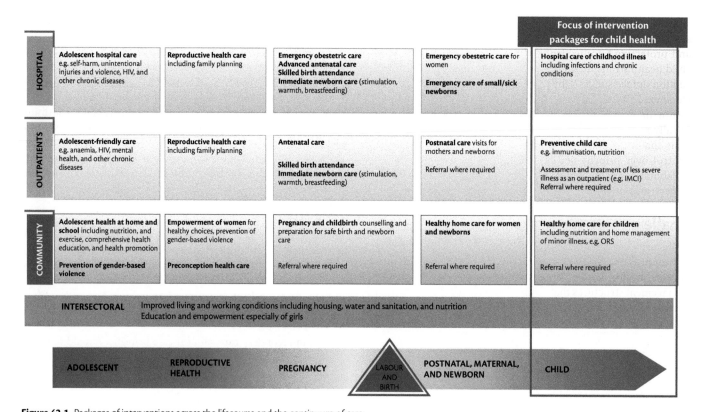

Figure 42.1 Packages of interventions across the lifecourse and the continuum of care.

Local action at the household and community level is important in addressing these broader child health priorities. Such initiatives will only succeed, however, within enabling economic and political environments created by fundamental intersectoral transformations at national and global levels.

Child health systems

The most important health system weaknesses limiting equitable access to child health services are: financial barriers to care; shortages or mismatched distributions of trained health staff and essential medicines; and governance structures that are unresponsive to local needs (Chapter 8).

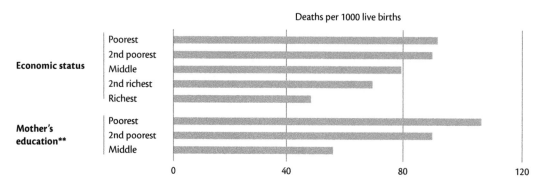

*Data from national Demographic and Health Surveys in 49 low- and middle-income countries, 2005–2012.
**Education data are not available for 10 countries.

Figure 42.2 Under-fives deaths by economic and maternal education status.

Increasing geographical coverage of quality child health services and removing user fees are both key to improving access and protecting families from catastrophic health costs. Where child health strategies do not reflect local concerns, health intervention uptake suffers. Child health strategies must therefore include explicit mechanisms that enable local adaptation of child health initiatives to address *both* local and global priorities. Locally responsive child health services also require health systems that are 'people-centred' and 'community-owned', where control over priority-setting is shared and negotiated within collaborative partnerships between policymakers, health practitioners, and citizens.

Challenges

Child health initiatives ought to be co-produced with families and communities. Barriers to this include sociocultural differences between health workers and their patients, hierarchical health management structures that restrict local adaptation, and governments with little incentive to change the societal power dynamics that brought them to power. There are, however, increasing examples of countries successfully overcoming these barriers (see case study).

Technical changes tend to be more readily achieved than social and political transformations. For example, IMCI became largely synonymous with improved clinical case management rather than the wider transformation of health and social systems that was originally intended. We need to ensure that the 'thrive' and 'transform' child health agendas are not eclipsed by 'survive' alone.

Future priorities

- Although there have been major advances in the reduction in overall child mortality, particularly related to infectious diseases, it is important to identify and prevent suffering in children in difficult circumstances, which includes trafficked children, child labourers, and those that are victims to child sexual exploitations.

- As countries undergo epidemiological transition, non-communicable diseases are becoming a larger proportion of the disease burden. Early childhood interventions including around exercise, diet, smoking, and alcohol use is a cost-effective primary prevention strategy that requires more attention.

Conclusions

A holistic and multi-sectoral strategy targeting primary, secondary, and community levels of care, as well as broader social determinants is central to improving child health and wellbeing. Child health strategies must actively engage with the complexity and context-dependence of health interventions when rolled out at scale. This is best achieved by more equitably balanced decision-making relationships between health professionals and citizens that champion local situational knowledge and priorities equally with global evidence.

Case study: Ethiopia halves its under-five mortality in nineteen years

Between 1990 and 2009, after two decades of severe political and economic instability and despite persistently poor economic growth, Ethiopia halved under-five mortality across all its ethnically and socioeconomically diverse regions. Major reductions were achieved in malaria mortality, undernutrition, and the numbers of families with poor access to water and sanitation. The 2003 Health Extension Program played a particularly important role in scaling up key health interventions delivered by large numbers of health extension workers.

Key factors underpinning these successes include:

- Coherent policy approaches across health priorities, contributing to 'horizontal' improvements in health system strengthening and household gender equality.

- Explicitly including health in poverty reduction and sustainable development policies.

- Adopting a health system governance model enabling local needs to be prioritised within national targets.

Questions

1. How does the global strategy differ from previous global child health initiatives?

2. What are the key differences in child health priorities currently facing Sierra Leone and Ethiopia?

Key publications

Bryce J, Victora C, and Black R (2013). The unfinished agenda in child survival. *Lancet* 382: 1049–59.
   Past challenges and future priorities in child health strategies.

Every Woman Every Child (2015). *The Global Strategy For Women's, Children's, and Adolescents' Health (2016–2030)*. Every Woman Every Child: New York, US.
   Provides full details of the global strategy.

Marston C, Hinton R, Kean S, et al. (2016). Community participation for transformative action on women's, children's and adolescents' health. *Bull World Health Organ* 94: 376–82.
   In-depth analysis of community participation, including key implementation challenges.

Bibliography

Balabanova D, McKee M, and Mills A (2011). *'Good Health At Low Cost' 25 Years On. What Makes a Successful Health System?* London School of Hygiene and Tropical Medicine: London, UK.

Banteyerga H, Kidanu A, Conteh L, and Mckee M (2011). Ethiopia—placing health at the centre of development. Chapter 4. In: Balabanova D, McKee M., and Mills A (eds) *'Good Health At Low Cost' 25 Years On. What Makes a Successful Health System?* London School of Hygiene and Tropical Medicine: London, UK.

Daelmans B, Black M, Lombardi J, et al. (2015). Effective interventions and strategies for improving early child development. *BMJ* 351: 23–6.

Government of Sierra Leone (2015). *National Ebola Recovery Strategy For Sierra Leone 2015–2017*. Government of Sierra Leone: Freetown.

Larson H and Schulz W (2015). *The State of Vaccine Confidence 2015*. The Vaccine Confidence Project, London School of Hygiene and Tropical Medicine: London, UK.

Shaw B, Amouzou A, Miller N, Tafesse M, Bryce J, and Surkan P (2016). Access to integrated community case management of childhood illness services in rural Ethiopia: a qualitative study of the perspectives and experiences of caregivers. *Health Policy and Planning* 31: 656–66.

Sheikh K, Ranson M, and Gilson L (2014). Explorations on people centredness in health systems. *Health Policy and Planning* 29: ii1–ii5.

UNICEF/World Health Organization (2012). *Care for Child Development Package*. World Health Organization: Geneva.

Wang H, Bhutta Z, Coates M, et al. (2016). Global, regional, national, and selected subnational levels of stillbirths, neonatal, infant, and under-five mortality, 1980–2015: a systematic analysis for the Global Burden of Disease Study 2015. *Lancet* 388: 1725–74.

Watkins K (2016). Longer lives and unfinished agendas on child survival. *Lancet* 388: 1450–52.

Witter S, Brikci N, Harris T, et al. (2016). *The Sierra Leone Free Health Care Initiative (FHCI): Process and Effectiveness Review. Final Report*. Oxford Policy Management: Oxford, UK.

World Health Organization (2016). *Towards a grand convergence for child survival and health: a strategic review of options for the future building on lessons learnt from IMNCI*. WHO: Geneva.

SECTION 8

Influencing policy

CHAPTER 43

Ethics and rights

Maureen Kelley

This chapter discusses the clinical obligations, public health ethics, and human rights in the context of women's, children's, and adolescents' health. It should be read in conjunction with Chapters 5 (Economic evaluation in global health), 6 (Social determinants of health), and 45 (Advocacy to improve health).

Key points

◆ Ethical arguments offer an important rationale for best practices in clinical settings and support evidence-based policies and programmes aimed at improving reproductive, maternal, newborn, and child health (RMNCH) regionally and globally.

◆ Healthy communities and populations depend on strong commitments to the value of women's, children's, and adolescents' health.

◆ It is important to recognise the inherent worth of all persons—as defended by an appeal to human rights.

◆ As we develop health and behavioural interventions, policies, and programmes in RMNCH we should be mindful of ensuring a fair distribution of benefits and burdens, and avoid unintended, harmful consequences.

Background

The lifecourse view of reproductive, maternal, newborn, child, and adolescent health, encourages a more integrated, intergenerational approach to improving maternal and child survival and morbidity, particularly in low-income settings. In addition to evidence-based appeals to efficacy, ethical arguments appealing to the value of promoting women's, children's, and adolescents' health along the lifecourse have also helped garner attention for much needed RMNCH investments, rather than thinking of women's health and child health competing with each other. In this chapter, we will reflect on those arguments and consider the ethical challenges that sometimes arise when considering ethical issues from the bedside to global priority setting.

Ethical considerations across clinical, public health, and global domains

A full account of ethics in RMNCH needs to offer guidance in the clinical domain—where health care is delivered to women, children, and adolescents. It also needs to attend to public health, the advancement of key country-level, regional, and global outcomes— like lowering global rates of death in childbirth or stillbirth, or ensuring equitable uptake of new interventions like human papilloma

virus (HPV) vaccine. Finally, ethical reflection in RMNCH should include consideration of the rights and dignity of patients, especially marginalised women, children, and adolescents. Together, the ethical principles applied across these domains offer essential tools for guiding clinical practice, evaluating wider health programmes or policies, and setting agendas for advocacy (Figure 43.1). In daily practice, clinicians may rarely consider the public health or global implications of care, whereas policymakers may rarely tangle with challenging ethical considerations at the bedside, but they both need to be aware of the full scope of ethical considerations.

Challenges

Ethical challenges in RMNCH tend to arise in three ways.

(1) Difficult ethical choices arise within each domain. In the wards (clinical ethics), when a clinician must decide whether an adolescent has the capacity to decide whether to discontinue life-sustaining treatment against her parents' wishes. At the societal level (public health ethics), when public health officials and sexual health experts must weigh parental refusals or community objections against population health benefits of expanding access to contraception and family planning in communities. At the global level (health and human rights), when an organisation like the World Health Organization evaluates implementation of a child nutrition programme and must prioritise between regions according to ethical principles—should they target the countries with highest child mortality, but low infrastructure for delivery, or those that have slightly lower rates of malnutrition but better health systems infrastructure? Which will be the most effective use of resources in terms of lives saved?

(2) Ethical questions also arise when we make decisions across domains. Consider a vaccination example: imagine you are a paediatrician within a country or state mandating Measles Mumps and Rubella (MMR) vaccination during a measles outbreak but you encounter a parent refusing to allow your patient to be vaccinated. Your clinical obligations to the child and parent are in tension with your awareness of the potential risk to other children in the community and wider public.

(3) The last type of ethical challenge in RMNCH arises when our ethical obligations to different persons conflict. In obstetrics, these might be conflicts between obligations to the woman as your patient, but also the developing baby—for example when the mother refuses chemotherapy to treat her cancer out of concern for her foetus, risking her own life to save her baby.

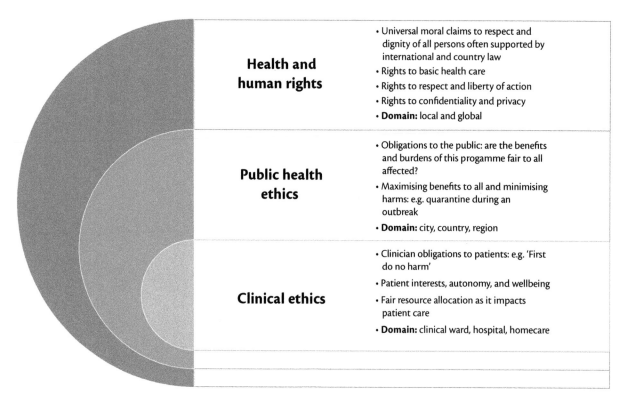

Figure 43.1 The domains of ethics and health care.
Reproduced courtesy of the authors.

Identifying unintended consequences of RMNCH programmes and policies

An important consideration in evaluating RMNCH policies and intervention packages is to be mindful of unintended consequences, such as stigma, blame, or inadvertent harm. It is not always possible to predict the way that public health messages may be received, or unexpected incentives may be created for harmful behaviour. Evaluation of pilot programmes and community engagement in design prior to implementation can help identify potential concerns. In child health, the research into the effects of severe child malnutrition on later adult health is critical to appreciating the risk of later illness for severely malnourished children and to help increase investment in research and interventions. However, it is important to be mindful of how we frame messages around scientific findings in areas such as child malnutrition, premature birth, and child neglect. There is a risk that children living in poverty will be viewed as irretrievably set back. The science does not support this view—environment, individual resilience, and other factors can still be effective in improving a young adult's health and future development despite severe setbacks in early childhood. For this reason, the lifecourse view should not be understood as deterministic. Moreover, ethically, adolescents and adults who have suffered such setbacks are more worthy of support and interventions to improve their health and wellbeing beyond 'critical windows' for intervention.

Health and human rights: an important tool for advocacy in RMNCH

Rights are moral claims, often backed by law, made against others such as governments or other persons, and offer a powerful tool

for advocating for those who often lack moral consideration in society—such as orphans, migrant children, or sex workers. A more foundational appeal to health and wellbeing as a human right, such as defended in the United Nations Convention on the Rights of the Child, is not contingent on whether upholding this right leads to the good of a society or overall health of a population. Such an argument asks us to commit to treating preventable diseases among women, children, and adolescents living in poverty because as human beings they deserve a dignified life, an education, safe childbirth, and a life free of domestic violence.

Pragmatic appeals for good outcomes for families, communities, and governments are effective arguments when made to those who must manage scarce resources—ministers of health, policymakers, governments, and communities who might otherwise find the human rights appeals on behalf of girls and women a threat to traditional values. However, without a strong reminder of the more foundational claims of girls, children, and women as human beings of equal worth and standing, we risk perpetuating the view that investing in the health of women, children, and adolescents can be subjugated to other more pressing public health needs because their lives are not of equal value. Lasting advances in alleviating the burden of disease for women, children, and families depend upon norms and laws supporting the health and social rights of women and young people.

Future priorities

- ◆ In the context of limited resources for research, policies, and interventions, any major decision needs to be viewed through an ethical prism. Inevitably, rights or values will sometimes conflict and there will often be unintended consequences; these must be carefully discussed and evaluated.

◆ Rights should be used as a tool for advocacy, particularly for the challenges that have been neglected, like improving adolescent health and reducing stillbirth, and for marginalised, vulnerable populations, like child sex workers that are difficult to reach.

Conclusions

One of the great strengths of the lifecourse approach to RMNCH is that it reflects a deep truth more accurately: the health and wellbeing of women, children, and adolescents are intimately connected, biologically and socially. Developing ethical arguments is an essential part of clinical practice and responsible policy. Ethical reflection can help us appreciate the integral connections in the social wellbeing and health of women, girls, and children over the lifecourse, while giving us the critical tools to carefully evaluate treatment decisions and programmes.

Case study: multi-level dilemmas of care in resource-limited settings

The most heartbreaking, hard choices are dilemmas of poverty. In many areas of the world, neonatal intensive care is not available, as facilities lack both adequate equipment and/or skilled staff to provide care to severely ill newborns. Many such units do not have ventilator support, continuous positive airway pressure (CPAP), or supplies of life-saving drugs such as surfactant. Low-cost CPAP has been developed as a bridge for respiratory management of preterm infants. Still, the lack of resources results in very difficult decisions about which babies to accept on the unit, which babies among several in respiratory distress to place on CPAP and for how long, and which to give scarce drugs like surfactant.

Consider the three domains of ethics (Figure 43.1) and the different roles and ethical responsibilities. At the global and country level, government officials and experts will adopt criteria for fair allocation of scarce resources and investment in neonatal respiratory care. Responsibilities in this role are to populations—it might be district level, country, regional, or global. Decisions for investment will typically be considered alongside the many competing needs within healthcare delivery (e.g. infectious disease, chronic disease, injury, health systems). Allocation decisions will also compete with meeting other basic needs such as education, security, housing, and employment. The prior decisions will impact the delivery of care at the hospital, ward, and bedside.

For example, the director of a hospital in rural Uganda and the head nurse of the Neonatal Intensive Care Unit (NICU) will need to decide how best to stretch a tight budget to restock surfactant, when, across the hospital, the paediatric ward is battling an outbreak of diarrhoea. The hospital director will need to think of the needs of all those served by the hospital, while the unit staff will want to advocate for the needs of their patients. Fair compromises across the wards are critical for a functioning hospital. Imagine that over the weekend three preterm infants are admitted, all with 'poor respiratory scores'. Prior agreement on the unit to a ranking of respiratory scores to guide interventions can help guide allocation decisions fairly. Discussions, training, and planning can help manage these ethical dilemmas prospectively. However, no amount of training will make it less heartbreaking when a clinician must face the parents of the baby who does not receive scarce respiratory support that night.

Questions

1. Can you identify ethical challenges arising in clinical, public health, and global health contexts in RMNCH—how does a shift in roles sometimes shift the ethical considerations?

2. What is the central ethical tension between the appeal to public health and appeal to health and human rights; and can you think of a way to reconcile this tension?

3. Can you identify examples of well-intended public health programmes or interventions that have had unintended harmful consequences? And, can you think of ways those harms might have been avoided or mitigated?

Key publications

Mann J, Gostin L, Gruskin S, Brennan T, Lazzarini Z, and Fineberg H (2013). Health and human rights. In: Grodin M, Tarantola D, Annas G, and Gruskin S (eds). *Health and Human Rights in a Changing World*. Routledge: New York, US. pp. 16–27.
A foundational essay, setting out the framework of the health and human rights approach and explaining the three ways that health and human rights are inextricably linked and should be linked when evaluating public health interventions, programmes, and policies.

Kass N (2001). An ethics framework for public health. *Am J Public Health* 91(11): 1776–82.
A helpful ethics framework for guiding priority-setting and evaluating the fairness and ethical appropriateness of RNMCH programmes and interventions in light of the impact on public health.

Persad G, Wertheimer A, and Emanuel E (2009). Principles for allocation of scarce medical interventions. *Lancet* 373: 423–31.
A thoughtful presentation of the sometimes competing ethical principles guiding fair allocation of scarce medical resources. This paper offers an excellent framework for discussing the case study.

Bibliography

Boama V and Arulkumaran S (2009). Safer childbirth: a rights-based approach. *International Journal of Gynecology and Obstetrics* 106: 125–7.

Braveman P and Gruskin S (2003). Poverty, equity, human rights and health. *Bull World Health Organ* 81(7): 539–45.

Farmer P and Gastineau N (2002). Rethinking health and human rights: time for a paradigm shift. *Journal of Law, Medicine, and Ethics* 30: 655–66.

Grodin M, Tarantola D, Annas G, and Gruskin S (2013). *Health and Human Rights in a Changing World*. Routledge: New York, US. pp. 16–27.

Kerber K, de Graft-Johnson J, Bhutta Z, Okong P, Starrs A, and Lawn J (2007). Continuum of care for maternal, newborn, and child health: from slogan to service delivery. *Lancet* 370: 1358–69.

Mann J, Gostin L, Gruskin S, Brennan T, Lazzarini Z, and Fineberg H (1994). Health and human right. *Health and Human Rights Journal* 1(1).

Melberg A, Diallo A, Ruano A, Tylleskar T, Moland K (2016). Reflections on the unintended consequences of the promotion of institutional pregnancy and birth care in Burkina Faso. *PLoS ONE* 11(6): 1–14.

UN General Assembly (1989) *Convention on the Rights of the Child*, 20 November 1989, United Nations, Treaty Series, 1577, p. 3, available at: http://www.refworld.org/docid/3ae6b38f0.html.

Wise P (2009). Confronting social disparities in child health: a critical appraisal of life-course science and research. *Pediatrics* 124: S203–211.

Wise P (2016). Child poverty and the promise of human capacity: childhood as a foundation for health aging. *Academic Pediatrics* 16: S37–S45.

CHAPTER 44

Translating research into policy

Elizabeth Mason and Blerta Maliqi

This chapter will address how research is used to develop policies, and gives specific examples of policy development and adoption.

Key points

- Policies in global women's, children's, and adolescents' health go beyond specific medical interventions, to health system and importantly to multisectoral action.
- Policy adoption is a dynamic process and, although there are global guidelines, each policy needs to be adapted to the country context.
- Policy adoption is not equivalent to policy implementation.
- Implementing policies in a health system requires consideration of the building blocks of the health system.
- Monitoring of policy implementation is critical for accountability.

Background

To improve women's, children's and adolescents' health, countries have to continuously review, develop, adopt, and implement new policies across the health sector. To address equity and move towards quality Universal Health Coverage (UHC), a number of core policies need attention.

The Global Strategy for Women's, Children's, and Adolescents' Health (2016–2030) (2015) sets a vision that looks beyond the survival of women, children, and adolescents, considering how they can thrive and transform in order to contribute to society and live healthy, happy lives. Health-specific and multisectoral policies are key to accelerating progress and achieving this vision. These policies are the basis upon which reproductive, maternal, newborn, child, and adolescent health (RMNCAH) interventions are delivered, how they are delivered and who should be receiving them. Figure 44.1 highlights core policy areas needed for a holistic approach to addressing women's, children's and adolescents' health.

National policy development and implementation is a continuous process which ensures policies are evidence-based, implemented, monitored and evaluated, and, ultimately, that new evidence is generated to improve policies in the future. This policy development cycle is shown in Figure 44.2.

Policy development

Evidence-based policymaking for public health is a systematic approach to the use of data and information to enhance clinical care and population health.

The policymaking process defines the healthcare benefits, who has access to these benefits, and under which conditions, as well as regulating people's relationship with the health system. Public health policies must address the health needs of diverse groups of the population and on a massive scale. As such, health policymaking requires considerations for a number of large and complex inputs, such as social, economic, environment, geographical, political, historical, and cultural factors. This is very important for policies related to the health of women, children, and adolescents as they define their ability to access and use services, while considering social and economic challenges, as well as resource requirements and sustainability.

An interesting challenge within evidence-based policymaking is the need for a range of interventions to address a single issue and maximising resources to ensure the most effective *set* of interventions. To address this, a more varied approach to evidence-based policymaking is needed. Widening participation in the policymaking process is central to this. Multi-stakeholder platforms and dialogues offer a way to bring stakeholders together at different levels (global, national, and regional) and across sectors to agree on action strategies for addressing issues. These platforms are spaces to build a shared purpose, agree on key issues, review evidence, and set a working agenda for next steps that are contextualised and feed into needs and demand.

The results of the policy development process at the country level depends on the champions, actors involved, resources, and accountability. At the global level, the World Health Organization (WHO) leads the process in developing evidence-based policies for global public health, including guidelines for maternal and child health. The GRADE (WHO, 2012) (grading of recommendations, assessment, development and evaluation) approach is used to develop these guidelines.

Policy adoption

Evidence-based guidelines need to undergo a process of contextualisation at the country level and adoption by stakeholders before they become implementable policies. In addition, engaging influential forums and key stakeholders is one approach to promoting the adoption of evidence-based policies.

Policy implementation

Implementing evidence-based policies is challenging to achieve. Shelton (2014) notes that: 'Public health decision making requires knowledge of not just whether something works under a particular circumstance, but also how, when, and why for broad applications'. This has been identified as the 'know-do' gap, and it remains a key roadblock to full implementation of policies for public health (WHO, 2006).

HEALTH SECTOR POLICIES FOR SUPPORTING DELIVERY OF REPRODUCTIVE MATERNAL NEONATAL AND CHILD HEALTH (RMNCH) INTERVENTIONS	
POLICY TOPIC AREAS	**POLICY ON:**
1. Constitutional and legal entitlements that facilitate universal access to health care in support of RMNCH programming	• Right to the highest attainable standard of health • Universal access to health care and services
2. Strategies, plans, and mechanisms to guide RMNCH programme implementation	• Integration of RMNCH into National Health Strategy and Plan • National RMNCH strategy(ies) and implementation plan(s) • RMNCH institutional arrangements
3. Human rights-based approach to maternal, newborn and child health, including related sexual and reproductive health issues	• RMNCH programming includes a human rights based approach • Access to sexual and reproductive health services • Legal basis for safe abortion
4. Mobilisation and allocation of financial resources	• Sustainable financing of RMNCH • RMNCH resource allocation and expenditure • Elimination of financial barriers • RMNCH resource reporting and tracking
5. Human resources	• Deployment and retention • Accreditation and certification • Authorisation of service provision and task shifting • RMNCH training curricula
6. Essential health infrastructure	• Essential health infrastructure and health facilities
7. Essential medicines and commodities	• Essential medicine, supply, and equipment list • Medicine and commodity security
8. RMNCH service accessibility and quality	• Adapting RMNCH essential interventions for local use • Standards on quality of RMNCH care • Standards for RMNCH referral care • Supportive supervision for all RMNCH health workers in the delivery of quality RMNCH care • Community participation • Community mobilisation and health education
9. Collection and use of data for planning and evaluating progress	• Birth registration • Death notification • Death reviews • Well-functioning health information systems, including logistics, and surveillance system for RMNCH • Defining key RMNCH indicators • National and subnational RMNCH targets • Data review process

Figure 44.1 A policy guide for implementing essential RMNCH interventions.

Reproduced with permission from Partnership for Maternal, Newborn & Child Health and WHO. A Policy Guide for Implementing Essential Interventions for Reproductive, Maternal, Newborn and Child Health (RMNCH): A Multisectoral Policy Compendium for RMNCH. World Health Organisation. Geneva, 2014. Copyright © World Health Organization 2014.

MULTISECTORAL POLICIES WHICH INFLUENCE SERVICE DELIVERY AND RMNCH OUTCOMES	
POLICY TOPIC AREAS	**POLICY ON:**
1. Inclusive economic development	- Eradicating income poverty and hunger - Reducing inequalities - Ensuring decent working confitions and opportunities and productive employment
2. Inclusive social development	- Adequate nutrition - Quality education - Social protection - Gender equality
3. Environmental sustainability	- Protecting biodiversity - Stable climate - Safe and affordable drinking water - Adequate sanitation
4. Peace and security	- Freedom from violence and abuse - Resilience to natural hazards - Conflict-free access to natural resources
5. Infrastructure for development	- Information and Communication Technologies and eHealth - Essential infrastructure
6. Obligations and duties	- The respect, protection and fulfilment of human rights - International standards of behaviour and practice - Efforts to improve development assistance and impact on development
7. Good governance	- Voice and accountabillity - Political stability and absence of violence - Government effectiveness - Regulatory quality - Rule of law - Control of corruption

Figure 44.1 (*Cont.*)

Effective healthcare systems are needed to implement policies and achieve high quality, equitable coverage of cost-effective interventions. Six 'building blocks' have been described by the WHO.

1. Leadership and governance

National leaders need to advocate for evidence-based maternal and child health policies, as well as planning, funding, and implementing them.

2. Health financing

The implementation of policies and provision of high quality maternal and newborn health services requires sufficient investment in all the health system. High out-of-pocket user fees in many countries prevents care-seeking, and indirect costs such as transport, being out of work, and the partner's/family's time contribute to the financial burden.

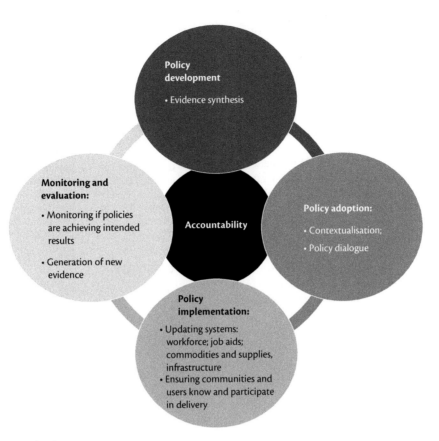

Figure 44.2 The policy developmental cycle.
Reproduced courtesy of the authors.

3. Health workforce

The workforce needs to be skilled, supported, motivated, and adequate in number and distribution. This is a particular challenge for interventions that require specialist skills, such as skilled birth attendance and inpatient neonatal care.

4. Health service delivery

This relates to the ability of the health system to deliver interventions of a high quality, as well as provide equitable access to care. For example, the presence of a skilled birth attendant is less effective without the availability of evidence-based interventions for care around the time of birth, such as equipment for newborn resuscitation, and a lack of sensitive care responding to a woman's needs and wants.

5. Health information systems

There is a lack of standardised global indicators, particularly in newborn and adolescent health, and currently few are included in national tracking systems. This leads to a lack of quality data for RMNCAH policies and interventions, impeding the ability to monitor and evaluate programmes at a facility, district, and national level.

6. Essential medical products and technology

Many settings experience a consistent lack of basic supplies, or poor quality supplies, hampering the implementation of policies and interventions.

Monitoring, evaluation, and accountability

◆ The monitoring and evaluation of a policy on a national level can be challenging, but should nonetheless be planned for at the implementation stage to ensure that baseline measurements are conducted and the required data is collected. This should include a cost-effectiveness assessment.

◆ Accountability is also essential to ensuring policies are implemented in practice. For example, Papp et al. (2013) showed in Orissa, India, the participation of local women and intermediary groups, health providers, and elected politicians, was shown to successfully accelerate efforts towards improving maternal health. These groups were able to increase demand for rights and services, leverage intermediaries to legitimise those demands (particularly of the poor and marginalised), and help to sensitise leaders and health providers to the needs and plight of women in their community.

Conclusions

Development and adoption of public health policies requires not only strong evidence of effectiveness, but must also take into consideration the broader context. Policies for RMNCAH are dynamic and need to be updated on a regular basis as new evidence of what works is made available.

Implementation of the policies is equally, if not more, important as their adoption. Monitoring of the policy implementation is key to accountability for results. The role of community action in monitoring policy adoption is increasing.

Case study: maternal death surveillance and response programme

The adoption of the Maternal Death Surveillance and Response (MDSR) by countries with medium and high maternal mortality is an example of policy implementation.

MDSR is an approach that sets out the essential information required to inform the design of targeted policies and programmes that work towards the elimination of preventable maternal deaths. Despite its importance, by 2010 only fifty-two low- and middle-income countries with high maternal mortality had adopted elements of MDSR policies and implementation. In 2011, the UN Commission on Information and Accountability for Women's, Children's, and Adolescents' Health advocated for 'better information for better results'. What ensued was a sharp increase in the number of countries adopting national policies to review maternal mortality. By 2016, 110 countries had adopted MDSR, although at varying levels of implementation. Assessing the corresponding reduction in maternal mortality is ongoing, but this case illustrates the importance of leadership in policy change.

Questions

1. Why is the evidence-base for public health policies more complex than for medical policies?

2. What are some of the issues countries need to consider in adoption of RMNCAH policies?

3. Is adoption of policies enough for action? If not what else is needed to ensure implementation?

4. Who is accountable for policy adoption and implementation and how can accountability be enhanced?

Key publications

A Policy Guide for Implementing Essential Interventions for Reproductive, Maternal, Newborn and Child Health (RMNCH) (2014). *A Multisectoral Policy Compendium For RMNCH.*WHO: Geneva.
    This book details the key policies for RMNCH, it includes policies across the different sections of the health sector according to the health system building blocks, also multisectoral policies relevant to RMNCH.

The Global Strategy for Women's, Children's, and Adolescent's Health 2016–2030 (2015). Every Woman Every Child: New York, US.
    The Global Strategy was launched by the UN Secretary General in September 2015. It contains the key strategies for improving women's, children's and adolescents' health up to 2030, and focuses on survive, thrive, and transform. It contains targets to be achieved towards the SDGs relevant to health and is accompanied by an implementation plan and accountability framework.

Victora C, Requejo J, Barros A, et al. (2016). A decade of tracking progress to maternal, newborn and child survival: Countdown—The 2015 Report. *Lancet* 387(10032): 2049–59.
    The Countdown to 2015 was key to tracking progress towards the MDGs in the seventy-five highest burden countries. The 2015 report presents global and country progress towards MDGs 4 and 5, and relevant health system and policy adoption country by country. The BMC Public Health

supplement on Countdown country case studies published in September 2016, is an excellent reference in country policy adoption.

Singh N, Huicho L, Afnan-Holmes H, et al. (2016). Countdown to 2015 country case studies: systematic tools to address the 'black box' of health systems and policy assessment. *BMC Public Health* 16(Suppl 2): 790.
    Evaluating health systems and policy (HSP) change and implementation is critical in understanding RMNCH progress within and across countries. Whilst data for health outcomes, coverage, and equity have advanced in the last decade, comparable analyses of HSP changes are lacking. The paper presents a set of novel tools developed by Countdown to 2015 to systematically analyse and describe HSP change for RMNCH indicators, enabling multi-country comparisons. These are the first HSP tools using mixed methods to systematically analyse and describe RMNCH changes within and across countries, important in informing accelerated progress for ending preventable maternal, newborn, and child mortality in the post-2015 era.

Bibliography

Every Woman, Every Child (2015). *The Global Strategy for Women's, Children's, and Adolescent's Health 2016–2030.* http://globalstrategy.everywomaneverychild.org/pdf/EWEC_Global_Strategy_EN_inside_web.pdf

Hunter D and Killoran A (2004). *Tackling Health Inequalities: Turning Policy into Practice?* NHS Health Development Agency. http://www.who.int/rpc/meetings/en/Hunter_Killoran_Report.pdf

Papp S, Gogoi A, and Campbell C (2013). Improving maternal health through social accountability: A case study from Orissa, India. *Global Public Health* 8: 4.

Partnership for Maternal, Newborn and Child Health (2011). *A Global Review of the Key Interventions Related to Reproductive, Maternal, Newborn and Child Health (RMNCH).* PMNCH: Geneva.

Shelton J (2014). Evidence-based public health: not only whether it works, but how it can be made to work practicably at scale. *Glob Health Sci Pract* 2(3): 253–8.

World Bank (2015). *Measurement and Accountability for Results in Health Summit.* 9–11 June 2015 World Bank Headquarters: Washington, DC, USA. http://www.who.int/mediacentre/news/releases/2015/health-measurement-accountability/en/

World Health Organization (2006). *Bridging the 'Know-Do' Gap Meeting on Knowledge Translation in Global Health.* 10–12 October 2005 World Health Organization: Geneva, Switzerland. WHO/EIP/KMS/2006.2. https://www.measureevaluation.org/resources/training/capacity-building-resources/high-impact-research-training-curricula/bridging-the-know-do-gap.pdf

World Health Organization (2010). Engaging Innovative Advocates as Public Health Champions Research innovation briefs. WHO: Geneva. http://www.who.int/woman_child_accountability/about/coia/en/index5.html

World Health Organization Handbook for Guideline development (2012). http://apps.who.int/iris/bitstream/10665/75146/1/9789241548441_eng.pdf http://www.who.int/publications/guidelines/handbook_2nd_ed.pdf?ua=1

World Health Organization (2014). *A Policy Guide for Implementing Essential Interventions for Reproductive, Maternal, Newborn and Child Health (RMNCH).* A multisectoral policy compendium for RMNCH. WHO: Geneva. http://www.who.int/pmnch/knowledge/publications/policy_compendium.pdf?ua=1

World Health Organization (2016). Time to respond: a report on the global implementation of maternal death surveillance and response. http://apps.who.int/iris/bitstream/10665/249524/1/9789241511230-eng.pdf?ua=1 http://who.int/maternal_child_adolescent/epidemiology/maternal-death-surveillance/progress/en/

World Health Organization Guidelines Review Committee (Web introduction) http://www.who.int/publications/guidelines/guidelines_review_committee/en/

CHAPTER 45

Advocacy to improve health

Tony Waterston and Delan Devakumar

This chapter will describe how to go from understanding the health issues of women, newborns, children and adolescents, to being an advocate for change.

Key points

- The combination of complexity of cause and lack of empowerment means that advocacy by health professionals is essential.
- Advocacy by health professionals working together with members of civil society has historic origins and should use evidence-based principles.

Background

It is essential for health professionals to speak out for improving women's, children's, and adolescents' health, to prevent injustices and to protect those who may not have a voice or are powerless. There is a long history of advocacy in public health, and there are multiple opportunities for advocacy. The health problems are complex and involve numerous causes, for example social determinants are prevalent and government policy on health may be inadequate. To achieve the targets described in this book requires advocates and champions. Neonatal health, for example, would not have been addressed without people highlighting the inequity in care and outcomes. In the field of child health, the underpinning principles for advocacy come from the United Nations Convention on the Rights of the Child.

What is advocacy? Advocacy can be defined as 'speaking out on behalf of a particular issue, idea, or person', acting as a catalyst for change. It can occur at all levels, from individuals to states, and includes all health professionals. The targets of advocacy have traditionally been healthcare focused, but wider determinants of health are essential. An understanding of social and political science is important when thinking of the best ways to advocate for and improve a situation. There are a number of steps involved in designing an advocacy strategy that are summarised in Figure 45.1.

Advocacy toolkit

An example of a 'toolkit' for effective advocacy, is described below:

1. Work together with others
   Coalition building is generally required for effective advocacy. This might be a professional association or a non-governmental organisation (NGO) that has links with the population.

2. Target decision makers
   Advocacy which does not reach its target is ineffective, so get to know how the system (health service or political) works in practice.

3. Use data, presented in a simple format
   A scientific evidence-based approach is fundamental to convince decision makers of the need for change. This has to be accessible and concise to get the message across.

4. Use the media
   If the advocacy message is to be taken up by the wider public then it needs to be disseminated. Increasingly, social media channels are more important than traditional methods. Training on communication can be essential.

5. Gain the support of the general public
   Support from the public, for example for an issue such as female genital mutilation, will play a large part in bringing about reform. This requires an understanding of cultural attitudes.

6. Be prepared for slow progress and accept small incremental improvements
   There are rarely quick solutions in advocacy. It took health professionals in the UK nearly fifty years to bring about a ban on smoking in public places, despite good evidence being available.

Challenges

The advocate can face sanctions from their employer and opposition from other staff, so courage is needed and, ideally, support from his or her professional association or union.

There may be strong cultural objections to concepts such as children's rights. Corporal punishment, for example, has quite strong support in many communities. Hence diplomacy is needed and collaboration with local members of civil society is essential.

Future priorities

It is important for advocacy to be evidence-based, both in what is recommended but also in the techniques used. Applying the scientific method to advocacy can help to improve its results. As part of this, we need to better understand the best methods to evaluate advocacy and define outcomes.

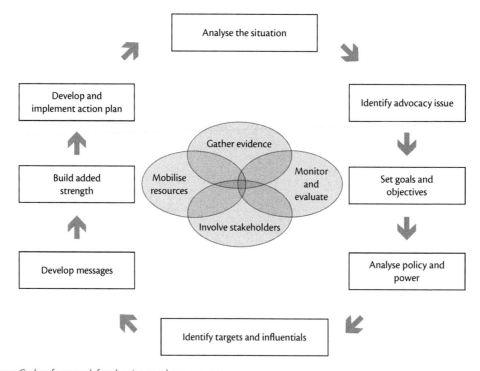

Figure 45.1 The Advocacy Cycle: a framework for planning an advocacy strategy.
Reproduced with permission from Save the Children, *Advocacy Matters: Helping children change their world*, 2007, The International Save the Children Alliance. Copyright © Save the Children.

Conclusions

Advocacy is an essential component of the work of all health professionals to ensure that services work better for the population and for patients. Effective advocacy requires diplomacy, persistence, an understanding of how systems work, and an ability to work with disciplines outside medicine. In the field of global health, advocacy is essential in tackling the heavy toll of death and disease and improving the quality of services, making them more responsive to individual and family needs.

Case studies

Case study 1: combating the commercialisation of infant feeding

The current decline in global breastfeeding rates is in part related to the commercialisation of infant feeding and heavy promotion of baby foods by multinational corporations. The promotion of formula feeding leads to increased infant deaths from diarrhoeal disease and malnutrition, as a result of the use of unclean water and insufficient milk powder, owing to high costs.

The World Health Organization International Code on Marketing of Breastmilk Substitutes was developed to regulate commercial promotion, but it is violated on a regular basis by prominent companies. The code has no specific enforcement mechanism and relies on organisations such as the International Baby Food Action Network (IBFAN), to enforce compliance. IBFAN is a network of groups which took action to implement the code and the subsequent resolutions of the World Health Assembly. Examples of practices opposed by IBFAN are: free donations of infant formula to hospitals and community health centres; the use of company staff to give infant feeding advice; misleading advertisements in the media and on product packs; and the sponsorship of paediatric associations.

IBFAN reports on breaches of the code annually. Of the 194 countries analysed in the report, 135 have in place some form of legal measure related to the code but only 39 countries have laws that enact all provisions of the code.

Many countries have their own national organisation which promotes implementation of the code. For example, in India, the Academy of Paediatrics has banned all sponsorship by baby food manufacturers, following the incorporation of the international code into law in India.

Case study 2: advocacy to improve the response to child sexual abuse

An estimated 40% of Indian women have suffered sexual abuse in childhood or adolescence. The figure for men is unknown. In 2012, the Government of India passed the Protection of Children from Sexual Offences Act (POCSO), which includes sections on sexual assault, sexual harassment, use of children for pornographic purposes, and abetment. In response to reports, the police are meant to ensure care and protection and record a statement and refer for medical examination.

Society for Nutrition, Education and Health Action (SNEHA) provides counselling and extended response services for survivors of violence. The programme brings together community activities, legal support, and works together with the police and health services. Partnership with Mumbai's public teaching hospitals revealed that a range of hospital teams and social workers were called upon in cases of child sexual abuse. This system had not previously involved non-government organisations and psychosocial counselling, meaning that child survivors of sexual violence were subjected to multiple interviews and examinations.

Advocacy involved collaborative research with one of the hospitals, interviewing women who have experienced violence. The results were shared with department heads, with the suggestion of starting outpatient clinics specifically for women, children, and adolescents facing family conflict. Sustained advocacy by counsellors, who met informally and formally with clinicians, encouraged them to refer women, children, and adolescents, and communicate their management plans. In addition, several public engagement events were held in the hospitals, using drama, poster competition, and games talking about gender-based violence and film screenings.

The hospitals instituted a response system in which clinicians contact in-house SNEHA counsellors, who coordinate attendance across specialties. The hospitals have mandated the inclusion of a SNEHA report (safety assessment, observation, home visit, consultation, and liaison with the Government Child Welfare Committee) when the police file charges.

Nayreen Daruwalla, Gauri Ambavkar, and Reshma Jagtap, Society for Nutrition, Education and Health Action (SNEHA).

Questions

1. Why is advocacy important for change in relation to maternal and child health?

2. What are risks of advocacy?

3. Can you give an example of some areas of maternal and child health where, in your experience, advocacy is needed?

Key publications

The UN Convention on the Rights of the Child (1989).
    This is the most rapidly and widely ratified international human rights treaty in history. It sets out standards for recognition and implementation of children's rights by national governments and is a valuable fundamental basis for child health advocacy.

Waterston T and Goldhagen J (2007). Why children's rights are central to international child health. *Arch Dis Child* 92(2): 176–80.
    This paper examines problems in child health from a child rights' perspective, including child labour, services for children with a disability, and violence against children; it looks at the role of health professionals in using the Convention on the Rights of the Child in prevention.

Waterston T (2016). Advocacy and the paediatrician. *Paediatrics and Child Health* 28(5): 179–84.
    This article examines the type of advocacy carried out by national paediatric associations and the training requirements of the successful advocate.

Bibliography

American Academy of Pediatrics CATCH program www.aap.org/catch/

Devakumar D, Spencer N, and Waterston T (2016). The role of advocacy in promoting better child health. *Arch Dis Child* 101: 596–9.

Isaacs D (2015). Advocacy. *J Paediatr Child Health* 51: 747e8.

ISSOP position statement on Sponsorship of Paediatric Associations by the Babyfood Industry. http://issop.org/index.php?option=com_content&view=category&layout=blog&id=33&Itemid=24

Marmot M (2008). *Closing the Gap in a Generation: Report of the Commission on the Social Determinants of Health.* WHO: Geneva.

Royal College of Paediatrics and Child Health (2008). *Advocating for Children.* RCPCH: London. Available from: www.rcpch.ac.uk

Waterston T (2009). Teaching and learning about advocacy. *Arch Dis Child Ed Prac* 94: 24e8.

CHAPTER 46

Current challenges and debates for women's, children's, and adolescents' health

David Osrin

Tremendous progress has been made in maternal and child survival over the last thirty years. Partly as a result, the agenda has expanded beyond survival to growth, development, and wellbeing. In a context challenged by population transitions and environmental change, disease-specific programmes have been relatively successful and have developed ways of measuring burden and success. The contemporary challenge, exemplified in the United Nations Sustainable Development Goals (SDGs), is to bring together women's, children's, and adolescents' health programming over the lifecourse and between sectors.

Key points

- ◆ Great improvements in survival worldwide, especially in maternal and child survival, need to extend to nations and groups who have been left behind. Key focuses include stillbirth, newborn death, and adolescent health. Including outcomes beyond survival is also important.

- ◆ Sustainable improvements in the health of women, children, and adolescents will benefit from a lifecourse approach to health programmes, intersectoral linkages—particularly with education and environmental health—and consideration of political and cultural forces beyond the health sector.

- ◆ Women's, children's, and adolescents' health is at the centre of universal health coverage. While specific interventions may vary, every woman and child should receive the essential packages in the continuum of care at community or facility level.

- ◆ Research gaps in specific topic areas would benefit from 'putting together the jigsaw' over the lifecycle and across sectors. One cross-cutting gap is for improved programme measurement, to drive quality of care as well as coverage and equity.

What has happened?

Transitions

The current Global Strategy for Women's, Children's, and Adolescents' Health (2016–2030) has three aims: survive, thrive, and transform. This vision acknowledges how far we have come, the continuing challenge of women's, children's, and adolescents'

survival, and our hopes for the future. One of this book's key messages is the immense improvement we have seen in women's, children's, and adolescents' survival. From a situation in which maternal and child mortality represented a largely unexamined mass of deaths of the unacknowledged, unregistered, and unequal, to a world in which under-five mortality has fallen by 52% between 1990 and 2015, and maternal mortality by 44%. How has this happened? Fundamentally, our expectations have risen on the basis of knowledge, social and economic change, opportunity to care for ourselves and our children, and transferable technologies that enable us to act preventively or therapeutically. As birth rates fall, mortality falls, families escape from poverty traps, and transgenerational health improves. Societies change, notably by allowing women to access education and move from reproductive to productive work. Population growth slows too, with implications for sustainability and planetary health.

The shift of attention from surviving to thriving is happening on a background of transitions:

The *demographic transition* describes falling mortality, especially of children, and an associated fall in fertility. Increased survival across the lifespan is accompanied by falling birth rates, loss of the demographic dividend, and expansion in senior age groups.

The *epidemiologic transition* is both a cause and an outcome of the demographic transition. At its simplest, it describes a fall in the proportionate burden of infectious disease and a rise in non-communicable disease.

The *nutrition transition* describes the replacement of diets dominated by low-density unrefined carbohydrate by diets rich in sugar, animal protein, and fats. This is currently manifesting as a double burden of malnutrition in which under and over-nutrition co-exist. Intimately connected with dietary sources is an environmental transition in which water scarcity, agricultural practices, air quality, and climate combine with urbanisation, trade, and migration to affect patterns of subsistence and lifestyles.

From holism to atomism and back again

The 'child survival revolution' followed shortly after the articulation of a vision of primary health care in the Alma Ata declaration of 1978. Although conceived holistically, it marked the first steps in disaggregated approaches to problems and measurement of progress. The most clearly beneficial components were the development and dissemination of oral rehydration therapy for diarrhoea and the consolidation and expansion of immunisation programmes. Other constituents included growth monitoring, female education, family planning, and food supplementation. Progress in these areas has been mixed and we cannot yet claim global success. There has been a tendency to decompose health into pieces and develop individual approaches and metrics of achievement. What we are seeing now is an effort to recombine them by bringing together services and programmes for women, children, and adolescents into a continuum of care. At the same time, we see a reconfiguration of helath care from a situation in which multiple vertical programmes coexist with weak infrastructure and deficiencies in human resource numbers, protocols, skills, equipment, and consumables into a framework in which health care is universal and of general quality. An important emerging challenge is to recombine therapeutic health care with prevention and to relocate health in a complex system that includes other sectors, politics, and the global environment.

What is happening?

Surviving

There is a huge amount of unfinished business. Preventable deaths remain unacceptably common in many countries and inequitably distributed within them. Nevertheless, attention is now turning to health and wellbeing over the lifecourse, including the neglected period of adolescence. The shift in focus is the result of qualified success. When child mortality across the world was high, mainly as a result of infections, the focus was on diarrhoea and pneumonia. As these relatively tractable causes at primary care level became less salient, newborn mortality contributed a growing proportion of deaths, now almost half of child deaths worldwide. As measurement and programmes address newborn deaths, and as institutional births increase, stillbirths are emerging as important. Like neonatal mortality before it, stillbirth is an example of a global health priority that is only now becoming visible. There are approximately as many stillbirths (2.6 million) as neonatal deaths (2.5 million), and the death of a baby around the time of birth has profound implications. First, it is enormously traumatic for parents and families and the emotional effects are lifelong. Second, stillborn babies have not been counted in global considerations of child survival. This invisibility is itself disheartening, and hides the high proportion of stillbirths that are preventable with effective antenatal care, particularly by addressing maternal infections and non-communicable conditions, and improved intrapartum care.

A similar sequence has been seen for maternal health: from mortality, to morbidity, to women's health, to intuitive linkage with existing reproductive health programmes. Maternal mortality is the tip of an iceberg of reproductive ill health. For example, for every woman who dies around pregnancy, 20–30 survive a complication. These complications often have sequelae that lead to lifelong ill health and effects on the family. At the same time, we have seen an incremental medicalisation of pregnancy—despite the fact that the history of evidence-based medicine began with a critical examination of obstetric practice—most visible in an epidemic of private sector elective Caesarean sections.

Thriving

Child development and disability are both health and social challenges. Their connections with perinatal problems such as preterm and birth asphyxia are manifest in the global disability-adjusted life-years (DALYs) burden, but this is only part of the story. Malnutrition remains an unacceptable global burden, both in terms of acute malnutrition (indexed by wasting) and chronic malnutrition (indexed by stunting). There have been substantial improvements in the management of acute malnutrition, from experience gathered in crises caused by flooding, natural disaster, and political upheavals. Consensus has not been reached on ready-to-use foods; the prevention of longer-term stunting remains a huge challenge and links back to low birthweight and the need for more focus on foetal and maternal wellbeing.

Our hopes of reducing stunting and increasing developmental potential within a generation have limits. Emphasis has been placed on intervention at certain points in the lifecourse—preconception, during pregnancy, and in early life—but the aetiology is trans-generational and tightly bound with gender concerns. The emergence of theory around the Developmental Origins of Health and Disease has implications for the way we think about the lifecourse. If a woman's health and nutrition around the time of conception have long-term effects on her child, and if environment and feeding in early life can affect susceptibility to ill health in later life, the effects of changes need to be seen over whole lives. Understanding this is made more complicated by the likelihood of influences over several generations. For example, treating malnourished young children becomes more complicated if we are concerned not to increase the risk of diabetes and hypertension in later life. And reducing child marriage may have benefits not only in terms of foetal and young child survival, but also in terms of adult health in offspring. Birth spacing and limiting through contraception, and abortion when required, improve the health of women and their families. Girls must be nourished and their illnesses treated; they should have access to school and higher education; and they should not conceive too young.

What should happen?

Transformation

Our expectations have changed with diminishing poverty, greater uptake of health care, and the spread of knowledge about health behaviours. Not all of this has been the result of purposeful programming. At least some of it has resulted from demographic transition and the availability of health care, both public and private, accompanied by better living conditions and an erosion of the sense of fatalism, as well as an aspiration for better lives. On the purposeful side, maternal and child survival advocates have emphasised understanding the numbers around the problem, including cause-specific mortality. Numbers have been used in three ways: as a means of bringing deaths out of the shadows and stimulating response, as a means of understanding the contributors to mortality in order to know what to address as a priority and to target intervention, and as a means of tracking whether they are improving. Measurement has helped us to see the problem, divide it into sub-problems, and address them. It has, however, given the persisting inequalities between and within nations an air of solubility through depoliticised incrementalism. Beyond survival and disability, people's idea of health—and their ability to achieve it—may be driven more by political atmosphere and longstanding structural violence than by an optimism that sees piecemeal translation of evidence into policy as the way to improve health and survival.

Assembling the jigsaw

If there is a theme to the last decade, it is putting together the pieces. For a number of reasons—including breaking a problem down to better address it—the obvious cyclical continuity between pregnancy, newborn infants, children, adolescents, young people, and adults was lost. The last few years have seen efforts to put it back together. To be deliverable, preventive and curative care over a continuum requires a strong platform of integrated services. The health sector needs to provide available, affordable, and appropriate contraception and abortion services, preconception care, antenatal care, skilled birth attendance, newborn care, immunisation, and treatment for illness. People will fall through gaps between these services if they are not harmonised, and if community-based activities are not connected with institutional care. The nature and delivery of activities to improve maternal, perinatal, infant, and child health is at a stage of development that makes it implementable and based on evidence of likely effect. This is not yet the case for adolescents, for whom particular challenges include undernutrition, sexual and reproductive health, mental health, risk taking, substance use, infections, non-communicable diseases, injuries, and violence. Similarly, although intervention to support early child development is a priority included in the UN SDGs and the Global Strategy for Women's, Children's, and Adolescents' Health (2016–2030), we are only beginning to assess the practicalities and potential effectiveness of strategies. There is considerable crossover and early child development is a prime example of something that should be seen within a continuum: from adequate nutrition before and during foetal development, to breastfeeding, parental leave, adequate infant and young child feeding, play and stimulation, environmental hygiene, water and sanitation, and access to education.

The problem of universality

If we are to achieve integration that addresses inequalities, transitions and generational continua, we need to achieve universal health coverage: promotive, preventive, curative, rehabilitative, and palliative health services available to all, of effective quality, and whose use does not expose people to financial hardship. There is agreement for this from the World Health Organization (WHO), the World Bank, and within the UN SDGs. Managing universal health coverage will be challenging for three main reasons. First, all countries are susceptible to resource constraints and periodic unstable governance. There is a debate to be had about reconciling the human right to health with prioritisation of provision, although reconciliation is possible under international law and principles of fairness. Second, the complexity of pluralistic care that mixes the private and public sectors is only beginning to be engaged with and will require more regulation than is currently in place.

Third, the argument for universal health coverage must contend with an ideological climate that is not particularly receptive. The child survival revolution appropriated a political word to describe a concerted effort to improve health. In doing so, it reflected a period in which global health came to be seen as apolitical. The tacit ideologies behind this were, however, political. They brought with them an emphasis on decomposing a problem, technology transfer, metrics, and managerialism that were echoed in other spheres over the latter half of the twentieth century. These convictions developed from a postwar liberal consensus which began to be replaced—around the time of the Alma Ata declaration—with a nascent neoliberal perspective. In the early days, this led to the heavy-handed diktats of structural adjustment. Later on, its libertarian turn supported the idea of community action, which paradoxically legitimised the retreat of the state while depoliticising the essence of local action.

Expanding the agenda

The influence of environment on health is profound. Poor housing and sanitation, dirty water, environmental toxins, unstable electricity supply, lack of outdoor places to play, and air pollution are particular concerns. More than half the world's people now live in cities and towns, in which access to balanced diets, water and sanitation, and clean indoor and outdoor air are particular concerns. Urban life also illustrates the nutritional and epidemiologic transitions. Reduced exercise, diets high in sugar, salt, and fat, and exposure to air pollution increase the risk of non-communicable diseases (NCDs), and urban density and mobility increase the risk of infectious disease.

Although addressing inequalities is part of this continuum, we struggle to cross the barriers between sectors. Three areas of particular importance are education, gender, and conflict. There is little doubt that education, to completion of school and beyond, is a best buy for women's, children's, and adolescents' health. But there is a degree of persistence of a segmented approach that makes health education central to programming rather than general education. This is a product of sectoral limitation. Similarly, gender tends to have been confined to approaches that (at best tacitly) equate it with female-centred reproductive health, viewing girls and young women as future mothers and ignoring the higher burden of NCDs and risk-taking behaviour seen in men. By extension, gender-based violence exacts a huge toll on women, children, and adolescents, and is legitimised and maintained by structural forces in societies. About one-third of women have experienced violence in their lifetime, be it physical, emotional, sexual, or economic. The public health toll is unquantified, since violence is associated with injury, sexually transmitted infection, unplanned pregnancies and abortion, stillbirth, low birthweight and preterm, harmful drug and alcohol use, common mental disorders, and transgenerational repetition of violence. Beyond the direct effects of conflict on health, indirect effects, such as food shortages, health service breakdown, family disruption, and displacement, are felt disproportionately by women, children, and adolescents and resound over generations.

Conclusions

This is a century in which we acknowledge complexity, in which individual and population health is affected by a system that encompasses the environment, politics and economics, food production, conflict, mobility, and gender. A range of needs have to be met if we are to ensure the best health for women, newborns, children, and adolescents (Figure 46.1). We need to fix health systems so that care of good quality is available to all, we have to join the components

What we want

Get appropriate, affordable health care

Get educated

Drink clean water and eat clean food

Breathe clean air

Live in a stimulating environment

Get exercise

Have rewarding and remunerative work

Be protected from violence, conflict, and disasters

Have safe, consensual sex

Be protected from the effects of drugs and alcohol

Plan the timing and number of children

Have a safe pregnancy and birth

Breastfeed and have a sufficient, diverse diet

Be protected from infections

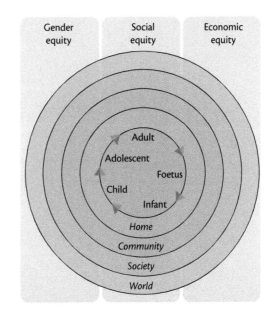

Figure 46.1 A wish-list for women's, children's, and adolescents' health.

together over the lifecourse, and we have to achieve communication between health and other sectors.

Questions

1. What are the barriers to improving women's, children's, and adolescents' health over the next decade?

2. Beyond the health sector, which sectors should be involved in health improvement?

3. How are education, gender, and conflict related to women's, children's, and adolescents' health?

Bibliography

de Bernis L, Kinney M, Stones W, et al. (2016). Stillbirths: ending preventable deaths by 2030. *Lancet* 387(10019): 703–16.

Devakumar D, Birch M, Osrin D, Sondorp E, and Wells J (2014). The intergenerational effects of war on the health of children. *BMC Medicine* 12: 57.

Dua T, Tomlinson M, Tablante E, et al. (2016). Global research priorities to accelerate early child development in the sustainable development era. *Lancet Global Health* 4: e887–e889.

Global Burden of Disease 2015 Child Mortality Collaborators (2015). Global, regional, and national levels of maternal mortality, 1990–2015: a systematic analysis for the Global Burden of Disease Study 2015. *Lancet* 388: 1775–812.

Global Burden of Disease 2015 Maternal Mortality Collaborators (2016). Global, regional, national, and selected subnational levels of stillbirths, neonatal, infant, and under-five mortality, 1980–2015: a systematic

analysis for the Global Burden of Disease Study 2015. *Lancet* 388: 1725–74.

Hawkes S and Buse K (2013). Gender and global health: evidence, policy, and inconvenient truths. *Lancet* 381: 1783–7.

International Food Policy Research Institute (2016). *Global Nutrition Report 2016: From Promise to Impact: Ending Malnutrition by 2030.* International Food Policy Research Institute: Washington, DC, US.

McPake B and Hanson K (2016). Managing the public-private mix to achieve universal health coverage. *Lancet* 388: 622–30.

Neira M, Fletcher E, Brune-Drisse M, Pfeiffer M, Adair-Rohani H, and Dora C (2017). Environmental health policies for women's, children's and adolescents' health. *Bull World Health Organ* 95: 604–6.

Patton G, Sawyer S, Santelli J, et al. (2016). Our future: a Lancet commission on adolescent health and wellbeing. *Lancet* 387: 2423–78.

Prüss-Ustün A, Wolf J, Corvalan C, Bos R, and Neira M (2016). *Preventing Disease Through Healthy Environments. A Global Assessment of the Burden of Disease from Environmental Risks.* World Health Organization: Geneva.

Richter L, Daelmans B, Lombardi J, et al. (2017). Investing in the foundation of sustainable development: pathways to scale up for early childhood development. *Lancet* 389: 103–18.

Rumbold B, Baker R, Ferraz O, et al. (2017). Universal health coverage, priority setting, and the human right to health. *Lancet* 390(10095): 712–14.

United Nations (2015). *The Global Strategy for Women's, Children's, and Adolescents' Health (2016–2030).* UN: New York, US.

UN Inter-agency Group for Child Mortality Estimation (UN IGME) (2015). *Report 2015: Levels and Trends in Child Mortality.* United Nations Children's Fund: New York, US.

WHO, UNICEF, UNFPA, World Bank Group, and the United Nations Population Division (2015). *Trends in Maternal Mortality: 1990 to 2015.* World Health Organization: Geneva.

Index

Note: Tables, figures and boxes are indicated by an italic *t*, *f* and *b* following the page number.